Springer Series in Neuropsychology

Harry A. Whitaker, Series Editor

Springer Series in Neuropsychology

Harry A. Whitaker, Series Editor

Richard E. Cytowic

Synesthesia
A Union of the Senses

With a Foreword by Ayub K. Ommaya

With 86 Illustrations

1989

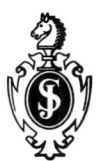

Springer-Verlag
New York Berlin Heidelberg
London Paris Tokyo

Richard E. Cytowic, MD
Capitol Neurology
7201 Wisconsin Avenue, Suite 360
Bethesda, MD 20814-4810, USA

Library of Congress Cataloging-in-Publication Data
Cytowic, Richard E.
　　Synesthesia : a union of the senses / Richard E. Cytowic.
　　　p.　cm.—(Springer series in neuropsychology)
　　ISBN 0-387-96807-5
　　1. Synesthesia—Physiological aspects. 2. Senses and sensation.
　I. Title.　II. Series.
　QP435.C97 1989
　152.1—dc19　　　　　　　　　　　　　　　　　　88-19064

Typeset by TCSystems, Inc., Shippensburg, Pennsylvania.
Printed and bound by Arcata Graphics/Halliday, West Hanover, Massachusetts.
Printed in the United States of America.

9 8 7 6 5 4 3 2 1

ISBN 0-387-96807-5 Springer-Verlag New York Berlin Heidelberg
ISBN 3-540-96807-5 Springer-Verlag Berlin Heidelberg New York

Show Off the Casket of Gems

I am a luminous being, a thousand points of light.

The light is strong. It casts out shadows, overwhelms lies, manipulations, and all that is evil and untrue. It is a light of truth, intoxicating beauty.

There are those starved of beauty. Like a seed that hungers for the warmth of the sun, they are nourished by the gem's beauty and power. Far, far outside the wall, the rumble of their cry—Show off the casket of gems!

Love comes from the magic of the stones. Hands reach out to rub and touch their surface. The warmth of touching stays to find a home in the heart and then shines back out through space and time.

Indentations in space and time focus the light like bowls of polished mirrors and shine it down as the light of stars.

My soul is full of stars; my heart of colored music.

Foreword

Understanding our own bodies and its functions has become in this age a major source of interest, research, and considerable effort. Nowhere is such curiosity in action seen with better clarity than in the work now in progress on the very source of our curiosity, that is, the brain and the mind. A paradox emerges when we try and grasp within an overall view what is now known about the way our brains work as revealed by the veritable avalanche of new facts and ideas discovered by the neurosciences. With superb precision we can now trace, for example, the course of a visual event initiated at the retina of our eye, through all the neural pathways in the brain, and postulate mechanisms for the building of a perception in the visual parts of the brain at the cellular and cell-groups levels. We can also do this for hearing and to some extent for touch and other sensations. We can describe in exquisite detail the workings of our brain systems controlling our motor actions. But nowhere do we find the mechanisms of integration at the highest level to which we can point and ask: "Is this how we come to understand?" In short, the discovery of how the mind and its conscious (as well as subconscious) functions are organized eludes us even as the sheer number of facts about the detailed workings of the brain threaten to overwhelm the neuroscientist as well as the layman. Obviously there is a great need for better theories with which some of these data may be organized and better understood.

It is within this context that I find Dr. Cytowic's book on synesthesia a fascinating and novel contribution. A moment's introspection will assure anyone that while we easily know that what we see and hear are distinct events, we are simultaneously capable of integrating these events in forming ideas and thoughts about the information such sensory inputs bring to our brains. In most persons, however, this integration is at a level of brain organization of which we remain unaware. In synesthetes, as clearly brought out by Dr. Cytowic, there is a conscious mixing of some of these sensory channels almost as if what is normally a subconscious mechanism is somehow bared to their consciousness. It is not surprising therefore that the cognitive skills of persons with synesthesia are uneven.

Although some may be able to display extremely powerful feats of memorizing and others use their modality crossing sensations as inspirations for creative work, there is a fair amount of evidence marshalled in this book to support the thought that synesthesia is bought at the cost of some degree of intellectual handicap. This is not to say that synesthetes are therefore doomed to a mildly impoverished extent of personal achievement. The incredible complexity and enormous range of human achievements in spite of physical and mental handicaps far greater than that posed by synesthesia is ample evidence that human minds can find ways to utilize handicaps or, in overcoming them, develop other talents to achieve their goals. While Luria's mnemonist could not become the concert violinist he wished to be or hold a steady job for long, his extraordinary feats of memory certainly ensured his livelihood and his place in history.

What is perhaps most important about this book is the stimulus it will provide to the imagination of the reader in pondering the rich feast of knowledge about a most fascinating part of ourselves. After all, synesthesia is what we all do without knowing that we do it, whereas synesthetes do it and know that they do it.

AYUB K. OMMAYA, MD
Professor of Neurosurgery
The George Washington University;
President, Foundation for Fundamental and
   Applied Neuroscience
Bethesda, Maryland

Preface

The idea that the senses can short circuit and that we can see sounds and taste shapes is inherently fascinating, strains our common sense, and appeals to our belief in magic.

Synesthesia came into my life in 1976, when I read A.R. Luria's book about a man with a photographic memory. It was called *The Mind of A Mnemonist* (Luria, 1968). During my later training in neuro-ophthalmology, I studied illusions and various distortions of vision with great interest. With this preparation, I knew I had stumbled on something extraordinary in running across two synesthetes within one month. They are VE and MW, 2 among the current 42 subjects of this book. The year was 1979, and I had no idea at the time how far those chance encounters would bring me. I am, of course, thankful to the many subjects who brought their condition to my attention. I am thankful too to the popular and scientific press for showing such an interest in this phenomenon.

Synesthesia has been known to the medical and psychologic community for over 200 years. The first medical reference to it was circa 1710, when an English ophthalmologist, Thomas Woolhouse, described the case of a blind man who perceived sound-induced colored visions (Castel, 1725, 1735). In 1704, Sir Isaac Newton tried mathematically to correlate the energy of sound and color, and the first practical application of this appears to be Castel's *clavecin oculaire,* an instrument that plays sound and lights simultaneously. Erasmus Darwin (1790) achieved the same effect with a harpsichord some time later. Correspondences with color are noted by Goethe in *Zur Farbenlehre* (Theory of Color) (1810). Thus, great minds have turned their attention to synesthesia and we should also note that many had either an artistic or a naturalistic disposition.

Those who know the term synesthesia through the literary symbolism of Yeats, Swinburn, Baudelaire, Hart Crane, Edgar Allen Poe, or Dame Edith Sitwell will not find any explication here. We are not talking about sound symbolism or metaphor, but a perception, a literal joining of the senses. However, the relation of synesthesia to art is discussed in Chapter 8.

I start with some historical background and then present synesthetes who tell in their own words exactly what it is that they perceive. They explain what it is like to have, in essence, a sixth sense. A review of theories follows with a new proposal that is consistent with the shift in conceptualization both of neural tissue and of cognitive function. In asking where in the brain synesthesia occurs, we look at things to which it is similar: the perceptions of eidetic memory, temporal lobe epilepsy, release hallucinations, sensory deprivation, and drug-induced synesthesia. Physiologic data are given to support my theoretical position. Following this, the neural substrate of synesthesia is examined in detail. I conclude that synesthesia resides only in the left hemisphere and that the hippocampus is an important node in the neural machinery that generates the parallel perception.

A shift in focus leads me to refute the idea that language has any role to play in the link between senses. It is unfortunate that early psychologists repeated the notion that synesthesia was merely a more intense form of metaphoric speech in which we all engage. This had a tendency, I think, to turn people away from what might be occurring in the brain of someone having a synesthetic experience. Even a partial answer to this question was not possible until the second quarter of this century, by which time both science and art had lost interest in the subject.

I present and review some familial cases of synesthesia and look into how this unique perception influences personality. We find that artists are not overrepresented among synesthetes and neither does it indicate great intellect or mental dullness. It is simply a rich additional way of perceiving the world.

I end by examining some closely held beliefs and showing that they are in fact illusory. This leads me to the delightful question, what is real? The reader is left to deduce the answer for himself. A disturbing but unintentional effect of analyzing how we create objects (that is, how we perceive them as being external in the three-dimensional Euclidean space we believe we have around us) has two sides: synesthesia no longer seems so unbelievable, but then reality no longer seems so real!

Why a book on synesthesia now, after so many years of disinterest, and why from a neurological perspective? As I mentioned above, the circumstances are partly accidental. Not long ago, it would have been difficult to give a satisfactory explanation for synesthesia in neurological terms. But we have learned more about the brain in the past 10 years than in the entire history of neuroscience. We have changed both our conceptualization of nervous tissue as well as our conceptualization of cognitive psychology so drastically since the heyday of synesthesia, that a coherent and convincing explanation of this remarkable condition is now possible. Review of the subject had been published in 1890 in French by Suarez de Mendoza (*L'Audition Coloree*) and in 1927 in German by Argelander (*Das Farbenhören und der synästhetische Faktor der Wahrnehmung*). But neither was able to approach the subject from a neurological basis. Because this current work represents the only book on the subject, it needs first of all to be addressed to a scientific audience and be as thorough as possible. In this, I think I have succeeded. But it is not beyond the interested lay person or the artist, although lay readers will find parts of this book too technical and reflective while scientists and philosophers will find other places too popular and artistic. Such are the predictable responses to any effort seeking to meet the challenge of writing the definitive work and of saying something reasonably reflective about a subject that has a fundamental appeal.

Although the present volume reflects 10 years of intermittent work, the majority of it was written at the Hambidge Center for Creative Arts and Sciences in Rabun Gap, Georgia. This is a unique facility in beautifully isolated countryside where there is a marvelous opportunity for artists and scientists to live and work together. My thanks for being a Fellow in the summers of 1987 and 1988. When I founded a private practice of neurology, Capitol Neurology, in Washington DC, I did not forsee that research would be something for which we would have a growing reputation. I thank my colleagues and staff of Capitol Neurology for the ability to take time away from the practice and also for accomodating the disruptions of television crews and reporters.

Harry Whitaker was a catalyst for developing this idea into a book. I want to especially thank Rey Aguirre of the Library of Congress for his friendship and valuable help, and Velora Jernigan and Anne Prussing of the Washington Hospital Center Library for helping track down obscure medical references. Thanks to Ray Pierotti, Executive Director of the Hambidge Center, for insightful discussions and an atmosphere for exchange between artists of all professions.

Hambidge Center   RICHARD E. CYTOWIC
Rabun Gap, Georgia

Contents

1
Introduction

Most people link their senses only by way of metaphoric speech, saying, for example, that red is a "warm" color, that a certain cheese tastes "sharp," that so-and-so is a "sweet" person. But there are a few who experience the phrase "I see what you're saying" as literally true.

What first strikes me is the *color* of someone's voice. [*Name*] has a crumbly, yellow voice, like a flame with protruding fibers. Sometimes I get so interested in the voice, I can't understand what's being said.

Spearmint tastes like cool, glass columns. Lemon is a pointed shape, pressed into my face and hands. It's like laying my hands on a bed of nails.

I enjoy music that has wavy metallic lines, like oscilloscope configurations. My favorite music has movement that extends beyond the peripheral vision.

I get so frustrated by advertisements because the letters and numbers are always in the "wrong" color.

These are examples of a parallel sensation called synesthesia. The word synesthesia comes from the Greek *syn* (union) and *aisthesis* (sensation), literally a joining of the senses. Synesthesia is an *involuntary* joining in which the real information of one sense is accompanied by a perception in another sense. In addition to being involuntary, this additional perception is regarded by the synesthete as real, often outside the body, instead of imagined in the mind's eye. It also has some other interesting features that clearly separate it from artistic fancy or purple prose. Its *reality* and *vividness* are what make sysnesthesia so interesting in its violation of conventional perception. Synesthesia is also fascinating because logically it should not be a product of the human brain, where the evolutionary trend has been for increasing *separation* of function anatomically.

Surely, this subject is fascinating by novelty alone. It is excellent material for cocktail party chitchat and has enormous appeal to those who unhesitatingly believe in flying saucers, psychokinesis, and astral projection. But could it be the stuff of serious science? Are there really people who can hear colors, taste shapes, see pain, and have their various senses filled with color? After collecting cases over a number of years, I conclude that the answer is unequivocally yes. One way to accentuate its validity as a perception is to say that synesthesia is a product of the brain and not the mind. Although synesthesia has been out of the literature for many years, it is still a charming perceptual oddity whose study has value today. Our conception of both nervous tissue and cognitive processes is dramatically different from the conceptualization of these processes at the turn of the century, when interest in synesthesia reached its peak. Synesthesia is more easily explained by our present understanding of functional anatomy, neuropsychology, and neurophysiology than was possible at the turn of the century when conflated psychological theories dominated the field of higher functions. As one might expect, exploring any oddity that violates the conventional rules of perception raises serious questions about our understanding of it.

Synesthesia is accepted as an absolutely real phenomenon by the medical community, if only because it has been independently noted by many investigators for over 200 years. Throughout those years, however, mechanistic explanations—particularly the search for universal correspondences among the senses—failed, and synesthesia was eventually left with a reputation, by the 1920s, as a psychological quirk without a basis understandable in terms of current neurophysiology. Despite this, it aroused inquiry in a wide range of disciplines. These included neurology, psychology, linguistics, comparative anatomy, artistic creativity, philosophy, and the mind-body problem. This characteristic of synesthesia to show its face in numerous disciplines is one clue to its nature. Each discipline has something to say about synesthesia from its own point of view.

Only recently have scientists been able to study regional metabolism, and thus function, in a living human brain while it is engaged in a specific cognitive behavior. This is elaborated in Chapter 4. Research on such metabolic changes during synesthesia shows that this rare condition is brain-based (perceptual) and not mind-based (such as imagery). On the basis of evolutionary and other lines of data, I have proposed, rather romantically, that synesthetes can be regarded as cognitive fossils in that synesthetic perception is a fundamentally mammalian (phylum-typical) attribute compared to language, which is uniquely human (species-typical).

It is not quite correct to say that a major task of this book is to *explain* synesthesia, since all explanations are transient, subject to change as our knowledge changes. A more accurate statement would be that this book will unfold what I call the Reciprocal Relationship between synesthesia as an isolated phenomenon and the disciplines to which it relates.One begins to see the underlying richness of synesthesia when one sequentially adopts the point of view of neurophysiology, perceptual psychology, language, music, and so forth, as well as those phenomena that share some similarities with synesthesia—hallucinations, temporal lobe epilepsy, Penfield's experiential responses from electrical stimulation of the brain, and eidetic memory, to name a few. As this strategy helps us understand synesthesia, we discover that we examine these overlapping areas in ways we may not have previously considered.

The result is serendipitous: we question some fundamental assumptions about perception along the way regarding what is real and what is illusory, some of which seems contrary to ordinary consensual experience as well as common sense. One example is the illusion of color constancy of objects in the varying spectrum of daylight, while another, to continue with the exemplar of color vision, is the complementary coloration of (physically white) colored shadows. In both instances, the color attributed to a light is different from what it "really is." It is different from what the physical properties of the light would lead one to predict and to perceive.

There can never be the expectation of definitive "answers" whenever one deals with fundamental questions that bear on the mind-body problem. The realistic hope is to make a little progress here and there, clarify an issue, rephrase a problem. Is the perceiver ever aware of raw sense data, or only the consequences of processes applied to that data? Synesthesia strikes most people as surprising, even bizarre. Perhaps it appeals to our appetite for magical thinking, as anthropological work on hallucinations and altered states of consciousness have suggested (Adler, 1972; LaBarre, 1975; Miner, 1956). Is synesthesia a real perception of a sense datum or just a projection? Is there actually the rare individual who can *really* hear colors and taste shapes? Yes, there is, and his existence does not rely on our wanting to believe the impossible. After looking at what I have termed the reciprocal relationship and scrutinizing illusions that are so common in our everyday life that they are taken for granted, synesthesia will no longer seem so bizarre. But then, reality will no longer appear so real either. The neuron, after all, is a storyteller that accentuates some features, completely ignores others, and is our fragile link to the physical world.

instruments filter reality (including neuron as instrument)

Historical Background

In looking at cases of synesthesia in the literature, one is shocked to find this phenomenon unexamined by neurologists. It has received essentially a psychological analysis (see references in Chapter 3). That it had its heyday in the 19th century is understandable in context of the tenor of the times. The French were particularly fascinated by it. Nineteenth-century French scientists were eager to discredit theological positions about the soul, and to translate spiritual mysteries entirely into psychological terms.

The dawn of the art movement kept some of this flavor. The late 19th and early 20th centuries saw the rise of both psychology and psychoanalysis; this was a time that paralleled the rise of surrealism, symbolist poetry, automatic writing, and other explorations of the newly discovered unconscious. "Know thyself" was the buzzword, and the method, "anything goes." Arthur Rimbaud (1854–1891), himself probably synesthetic, and stimulated by hashish and absinthe, was a prime mover in the symbolist movement and helped awaken public awareness of synesthesia in his time. His writings contain direct reference to his synesthetic perceptions, the best known example being *Le Sonnet des Voyelles* (1871):

> A Black, E White, I Red, U Green, O Blue—O vowels,
> I shall tell someday your latent birth.

Like eidetic imagery and other more introspective subjects, synesthesia ceased to interest psychologists after a time and fell into obscurity as the science of psychology turned to more "objective" topics. Synesthesia was never doubted as a real phenomenon, nor did its disappearance from the professional scene reflect a successful solution of the clinical problem. Historical developments and the shift of the professional climate toward more objective topics just signaled its demise. The sense that psychology had taken the phenomenon as far as it could was paralleled by a pressure in the visual arts and humanities to be "scientific."

This parallel development in the arts occurred over a 15-year period, the actual work displayed and the public's awareness reflecting ideas that were considered hot and timely by the artist 10 to 15 years earlier. The 1920s and the early 1930s saw the development of the American Art Deco and Art Nouveau movements, although those Americans actually studied abroad with European designers. The impact of the Fauvists, which had a lot to do with bestiality and going back to the senses, was coming to a close. (The French *fauve* means she-wolf or a pack of small wolves; the movement represented going back to nature, not in the sense of Rousseau, but in the sense of going back to the really deep-seated psychological nature of man, the animal in man—the irrational, the uncontrollable.) Symbolist poetry and automatic writing did not last long as artistic movements, either.

At that time the explanations of synesthesia were all psychological and were based on "associations," "meanings," and "feelings," which was the predominant focus of psychology at that time. This "feeling" point of view in the arts was considered very romantic; Cole, Constable, Turner, Beethoven, Schumann, and Mahler were all very romantic artists. The shift away from the romantic emphasis was represented by the Impressionist movement, which is actually quite scientific. The Impressionist movement began in the early 1900s and ended in the early 1930s with the American Impressionists, following which there was a gradual shift to more abstract paintings. Thus the visual arts turned away from the romanticism of feeling that synesthesia represented and adopted a more scientific view of looking at elements such as illumination, color, and shape.

Today's New Age, with its emphasis on spiritualism and its distrust of orthodoxy, will doubtless find synesthesia appealing. That it will be oversimplified and have more meaning attached to it than is warranted is certain. Of course, even today when one talks about synesthesia it is doubtful whether many people really grasp what is meant. They immediately try to associate it with the idea that "I'm hearing this piece of music and I see a beautiful landscape," which is not synesthesia at all, but merely imagination. An understanding of synesthesia was wanting 80 years ago as well. It certainly had no support from other disciplines we would consider essential today. A new point of view was needed, preferably one that related neuroanatomy and neurophysiology to cognition.

DEVELOPMENT OF NEUROLOGY

Although trephining and contralateral representation of movement were know since antiquity, what we consider modern neurology was in its infancy in the 19th century. One can regard the birth of modern neurology with the founding, in London, of the National Hospital for Nervous Diseases in 1860. The agenda of early scientists who contributed to the development of the new field of neurology was not commensurate with the study of so odd and subjective a phenomenon as synesthesia. It is almost impossible to find any references in the older neurologic literature, a situation that has scarcely improved in the 20th century.

Neurologists today know nothing of the subject. At times, if they try to guess at the neural basis of synesthesia, they liken it to a hallucination. The paper usually quoted in support of this view is David Cogan's (1973). But Cogan's simple paper on release hallucinations is no explanation at all and actually only an approximation at best. Less frequently, neurologists refer to "experiential hallucinations" and cite Penfield's work on electrical stimulation of the brain. However, it is impossible to find in-depth investigations or even a tentative suggestion of what might be happening in the brain of a synesthete. Instead, neurologists have shrugged their shoulders and gone back to paralysis and other gross derangements of function.

In truth, neurologists have never been interested in the working brain. That statement seems like an oxymoron, a pointed stupidity. Although Freud—who began his career as a neurologist tracing circuits in the brain—is often cited in the argument against this statement, Freud was, in fact, extremely antibiological. The history of neurology is very much concerned with movement, reflexes, integration of spinal cord pathways, and other elementary functions, while leaving disorders of thought and emotion to the realm of psychiatry and philosophy. As an outgrowth of psychiatry, neurology developed as the category for disorders for which an obvious physical abnormality of the nervous system could be found. Furthermore, the emphasis was always on gross derangements. Thus the modern division between mind and body grew in the past 130 years. As recently as the past decade, disorders of cognition and behavior that did not fit under the theoretical constructs of psychiatry were lumped under the single neurological category of "organic brain syndrome," a term that simply meant that "something" must be wrong with the patient's brain.

It is hard to name more than a few neurologists who have studied the highest levels of cognition. Even Hans Berger, inventor of the electroen-cephalograph (EEG), was a psychiatrist. In the United States the most interesting work on neurotransmitters, psychopharmacology and what is often referred to as behavioral neurology, neuropsychology, or neuroim-munopsychiatry, has come from the psychiatrists at the National Institute of Mental Health rather than the neurologists at the National Institute for Neurological Diseases, Communicative Disorders and Stroke. The system seems to be stuck in an antideluvian paradigm of orthodoxy that grinds and squeezes out imagination and creativity in the quest for conformity.

Neuropsychology, too, developed rapidly after the war thanks to the influx of doctoral-level researchers into the field. The unfortunate ar-rogance of physicians, however, prevented even the superlative Ph.D. neuropsychologists from making a greater impression simply because they were not physicians. Medicine does not like to deal with the mind. Doctors want to fix things that are broken, not contemplate how these things work. The farthest neurologists got into "cognitive" problems were the aphasias. The mind was for philosophers. I do not mean to be a harsh critic, but only to highlight the political separation of territory that developed and still remains in this century. It took neurologist Norman Geschwind 20 years of persistent effort to get his colleagues to think about behavior in terms of anatomy. His ideas were not readily accepted when introduced, but now that he is dead, these same skeptics lionize him.

I mentioned that synesthesia has been unexamined by neurologists, receiving instead a psychological analysis. The historical background of neurology may explain this curious fact. It also explains why most physicians have an overwhelming indifference to cognitive functions and why even neurologists—those physicians who claim the brain as their territory—have only recently developed an interest in this field. Let me give an example from the recent past.

In 1962, *Interhemispheric Relations and Cerebral Dominance* was published, edited by Vernon Mountcastle, a world-class neurophysiolo-gist at Johns Hopkins. The first chapter, by the anatomist Von Bonin, speculated if there were anatomical asymmetries that could account for cerebral dominance. His conclusion was that some "subtle" asymmetries had been described but were not clear enough to account for the functional differences between the two hemispheres. That became the standard gospel. Indeed, every time someone suggested that behavior was related to some particular structural organization of the brain, the invariable response was, "That is almost certainly not true." If, 10 years ago, one wanted a research grant to look at the brains of dyslexics, he was told by NIH that "everybody knows that dyslexics have normal brains." It should have seemed obvious that they did not. If they had normal brains, then why were they dyslexic?

There was, therefore, a powerful tendency to dismiss behavioral and intellectual abnormalities as having anything to do with the brain. Even today we hear that schizophrenics have normal brains and papers claim to have proven this to be so. Evidence mounts that this is false, as has been proven for the dyslexics.

If one actually reads Von Bonin's chapter, he learns not to trust review articles. We tend to respect an authority who has read and summarized all the literature but we never consider that he may have read it in a most curious way. Among the articles cited by Von Bonin there indeed was evidence of gross asymmetries in the human. This led to Norman Geschwind and Walter Levitsky's study (1968) showing that not only did these "subtle" asymmetries exist, but that they were readily visible to the naked eye and could be measured with rulers.

Heshl and other early neurologists pointed out anatomical asymmetries in both humans and animals. In the 1920s, asymmetries in fish—the cod, lamprey, and carp—were well known. The curious thing is that all this was forgotten. The reason for this dark age is that there was a tremendous revulsion following World War I to the notion that the brain had anything to do with behavior. Most people are unaware how powerful that revulsion was.

Norman Geschwind related to me that in 1942, at Harvard, professors joked that there were people who thought the brain might be related to behavior, but postulated that it would be hundreds of years before anything came of it and that it was a nonsensical speculation to consider this area. What a weird notion! Even in Geschwind's medical school, the brain was thought to be involved in twitching toes but nothing more. Every neuroscientist of the period participated in this collusion. Karl Lashley, a man of major eminence, did great disservice trying to prove that the brain was not involved in behavior, even though he spent his life working the field. One can only wonder what was going on his mind during that time.

I mention this history by way of introducing the fact that my study of synesthesia is a complete accident. I trained at a stroke center at which territory was clearly demarcated. Tuesday afternoon was set aside for an interdisciplinary conference in which everyone participated: neuro-logy, -pathology, -radiology, -surgery, and a basic neuroscience. The section of neuropsychology rarely spoke since it did not have any "real doctors."

Part of my internship was devoted to ophthalmology, with emphasis on neuro-ophthalmological disorders. It was here that I came to understand that physicians are interested in vision but not blindness, that vision is a psychophysical phenomenon, and that there were limits to organic assessment by Snellen charts, slit lamps, and Hruby lenses. Visual symptoms that had no visible pathology were ignored or dismissed out of hand. Yet I found references to unusual visual disorders in standard ophthalmological texts. It is as if these things had been forgotten. A paragraph here and there was enough to whet my appetite. I learned about palinopia, polyopia, afterimages, and color vision and particularly enjoyed discovering the causes of monocular diplopia. This condition was supposed to be impossible on an organic basis, we had been taught, and was therefore an infallible sign of conversion hysteria. How surprising to discover that its causes included dislocated lenses, macular disease, keratoconus, high astigmatic error, retinal degeneration, and cerebral lesions (Bender, 1945; Fincham, 1963; Rubin, 1974).

In neurology, "localizing the lesion" was an end in itself, and often a primary occupation. I detested neurology in medical school. In a fit of pique while studying for an examination, I threw my entire notes off the balcony, proclaiming that the subject was incomprehensible and that no one should be forced to learn such endless arcane facts that served no purpose.

My change of heart was precipitated by two events. One was the transition to seeing real patients and the influence of a teacher, Dr. William McKinney. He was the first physician I had ever seen sit down on the bed, take the patient by the hand, and actually talk to him. In the clinician's hands, neurology was no longer a collection of arcane facts but a method. Dr. McKinney suggested neurology would suit me and later arranged for me to go to the National Hospital for Nervous Diseases in London, an institute more commonly referred to by its address, Queen Square. The British have a much higher appreciation for higher functions that we do in the United States. The second event was my discovery of aphasia and the revelation that one could have a loss of language with preservation of more elementary functions. This was my introduction to the concept of higher functions and I thought it elegant.

The music critic Harold Schonberg mentioned that Maurice Ravel had aphasia, so I did what I could to investigate his illness personally. This included a correspondence with Ravel's physician Theophile Alajouanine (Cytowic, 1976b). Perhaps this single event stimulated my interest in how disease affects artistic realization, just as my interest in Chekhov began an interest in the relationship between medicine and the humanities (Cytowic, 1975, 1976a). The exploration of Ravel led me to read about "the other side of the brain" and split-brain research (Bogen, 1969a, 1969b, 1969c). Here another wonderful paradox was revealed: that the "person" who speaks is not the "person" who perceives or solves problems. They are separate but usually unified by the cerebral commissures.

Critchley's book on the parietal lobes and MacLean's papers on subjective experiences in temporal lobe epilepsy, psychosomatic medicine, and the reptilian brain were again another world, fascinating but unrelated to what was being taught at the bedside on teaching rounds or in the conference rooms. The chain seemed broken somewhere to me, and no one seemed interested in what Dejerine or Gowers or Yakovlev thought was important, nor did anyone suggest that such history should be learned. The relevant books had not been checked out of the library in years. What was taught was "new" and the most scientific. This state of affairs was hardly unique to my medical school.

I read Luria's *Mind of a Mnemonist* (1968) and already knew of hyperlexia, hypercalculia, and other elevated functions. No neurological explanation for any of these elevated functions existed, merely description, and what description there was was limited to case studies. These kinds of perceptual phenomena were better explained in the older non-American literature. It was interesting to read these works and compare them to the biological model of the National Institutes of Health that dominated medical thinking. Even the classics such as Alajouanine's (1948) analysis of aphasia in artistic realization had an enormous appeal to me. Its style and method were quite alien to what I had been exposed.

This is some of the background, then, on the circumstances that led to my interest in the more arcane aspects of medicine. It is a background that I hardly regret.

METHODOLOGICAL PROBLEMS

The prospect for making some headway in synesthesia seems difficult. Most of the studies will have a population of one. The "data output" of patients—their subjective experiences—do not correspond between subjects. There are no "objective" measures of their experience, no machines to attach to patients or to put them into that will give numbers on which to perform statistical analysis.

Does the prospect of complexity mean that one should abandon the search of trying to understand this unique perceptual phenomenon? I think not. One learns the most when seeing things that he cannot readily explain. If we see things we can explain right away, then we have not learned very much—we probably already knew it.

The reader expecting a "definitive" answer to the curiosity of parallel sensation will be disappointed. The field is at the beginning of a new stage of investigation, similar to when medical sciences were stuck in nosology and it was enough to describe the clinical features of a hitherto-unencountered disease. A study of synesthesia is, in a way, a trip back in time. When we review theories we will look at thoughts of psychologists and physicians from the 19th and early 20th centuries, scientists who are all too easy to dismiss as old-fashioned or passé. The review of this material has merit beyond its historical significance. This was a time full of ideas and theorizing as opposed to biotechnology. Geschwind drew on the work of Leipmann, Flechsig, and others in the century before him in formulating his "new" ideas on disconnection syndromes, now widely accepted. We too can draw on the past to stimulate creativity in the present. Consider the enormous contributions of Ramón y Cajal in numerous areas of medicine, particularly neuroanatomy and embryology. His scientific output is outstanding considering the circumstances in which he worked. Many students working today with superior preparations and high-technology probes cannot match their materials with ideas as well as men and women of Raymon y Cajal's era could.

How This Work Got Started

This work is the result of both my curiosity and my compulsiveness. For 9 years now I have been slowly collecting material as it came to me, and as word has spread of my interest in this subject, the pace has picked up. It now has come to the point that I never know what the postman is going to bring.

   I was chatting with a woman, VE, one afternoon during my fellowship in neuropsychology. As often happened in this environment, my beeper went off, producing a series of three shrill tones. Immediately, VE put her hand to her forehead, gesturing for me to silence the device. "Oh, those blinding red jaggers, turn that thing off!" I asked her to explain. She proceeded to relate that sounds made her see colors and that particularly high-pitched or loud ones could be painful. In the case of my beeper, the three beeps caused her to see red jagged lines "like lightening bolts." Each was accompanied by a stabbing pain in her forehead.

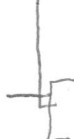

   This was the first instance of synesthesia I had encountered. Further discussion showed that she was polymodal, although seeing colored photisms in response to sound remained her dominant mode. An impromptu pilot experiment with a faculty member showed that her drawings in response to spoken Czechoslovakian words were quite different from those of a nonsynesthete, whose drawings paralled the rising and falling intonation at best. She also perceived color in response to smell and taste. "You know how strychnine smells pink?" she asked, assuming that I would. "It tastes the same pink that my angel food cake does." This explanation was of no help in understanding what she was experiencing. Luscher color cards produced different smells for her and bewilderment for the rest of us. The diagnosis of synesthesia was thus made and we discussed its relationship to Luria's patient and let the matter rest.

Several months later some acquaintances were at the home of my neighbor, MW, for dinner. MW taught theatrical lighting design at a conservatory. The residence was an open loft, and we were called to table, which was contiguous to the kitchen, in anticipation of the momentary arrival of the meal. During final preparations, MW announced that dinner would be delayed a few moments because there were "not enough points on the chicken."

With that casual remark he turned around, his face beet-red with the realization that he had disclosed some horrible secret. "Oh," he said with great embarrassment, "you don't know. Only Tony knows. He's the only one of my friends I've told," as he tried to extricate himself from his faux pas. Perhaps I would understand, he thought, appealing to the fact that I was a doctor. But his explanation only made the situation more bizarre. MW struggled to explain that taste had shape for him and that he cooked according to the shape of foods rather than their taste. He was disappointed that the chicken was "too round," a lackluster taste. He had intended it to have "points" in order to make it more appetizing, he explained, as he did some last-minute seasoning to the sauce.

While his other friends ribbed him, I realized that I had my second case of synesthesia and that they should both be looked into further. Fortunately, MW's undergraduate degree was in botany, and he understood the scientific method and the need for experimentation. He graciously consented to undergo the tedious psychophysical experiments, examinations, and invasive procedures that are documented throughout this book. He is the subject who has been studied the most thoroughly. I had no idea at the start how rich would be the outcome of studying this one person in detail, nor where it would lead.

How to approach the problem? One way of looking at synesthesia is to question the other side of the coin: "normal" perception. The one property generally considered to characterize perception is providing the organism with information about the environment. Information is the knowledge acquired through the presence of a stimulus. When we examine the thoughts of philosophers, neurologists, physiologists, and psychologists on the issue of perception, however, we see that the difference between "sensory fact" and "thought" is not so apparent. In fact, when one looks at the historical haul, it seems surprising that synesthesia is taken as an exception at all. Much thought on perceptions assumes a unity of the senses (see L.E. Marks, 1978, and Boernstein, 1970). Bertrand Russell quotes A.N. Whitehead as saying, "So far as reality is concerned, all our sense perceptions are in the same boat and must be treated on the same principle."

The bias in such an assumption that the process of perceiving is identical (aside from its contents) with the process of thinking led to the further assumption that the study of one (any one) sense can permissibly be applied to the physiology and psychology of the rest. This bias is operative by the fact that our understanding of perception has come about through reliance exclusively on one sense, vision. By virtue of being done in the laboratory, much of the work is also conducted under "optimal" circumstances that do not mimic real-life situations. The large amount of data on iconographic memory is such an example, and the demise of the icon is convincingly argued by Haber (1983).

Anyone who attempts to study synesthesia will invariably have to deal with kooks, cranks, and artistes. Some are most apparent, quoting verbatim descriptions of my work that they have obviously read in the popular press but that are supposed to represent their own visions. Whatever these visions may be, they are not synesthesia, and we have to reconcile ourselves that there are persons whose frame of reference is incommensurate with the majority. The need for these individuals to be "special" gives evidence of their lacking sense of individuality and self-esteem.

Next, there are those with "cosmic" personalities or those who profess psychic abilities. For them, synesthesia strikes a resonant chord in their souls. They are—alas—magnetically drawn to the researcher, compelled to share their life stories (which are long). Most people simply do not understand what synesthesia is and immediately try to associate it with imagination. Once they understand, however, they quickly explain that what they were describing is imagination and not a sensory experience. However, the occasional use of similar language raises the possibility of an overlap or continuum with imagery. The problem is where to draw the line; my solution for the time being is five defining criteria (see Chapter 3).

The number of subjects is small and they are geographically dispersed. Although excited to discover they are unique, few are enthusiastic about being examined or participating in the more tedious psychophysical or neurophysiological experiments.

 No florid personality disorders have been apparent either historically or in the current patient group. Results of the Minnesota Multiphasic Personality Inventory (MMPI) are singularly unimpressive. More sophisticated assessment of personality would probably be fruitful. Finally, more work on familial cases, perinatal history, and early development is needed.

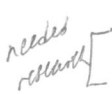

Criticism of Experiential Responses

Synesthesia is subjective, but science, despite all its pretenses toward objectivity, also reflects individual, cultural, and philosophical biases. The average person finds phenomenal experience in himself (and often in others) mundane. These experiences are self-evident and private. Only rarely do people such as Shirley MacLaine (1983) shout from mountain tops. Others are more like Peggy Lee, asking simply, "Is that all there is?"

Many oddities in neuropsychology come to attention by accident and often with considerable coaxing of the patient, who feels embarrassed or ashamed by what he has been taught is "not real." From here arises a fundamental objection that research based on experiential reports is "unscientific."

Verbal responses are the bread and butter of clinical assessment in neurology and neuropsychology. It is the only means in classical neurology to assess any sensory quality. Verbal reports often go beyond the metrication capacity of science to analyze a phenomenon physiologically. For example (Weiskrantz, 1986), testing with the same psychophysical methods with suprathreshold stimuli for orientation, movement, or detection in blindsight can give identical results (sometimes perfect performance) compared to testing in the intact visual field, and yet the subject insists that the perceptions in each test are worlds apart in quality. He "sees" the stimulus in the intact visual field but sees "nothing at all" in the blindsighted field. Unlike the scientist, however, he does not say, "I can make a verbal response to one but not the other," but insists that the experiences are completely different.

There are other examples where experiential reports alone have changed our concept of neurophysiology. The obvious example is dreaming during the rapid eye movement (REM) sleep stage. If no one had awakened sleepers during different EEG phases and asked them what was happening, the meaning and clinical correlation of this phasic EEG activity would have remained undeciphered. Worse yet, it might have been assumed to have no meaning at all. Verbal reports are often the neurologist's Rosetta stone. There are, of course, two sides to that stone. Experiential reports have advanced neuroscience; neuroscience should be able to help us better understand experience. This kind of support is essential in the analysis of synesthesia. One purpose of this book is to show that perceptual processes can occur on widely different levels of awareness in the individual. Blindsight research, for example, shows that verbal reports severely underestimate visual capacity, and work with split-brain patients shows that verbal reports may be actively misleading. No doubt there are complex issues in trying to disentangle the how and why of synesthesia, but it can in principle be understood just like any common experience, except that there is no shared referent.

Look at synesthesia epistemologically. One of the things that distinguishes basic from applied science is an appreciation for the potential importance of the little quirks of nature, something not immediately relevant to the solution of a practical problem. Basic science is so named because it does not require proof of relevance before phenomena are

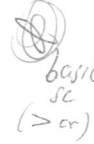

studied in the laboratories or discussed in theory. Things that do not lead to consumer goods, practical solutions, or the elucidation of some arcane theory can be extremely useful in helping us understand the nature of ourselves.

Synesthesia has no practical utility except to those who possess it, and even then not much, but it does teach us something about the nature of our perceptual experience that had been obscured. It teaches us to question many assumptions about our perception. If that is not a valid argument for studying the phenomenon, then what is? The progress of science requires that we go out of our way to examine what seem to be "irrelevant" abstractions of reality in order to make progress in understanding what we do think is relevant.

Modern science is based on the method of detailed analysis of Rene Descartes, which breaks down complex problems into their component parts in order to be examined. This examination by analysis is done simply because things are too complicated to be studied as wholes. Although we may lose information on interaction among the parts, we gain accessability to those parts. In this spirit we use preparations like *Aplysia* and *Limulus* in neurophysiology, and stimuli that are but suggestions of real scenes as models of full-blown reality in psychology. In perceptual psychology, these abstractions, charmingly referred to as "perceptual fruit flies," are ubiquitous.

For example, we are surprised at metamorphopsia, an illusion of movement in which objects advance or recede, change size, or otherwise have a fluid, dynamic alteration of characteristics that we ordinarily perceive as stable. Yet metamorphopsia can also be viewed as a normal mechanism operating out of context. Suppose you are playing tennis, accurately hitting the ball back and forth. As you play, the ball maintains a constant size regardless of its proximity, although the retinal image is much larger when the ball is close up than when it is in your opponent's court. As you volley the ball, you do not have an illusion that it shrinks and expands; rather, the parietal lobe (we assume) provides an illusion of constancy of size by in fact contracting and expanding the psychophysical size of the ball inversely to the "real" size, which is dependent on the geometry of foveation on the retina. It is only when metamorphopsia occurs with objects that we know should be stationary that we think that something is wrong. This phenomenon is just a release of a normal cognitive process in an incongruous situation.

The Ghost in the Machine

At some point we will need to review the history of various theories—philosophical and neural—that explain "how we do it." As all neuroscientists know, this discussion can easily get out of hand. But neuroscientists also know that one cannot discuss oddities of perception without dipping his toe in this vast ocean.

The question has stirred many minds greater than mine and for the same reason: the perception of "hard" reality (this book, the shoes on your feet, mountains) is not really as immediate or direct as it seems. Just as gravity describes the relationship between masses, so too do "mind," "consciousness," and similar terms refer to relationships between the organism and its environment. This theory holds that we will not discover the mind either by probing the brain as the neurophysiologists hope, or by searching the environment as the behaviorists do. Eccles is separate in seeing mind and consciousness as everywhere, surrounding us as a suprastructure.

Jesuit theologist and paleontologist Pierre Teilhard de Chardin suggested a mind principle, a spiritual inevitability, hovering over the process of evolution. Perhaps we invent such a principle because our minds are capable of spiritual experiences, projected onto the universe. The corollary is that one would not have a brain capable of spiritual experiences if there were no spirituality in the universe. Others have woven evolution into their explanation of how the conscious mind has a resident prestructure that the senses model to perceive an object. This is called phylogenetic learning.

The triune brain of Paul MacLean (1973, 1985) championed a vertical view, but not necessarily a hierarchical one like that of Hughlings Jackson. Many of MacLean's ideas (1949) were inspired by Papez (1937) and Yakovlev (1948, 1970).

In the 18th century it was held that the brain was equipotential, a concept dropped in the 19th century with the advent of the localizationists and the diagram makers. But the mass effect of Karl Lashley (1949), at least as based on its effect on memory, burst that balloon. Permeating all this, thanks to Hughlings Jackson (1898), was the hierarchical theory of brain function, which assumed that orders from "higher centers" percolated down to basal structures that just did what they were told and had no "mind" of their own.

The behavioral psychologists of the 1930s treated monkeys and men as behaving machines. Behaviorism of the 1940s and 1950s came out of logical positivism philosophy and produced numbers. Although behaviorism had the technology and methodology of "real science" it ran the other way from concepts such as awareness, consciousness, and perception.

Equipotentiality died with Lashley. In the 1960s the pendulum had completely swung the other way. Feature detection was the rage, in which a single neuron responds to a particular feature such as edge, orientation, shape, or movement, and these features are put together (somehow) to form a whole image. The somehow was suggested to be a wavefront by Eccles and a hologram by Pribram, both of whom drew a bit from network theory, and Eccles also on the modular organization of Szenthagothai.

Today, localization in neuropsychology is probably at a high watermark because holistic theories failed to explain more. In the holographic order, everything is enfolded and perception unfolds from the brain constrained accurately, one hopes, by sensory input to it. There is no boundary between mind and brain, only energy potentials converted into work. The ancient question of where the mind (*psyche, Seele*) interacts with the physical brain is the problem of downward causation. It has been easy to see how psychological properties can emerge from brain organization, but how mind operates on brain remains opaque.

The brain does change in response to external stimuli. This is called learning. Mental experience actually does affect physical and chemical structure. We believe that both sensation and thinking (whatever that is) redistribute the flow of nerve impulses (somehow) and synaptic strength (we assume) and probably neurochemistry too (why not?). Some find the connection between facilitation and habituation in *Aplysia* natural; others see it as a great leap (Kandel, 1979).

"Where is the ghost in the machine?" is a question particularly applicable to phantom vision and blindsight. Enucleated patients and those with striate lesions can perform a number of visual tasks in their "blind" field. When asked what they saw, they report "nothing;" when asked how they did it, they say, "I was just guessing." This feeling that "*I* didn't do it" is characteristic of synesthetes, too, who have a conviction that what they see is "out there," a property of the physical world. They are astonished if told that what their senses inform them of is "not real." "But how does everybody else think?" is a typical response. "How could you calculate if you can't *see* the numbers?" "How can you remember if there isn't any color?"

This all being said, what point of view shall we take in examining synesthesia? The answer is that we will probably not be consistent at all, but will take our cue from Debussey in responding to a critic: "Tell me, Mr. Debussey, what *rules* do you follow in composing?" "Mon plaisir."

MACHINE ANALOGIES OF BRAIN ACTIVITY

Ever since man began thinking about the brain and the machinery of the mind he has described it in term of the latest technology, as a machine. Aristotle did it, Descartes did it. We do it.

One cannot be impressed by machine analogies and neural activity, such as popularized by cybernetics, despite their prevalence and popularity. There is a long history of parallelism in neurological theory that seems to keep pace with current technology. In Mesmer's day, the paranoid was persecuted by malicious animal magnetism, his successors by galvanic shocks, then by the telegraph, radio, radar, and now the extraterrestrial beacon. Descartes was impressed by the hydraulic figures in the Royal Gardens and developed a hydraulic theory for the action of the brain. We have since had brain theories based on telephone wiring and electrical field theories, with the latest being based on computers and quantum physics.

The computer analogy is particularly poor, since the brain is a parallel processor, not a serial one. Another poor analogy sees the brain as the hardware and the mind as the software. Parallel-distributed processing is all the rage now. Answers are more likely to be forthcoming by studying the brain itself and the phenomenon of behavior than by making physical analogies. Such comparisons result in oversimplification of problems of behavior. Assumed machine analogies of brain function underlie the most common lay explanation for synesthesia, namely that of "crossed wires" among the senses. These false assumptions rest on the notion that a unique "sense datum," one that faithfully measures some physical property of our environment, travels unmodified and in isolation from a peripheral sense receptor to the higher levels of the brain.

How Does Mind Arise from Matter?

When one asks questions such as this, the investigations and partial answers discovered force him to reconsider the presumptions on which the question itself is based. Classical physics has taken for granted the separation of the world into mind (res cognitans) and matter (res extensa). Delbrück (1986) suggested that the significance of quantum physics is to force us to view mind and matter as aspects of a single system. It is our evolutionary development that has come to regard the mind as an independent, nonmaterial entity. Although the mind-matter dichotomy may make it easier to order our experience—such as perceptions such as size, color, position, shape, time, space, and causality—it may be no more than a practical illusion.

The world as seen through the uncertainty principle is remarkably similar to that of the infant who has not yet acquired the categories of adult cognition.

Since each of us made the transition from the infant's world, in which there is no clear distinction between subject and object . . . it is not wholly incongruous that in our rational thought processes we should be able to reverse this process (Delbrück, 1986).

There is no pure objectivity or subjectivity. Quantum theory shows that matter is altered by perception (it is not purely "objective") and biology shows that mind is certainly a product of the material world (it is not purely "subjective"). Why, then, should one wait for science to produce a coherent explanation of mind? It has not yet produced a satisfactory explanation of matter, and the end of that research is not in sight.

Consider that experiments in quantum mechanics in the early 20th century led to the conclusion that physical phenomena are shaped in fundamental ways by our perception of them. Although it is impossible to observe the wave and particle nature of light simultaneously, the dual nature of light is irrefutable. This duality is intuitively incompatible. Our common sense tells us that a wave is a wave and a particle is a particle, and that nothing can be both. We hold similar intuitions about our impressions—sound is sound, shape is shape, and color is color—and believe that these qualities belong to one sense and not another. Neils Bohr developed the idea of complimentarity to resolve the particle and wave paradox, proposing that both are related aspects of a single reality that could not be fully observed from any perspective, and that any experiment that demonstrates one aspect will inevitably interfere with the other. So too in our analysis of perception and perceptual deficits that are better understood than synesthesia (or at least more accepted because of their commonness), we will see how aspects of objects—color, shape, movement, texture—can detach from the object and be perceived separately or incongruously with objects from other senses. We must change the way that we conceive the questions, "What is perception?" and "What is real?"

Although it may be a product of evolution, the human mind actually has become what most of us presume it to be: an ideal entity that exists independently of the world it perceives. When we start looking at what actually happens when we perceive the world our presumptions about the nature of mind and reality begin to break down; we will look at some of these in this book.

For example, when we investigate visual mechanisms closely we find that it is our brains that construct much of what we take to be "objective" visual data. Color, for example, is not due to the wavelength of light reflecting off a surface, nor is it related to any obvious physical quality at any point on an object. What we see when we look at our surroundings is largely our own invention.

Take, for example, the detachment of shape. We have no difficulty recognizing a real tree from an artist's sketch of the same shape or a photograph of a tree, despite the enormously different images that each of these three examples casts on the retina. That we do not rely on "bits of data" from individual photoreceptors in constructing form is an obvious conclusion that can be logically developed into the premise that shape can detach from objects. A less apparent conclusion is that there is no such thing as sensory data.

This, of course, is Kant's idea that the conscious mind receives information from the senses in a prestructured form (*Critique of Pure Reason,* 1781). He argued that we experience sensory impressions only after interpreting them in terms of a priori categories such as time, space, object, and causality, all of which reside innately in the mind.

At the risk of belaboring the point of relativity (although it is necessary to do so to avoid questions such as, "What is it really?" and explanations such as, "It's just an illusion"), recall that to a single observer in a limited spatial domain, time and space seem reliable. However, time does not pass on a clock traveling the speed of light and a yardstick shrinks to zero length. Time and space mean nothing except in relation to each other. Neither is universal. Without universal time, other seemingly self-evident truths, such as causality, lose empirical validity as well. As we go on in subsequent chapters, the careful reader may consider the idea that objects are not objective. It is an inevitable and tantalizing thought, but I will not be on hand to extricate him from this dilemma. In some manner, synesthesia could not occur unless the properties belonging to one sense were sufficiently *modular* to detach and then reattach in another sense modality.

How Materialism Transcends Itself

We think we believe that relations between the brain and the mind are fixed. That we consensually agree about so much of the everyday world around us is a compelling argument for this point of view. Since the brain is a material object, we feel comfortable assuming that it operates according to fixed rules. The senses that are given to us by our brains must also be fixed and therefore faithfully reflect the real world as it exists.

We do not claim any active participation in interpreting the world, but accept it as given. The materialist view of brain qua machine does not permit us to be aware of a great deal of the transformation and unconscious interpretation that occur at the afferent end of the nervous system or at those parts of the brain that are inaccessable to conscious awareness. A nice example of a passive self in self-observation is given by Aristotle, illustrating that we are completely dependent on what the central nervous system delivers. When pressing an eye while looking at an object, the object *seems* to move with increasing pressure, but we are so aware of the causal connection that we are not deceived. We are aware of the subjective nature of the experience. Such an example, in which we are conscious of having an illusion and being unable to prevent it, illustrates the fact that we *can* sometimes distinguish between what is delivered to us by the brain and our active efforts at interpretation.

Many of the difficulties of the mind-body problem arise from our penchant to ask "what is" questions. We expect that we will one day really find out what the mind is. We have this expectation despite the fact that we do not know what matter really is, although we know a great deal about the physical structure of matter. We do not yet know whether elementary particles are "elementary" in any relevant sense of the term.

Similarly, we know a great deal about the structure of the mind, although we know nothing about the essence of the mind. Just like Newton, who sought an ultimate explanation for mechanical phenomenon, we too wrongly look somehow for an ultimate explanation. Mind is a process. It is a phenomenon of life of higher organisms, and almost all we know (especially the great unifying fact of the genetic code) is even less unified that our pluralistic knowledge about matter.

In his discussion of how materialism transcends itself, Popper (Chapter P1 in Popper & Eccles, 1977) begins with an extension of La Mettrie's book *Man A Machine* (1747), tracing the view of men as robots to the view of men as electrochemical machines. Both atomism and quantum physics started from the theory that matter, in the sense of occupying space, was ultimate, a substance neither capable of nor in need of further explanation. Matter is a principle in terms of which everything else had to be, and of course could be, explained. As knowledge progressed, however, the law of conservation of matter and mass had to be discarded. It turned out that matter was not a "substance" since it was not conserved but could be destroyed and could be created. Even the most stable particles can be destroyed by collision with their antiparticles as their energy is transformed into light. It turns out that matter is highly packed energy, something in the nature of a *process* since it can be converted into other processes such as light, motion, and heat.

The outcome of modern physics dictates that we *give up the idea of a substance or essence*. There simply is no self-identical entity persisting during all changes in time. There is no essence that is the persisting carrier or possessor of the properties or qualities of a thing. The universe appears to be not a collection of things, but an interacting set of events or processes.

Although the quest of science may be for simplicity, it is a real problem, particularly when we discuss things such as sensation, whether the world is itself quite so simple as some scientists or even philosophers think. The simplicity of Descarte's and Newton's theories of matter clashed with the facts, and these theories are now gone. The electrical theory of matter suffered the same fate, and the present quantum mechanics is not only less simple than one might have hoped but also clearly incomplete. So even in physics, appeals to simplicity can hardly be accepted as decisive. I use the example of physics since it is supposedly more "objective." The same arguments can be made of the messier phenomenon of human perception and the senses. But we should not deprive ourselves of interesting and challenging problems, such as what we really mean by "sensation," because such problems indicate that our knowledge and best theories are incomplete. Nor should we "explain away" the interesting problems by philosophical analysis or by persuading ourselves that the world would be simpler if they were not there. It is first necessary to get a full grasp of the problem to be solved in order to even attempt a scientific reduction. Then there is always the danger that we might refuse to admit any ideas other than the ones we happen to have at hand. Materialist theories, as intellectually satisfying as they may be, are not compatible with the facts. Hence the facts, difficult as they may to absorb, are intellectually challenging. So the decision seems to be between intellectual ease and dis-ease.

Synesthetes as Cognitive Fossils

Something as interesting as synesthesia deserves a romantic explanation. I offer one without apology. Synesthetes represent cognitive fossils in that synesthesia is a fundamentally more mammalian attribute than is language, which is more species-typical. I do not want to be misunderstood as considering synesthesia to be vestigial, more primitive or atavistic, nor comparable to animal psychology, which might infer that animals might not separate their senses. Nor do I even want to hint that it is perhaps how early man perceived in his prelinguistic phase. This would confuse us with scale of nature questions.

Synesthesia is more mammalian not because it could be more primitive, but because the *sensory* percepts are closer to the essence of what it is to perceive than are semantic abstractions, and thus more closely related to the adaptive demands of living in this world.

Synesthesia is evolutionarily earlier. A synesthetic perception is more fundamental to what it means to be a mammal in this world than is ascribing high-level semantic meaning to things. It is more phylum-typical behavior. Language is species-typical behavior for humans. In a way, we could welcome the synesthete among us as a representative of what it means to be not only human, but mammalian.

This notion is very romantic, of course, but to get right down to it the human brain does not configure itself, with all of its neocortical expanse, as a replacement for the emotional limbic brain, as we will discuss in Chapter 5. *The neocortical mantle is not a higher rung on the ladder, completely suppressing everything below it,* but is built as a detour in the ladder, interposed between brainstem and limbic brain.

The limbic system in the advanced mammal, such as the human, retains its status as the terminal stage of information processing, that stage for suppressing automatic preexisting biases in favor of newer alternatives to express themselves and where value, purpose, attention, and memory are calculated. This organ for calculating valence, to use a more neutral term, could have had either of two fates. It could have been replaced and suppressed by neocortex, which is to say that one's calculations of value and bias are now to be suppressed by higher calculations, a "better" organ for determining meaning and purpose. That seems to be the quintessential delusion of the intellectual in our midst. He thinks that the goal of thought is to suppress limbic system functions—to suppress emotion. But the cortex does not calculate emotion or valence. It just calculates.

The other way the limbic system could have evolved is the way that it did—and this is often misunderstood. The limbic brain has retained its functions as the decider of valence, those functions that remain the most important processes in the human brain. But it needs better data upon which to decide valence—the kind of data beyond those that are immediately at one's whiskers or in one's mouth. What the cortex, this brain machinery that makes us different from lower animals, does is only provide more highly calculated data about what is going on in the environment so that the limbic brain can decide questions of valence.

If one's environment poses the making of correct choices as the problem in life, then he has to have a limbic system. The choices boil down to fundamental ones about what it means to be a living organism. People who make their choices "emotionally," as we say, are more human than those who make them rationally exactly for this reason. One should permit his intellect only to inform his choices, not to override the fundamentally emotional ones. Synesthesia is a short-cut way of calculating realities, of attaching significance to things.

2
Synesthetes Speak for Themselves

In this chapter we will learn about the world of synesthetes through their own voices as they tell what it is like to have, in essence, a sixth sense. There are many permutations, and the range of synesthetic performance in clinical experience is broad. One patient may have a highly restricted form of colored hearing, for example, in which only a particular voice or particular kind of music will elicit photisms. The opposite extreme is the pentamodal patient: stimulation of one sense causes synesthesia in the remaining four. Such a vigorous type is best represented by Luria's famous patient, S (Luria, 1968).

Most often the trait is said to have been in existence as far back as the patient can remember. As children, synesthetes quickly discover that others do not perceive the world as they do. Keeping their special talent to themselves, they retreat into a secret world to avoid ridicule and disbelief, even from their own families. This must have an enormous influence on personality. Despite the emotional burden that being synesthetic imposes, as well as the practical trouble it can cause in school or social situations, synesthetes would not for a moment part with their special ability. They have an unshakable sense of conviction that what they perceive is real and valid, and their synesthetic associations are constant over their lifetime.

The experiences documented here raise rather disturbing questions about reality and what we assume to be a fairly stable understanding of perception. One obvious question is, "Where does perception occur?" Although we know a great deal about the functional architecture of the retina and segregation of visual and nonvisual outflow to the geniculate, colliculus, cerebellum (yes, visual fibers go to cerebellum), and other subcortical structures, and an enormous amount about ocular dominance columns, feature detection neurons, and so forth, we have no idea *where* or *how* perception occurs. We only know something about the neuro-anatomical substrates that are responsible for derivative aspects of perception. How it all comes together is a mystery. An equally difficult question is, "When does a physiological event become a psychological one?" When does all this brain activity reach consciousness?

Synesthetes Speak for Themselves

I remember most accurately scents. We were preparing to move into the house I grew up in. I remember at age 2 my father was on a ladder painting the left side of the wall. The paint smelled blue, although he was painting it white. I remember to this day thinking why the paint was white, when it smelled blue [Figure 2.1].

Colors are very important to me because I have a gift—it's not my fault, it's just how I am—whenever I hear music, or even if I read music, I see colors.

When I taste something with an intense flavor, the feeling sweeps down my arm to my fingertips, and I perceive that object [*weight, shape, texture, and temperature*] as if I'm actually grasping it [Figure 2.2].

When I listen to music, I see the shapes on an externalized area about 12 inches in front of my face and about one foot high onto which the music is visually projected. Sounds are most easily likened to oscilloscope configurations—lines moving in color, often metallic with height, width and, most importantly, depth. My favorite music has lines that extend horizontally beyond the "screen" area.

Something very strange is going on here. The speakers above are all intelligent, responsible people. They are not being "artistic," are not on drugs, and are not insane. Yet the incongruous adjectives and nouns come

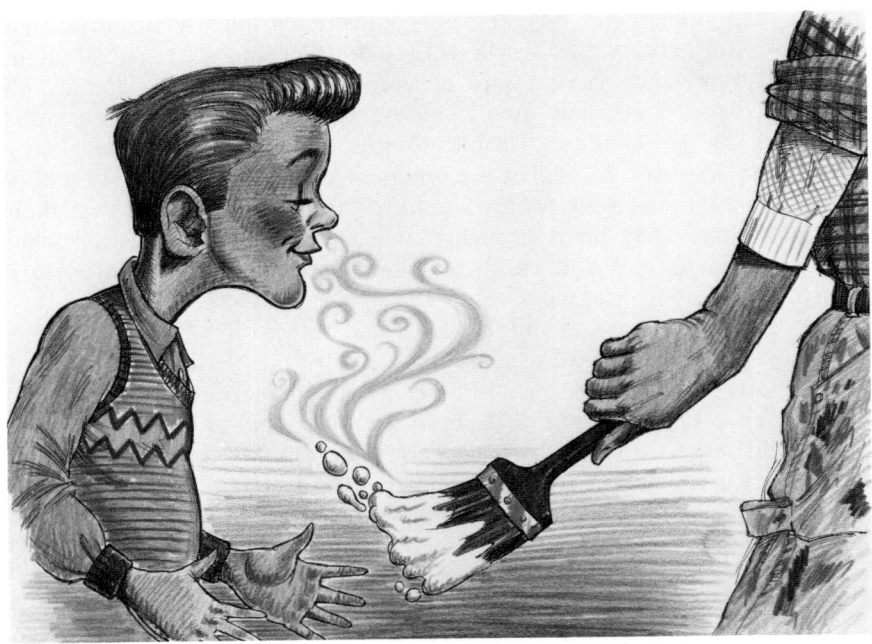

FIGURE 2.1.

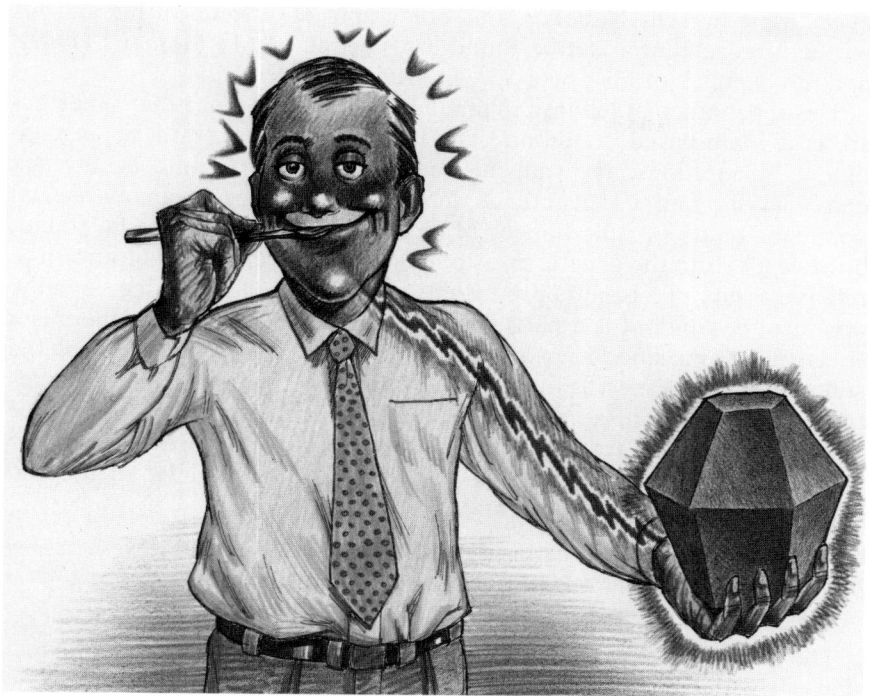

FIGURE 2.2.

tumbling out with conviction and reflect typical synesthetic sentiments. The speakers have never met, yet their stories are remarkably similar. All apologize frequently. "I know this sounds crazy, but . . . ." They also learned to stop talking about their green symphonies, salty visions, and tastes that feel like glass columns, long ago in childhood when they realized that they were different, and that no one else understood.

My parents thought I was very strange. They thought I was making it up to get attention. Everyone was always jumping in with psychological explanations: I had an overactive imagination, I was spoiled and wanted attention, a whole slew of things.

My mother was the only person that believed me, and I'm sure she was not truly convinced that what I experience is [sic] real.

Other parents may be more sympathetic. When Soviet writer Vladimir Nabokov, as a toddler, complained to his mother that the colors on his wooden alphabet blocks were "all wrong," she understood him to mean that the colors painted on the blocks did not correspond with his own letter-color associations. His mother understood this because she was synesthetic herself. Nabokov's autobiographical account of his and his mother's synesthesia can be found in "Portrait of My Mother" (1949), and in chapter 2 of his novel *Speak, Memory* (1966).

The appearance of the trait in families is strong evidence that synesthesia is a brain-based condition. The occurrence of synesthesia in contiguous generations, the transmission from parent to child in any sex combination, and its occurence in siblings all suggest an autosomal dominant mode of inheritance. More familial cases need to be found, however, before the genetic basis of synesthesia is clear. Penetrance (the relative ability of a gene to produce its specific effect in any degree in the organism of which it is a part) may explain, for example, why there is a spectrum of synesthetic performance—from restricted forms in which the stimulus is highly specific to the indiscriminate activation of all five senses by a wide variety of stimuli. In a restricted form, the subject may see colored shapes in response to *spoken* words only, whereas in the polymodal synesthete voice, music, environmental sounds, sights, and smells might all be seen, felt, and tasted:

I heard the bell ringing . . . a small round object rolled before my eyes . . . my fingers sensed something rough like a rope . . . I experienced a taste of salt water . . . and something white (Luria, 1968).

The examples above illustrate two points. First, although any combination or multiple combination of the senses is possible, the most common yoking is sound with sight, called colored hearing or *chromesthesia*. Another common form of synesthesia is colored numbers and letters. The second point is that color figures quite prominently in the various synesthesiae [colored hearing; colored olfaction; word-, number-, and name-color associations; colored taste (Downey, 1911); and colored music]. Why this should be so is not clear.

The following features of synesthetes and synesthesia are examined in some detail.

> Similarity of stories
> Spectrum of performance
> Synesthesia as an unelaborated sensation
> Validity, constancy, and limits of manipulation
> Personality and psychological stigmata
> Hypermnesis
> Familial cases

My first two subjects, MW and VE, were discovered by chance. The rest have brought themselves to my attention as a result of newspaper or magazine articles and radio and television programs that sometimes follow my presentations to professional scientific audiences. The popular press and television have been limited to North America and France; a Voice of America radio program was broadcast to 120 countries. The growth of cases has been exponential. Over the 9 years that I have collected cases, the bulk have been added recently as interest of the press has spread.

The following letter is typical of an unsolicited response:

Dear Dr. Cytowic:

I read the article (copy enclosed) from [*a particular newspaper*] concerning your work with synesthesia. It's an affirmation that I am not nuts and whatever my other problems may have been, being crazy was not one of them.

I am a sight/sound synesthete, most often seeing sound as colors, with a certain sense of almost pressure on exposed skin when sounds are very light or colors very bright. [*MM*] is quoted in the article as stating that it's sort of like a clear overlay, which is exactly right. You have no idea (or maybe you do at that!) how exciting it is to read someone else's description— and from a total stranger—of an experience that I have never been quite sure wasn't the result of my imagination or being insane. I have never met anyone else who saw sound. When enough people tell you that you are imagining things it's easy to doubt yourself. I've never been quite sure that I'm not crazy.

It's definitely colors, but I'm not sure that "seeing" is the most accurate description. I am seeing, but not with my eyes, if that makes sense.

I love my colors, can't imagine being without them. One of the things I love about my husband are the colors of his voice and his laugh. It's a wonderful golden brown, with a flavor of crisp, buttery toast, which sounds very odd, I know, but it is very real.

Would it be possible to meet others [*synesthetes*]? As I said, I have never met anyone else who does these things, and would very much like to, as much for the reassurance as anything else (RP, 5/1/87).

Table 2.1 summarizes the pertinent demographics, types of synesthesia, presence or absence of certain cognitive characteristics, and pertinent comments for the patients who are described in this book. This table contains current subjects only, and not historical cases. Most have been examined in person, a few by correspondence and telephone. Patients will be referred to throughout this text by the initials indicated in the table. The reader will wish to refer to this table throughout his reading of this book.

Similarity of Stories

Synesthesia has an ineffable quality, a quality William James defined in *The Varieties of Religious Experience* (1901): "The subject says that it defies expression, that no adequate report of its content can be given in words. It follows from this that its 'quality' must be directly experienced, it cannot be imparted or transferred to others."

There is a general social taboo against inner knowledge, the individual need to know, and the fear of knowing. Biases exist in our scientific and social systems against examining higher creativity and what society says

TABLE 2.1. Current synesthetic subjects with a brief description of their type of synesthesia.[a]

Tag	Age	Sex	Educ	Hand	FMLH	Type of synesthesia	?Proj	?Gmem	?Gmath	?Ggeog	Notes
AB	17	WF	12	L	N	Polymodal, letters, & numbers	Y	Y	N	N	Music, eating—colors and textures. Memory at 2 years old.
AC	30	WF	24	R	N	Number form	N	Y	Y	Y	Brother autistic.
BB	38	WM	14	R	N	Simple synesthesia, auras	Y	Y	N	Y	Spelling errors. No synesthesia with LSD.
CS	23	WF	16	R	Y	Number form	Y	Y	Y	Y	
CSc	21	WF	18	R	N	Musical tastes & smells	Y	Y	Y	N	
DB	26	WF	16	R	N	Number form, colorless	Y	Y	N	Y	TV producer. Highly organized.
DH	46	WM	16	R	N	Colored hearing	N	Y	N	N	No synesthesia with LSD.
DI	31	WF	16	M	N	Letters, words	N	Y	N	N	Memory at 4 years old. Color of a word not predictable from the color of individual letters.
DS	33	WF	18	R	N	Colored hearing, number form	Y	Y	N	N	Family history dyslexia. Acalculic. Memory at 2 years old.
DSc	32	WF	18	L	N	Letters and words	N	Y	N	N	Speech pathologist. Right-left confusion.
DSh	28	WF	18	R	N	Colored hearing	Y	Y	Y	Y	Hypercalculia. Cannot learn languages.
EW	62	WF	16	R	N	Colored hearing, number form	Y	Y	N	N	Four generations.

FKD	59	WF	18	R	N	Colored words, names	Y	Y	N	N	Niece is synesthetic. Romance language teacher.
GG	54	WF	16	M	Y	Colored numbers & letters	N	N	N	Y	No number form. Ludiomil: no change. Medical illustrator.
GH	31	WM	16	R	N	Colored hearing	Y	Y	N	N	Voices, music, environmental sounds. Geometric colored photisms. "Doesn't obscure my regular sight." Memory at 2 years old. Pilot, computer programmer.
HC	50	WF	14	R	N	Colored numbers & letters	Y	Y	N	N	Paints. "Always think in colors."
JB	66	WF	15	R	N	Simple synesthesia	Y	Y	N	Y	Paints her photisms. Sees form constants.
JL	13	WM	7	R	N	Colored numbers	Y	Y	N	N	Colors have moods.
JM	61	WF	14	M	N	Letters & numbers	N	Y	N	Y	Polyglot. Consistent in Latin alphabet. No number form.
LF	34	WF	16	R	N	Colored hearing	N	Y	N	N	Cousin of MT.
LH	61	WF	16	L	Y	Letters & numbers	N	Y	N	Y	Sister synesthetic. Son dyslexic, red–green, color blind.
MF	81	WF	16	R	N	Colored letters & numbers	N	Y	N	N	Clairvoyant. Has asthma & migraine.
MG	24	WM	18	R	N	Visual smell	Y	Y	N	N	Clairvoyant.
MLL	58	WF	13	M	N	Colored music	Y	Y	N	N	Clairvoyant.
MLP	32	WF	18	R	Y	Number form	N	Y	N	Y	Sister dyslexic; brother's 2 children left-handed & dyslexic.

(continued.)

TABLE 2.1. (*Continued*)

Tag	Age	Sex	Educ	Hand	FMLH	Type of synesthesia	?Proj	?Gmem	?Gmath	?Ggeog	Notes
MM	37	WM	14	R	N	Colored hearing	Y	Y	N	N	Music, words have shape and color, "like a transparency." LSD made more intense. Trouble with poetry. Computer programmer.
MMO	44	WM	20	M	N	Polymodal	N	Y	N	N	0 drugs. Toy designer. Probable transition between synesthesia and imagery.
MN	36	BF	18	L	N	Audioalgesic, smell	Y	Y	N	N	Cannot stand to hear foreign language. Marijuana: no change.
MT	34	WF	18	R	N	Letters & numbers	Y	Y	N	N	Three generations. LSD. Graphic representation causes it. Gender & personality. No number form. "Optical illusion that never goes away."
MW	43	WM	18	R	N	Touch, taste, smell	Y	Y	N	N	Acalculia. LSD 1971. No number form.
NM	46	WF	16	R	N	Letters, numbers, music keys	Y	Y	N	N	Sister synesthetic.
PO	41	WM	20	L	Y	Colored numbers, number form	Y	Y	Y	Y	No change after ruptured R MCA aneurysm.

Subject	Age	Race/Sex	Educ	Hand	FMLH	Synesthesia	?Proj	?Gmem	?Gmath	?Ggeog	Notes
PP	43	WF	16	R	N	Colored hearing	Y	Y	N	N	Artist. Colors sometimes opaque, sometimes transparent. Music, letters, numbers, words.
RB	49	WF	14	M	Y	Shaped pain	Y	Y	Y	N	Scot. 0 family history. Sister left-handed. Awkward dexterity.
RF	49	WM	14	R	N	Number form, colored	N	N	Y	Y	
RP	37	WF	18	R	Y	Colored hearing, touch, taste	Y	Y	N	N	0 drugs. Right-left confusion, poor speller, often transposes letters. WAIS IQ 135.
SO	42	WF	18	R	Y	Colored hearing, letters, numbers	Y	Y	Y	N	Father and left-handed sister synesthetic. 0 number form. Music has shape.
SP	39	BF	12	L	Y	Letters & numbers	N	Y	Y	Y	Sister with letters and numbers.
SdeM	48	WF	20	R	N	Numbers, number form	N	Y	N	N	Olfactory trigger.
TP	24	WM	12	R	N	Sound, taste, numbers	Y	Y	N	N	Reproduced number & letter list years later with mother. Dyslexic, reversals, spelling. Clairvoyant.
VE	42	WF	20	R	N	Polymodal, colored hearing	Y	N	N	N	
WW	46	WM	20	R	N	Colored hearing	Y	Y	N	N	Son of EW.

[a] Y (yes) or N (no) indicates the presence or absence of the trait indicated in the heading under which it appears. Educ, education (years). Hand, handedness (R, right-handed; L, left-handed; M, mixed dominance); FMLH, family history of left-handedness; ?Proj, synesthesia perceived externally; ?Gmem, good memory; ?Gmath, good mathematical aptitude; ?Ggeog, good sense of direction.

is not "normal." It can be difficult to get synesthetes to talk about their experiences because of previously encountered disbelief. "Nobody understands." "People look at me like I'm crazy." "I don't want to be a freak." True synesthetes are reticent; weirdos will talk about their "visions" at the drop of a hat.

The initials identifying the quotes that follow are keyed to the demographic and other data found in Table 2.1.

MN

I read with interest the article in the [*newspaper*] . . . as since early childhood I have thought I was the only person in the *world* with this.

GG

I realize that I, *almost alone,* possess this mnemonic device of seeing colors of the alphabet and numbers.

BB

The synesthete BB has simple synesthesia and auras around objects. Note the spelling errors. His synesthesia and dyslexia are discussed in a later chapter.

I have never communicated to anybody of seeing additional colored light. For one, I have failed to understand it myself, and to try to explain it to somebody else would leave me no better off. I was so happy to see that my experience is shared and acknowledged by others. I am 35 years old and work in the construction industry. Fear of ridicule has held my secrete [*sic*].

DS

I nearly fell over when I saw the article about you in [*a magazine*]. I ran to my husband, shouting "See! This is me! I told you it's real. I'm not nuts!"

MM

I see shapes and colors in response to sounds. I enjoy electronic music because it evokes such wonderful shapes and colors in my visual perception area. I feel for the first time that I am not nuts! The colored shape is seen as if I were looking through a plastic transparency which is in front of my eyes. If I shut my eyes, or if it is at night in the dark, then the shapes are the only thing in the field and are therefore more intense.

However, there is a secondary path. Sometimes when I hear words I will see shapes. This second one is the one that makes me feel silly. You will notice the shape which your last name evokes below [Figure 2.3]. I'm not much of an artist. This is the first time I've written something like this down, but it's accurate.

I have trouble putting into words some of the things I experience. It is like explaining RED to a blind person or Middle C to a deaf person. These connections have been with me essentially since birth and are so natural that they are hard to set down on paper. I find it a wonderful addition to life and would hate to lose it (10/21/83).

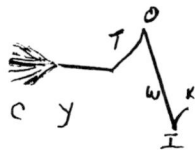

FIGURE 2.3. Shape of the author's (misspelled) spoken name, drawn by MM.

Range of Synesthetic Performance

The parallel sense of synesthesia is itself always simple and unelaborated. It is the kind or multiplicity of stimuli and the opportunity for multiple sensations in different modes that can make the synesthesia a compound sensation. It only seems more complex when, failing to find words to describe his sensation, a synesthete resorts to metaphor or analogy. This is how the uncritical mind may erroneously conclude that the parallel sense is a "mere association."

I call the simplest kind of synesthesia "simple synesthesia." These are colored auras or blobs that arise spontaneously. The stimulus may not be readily apparent.

SIMPLE SYNESTHESIA AND COLORED AURAS

BB sees "additional" colors bordering objects. They can parallel a boundary, come in "soft splotches" lacking orientation, or appear as a color wash over part of the object. Physical sensations of numbness, flushing, exhilaration, fear, and happiness accompany seeing the colors. At times they obscure the real object, for example, turning to face someone and "not seeing her but a small white center surrounded by black and a large green masking any feature of this person."

For BB, there is a green haze or outline, like a transparency, over the Golden Gate Bridge (which is actually painted orange). Colors can change with the same object (i.e., the bridge is not always green).

Whether his synesthesia is internal or projected may be moot. When BB is asked where he sees the colors, he replies, "In my mind, I am convinced of it." But he admits this only because he "knows" it is "really" not there. That is, because no one else can see it he doubts his own senses. "It's real to me. Only two people know about it. If I told anyone else they'd think I'm crazy."

Flashing light patterns, vivid and clear, seem like snow or halos. The colors he sees are primarily green, red, brown, and amber, singly or in a mixture. They are so subtle that the colors "sort of like float across your eyes."

Another subject describes her simple synesthesiae:

DS: My mind does not stop processing and usually I need to bore myself to sleep. Sometimes when I am really exhausted I see what I call "sleep designs." These are involuntary patterns, usually geometric, sometimes floral, always in color and similar to bolts of fabric or bedsheets. They change into different designs without any conscious effort on my part (3/1/87).

Strong emotions can produce an aura in patients who have some other somatic synesthesia. I have never seen it in isolation. Anger or the flash of insight may trigger a simple colored aura. Kissing and sexual intercourse is a reliable trigger in some subjects, causing colored photisms, tactile shapes and textures, and tastes (DS, DSh, MW).

DS: People say that anger is red, but I see purple. If I'm really upset at my kids and I'm yelling at them, there will be a purple background behind them. Where their head meets the background, its like an aura, a yellow luminescence going into purple. It dissipates slowly.

Figure 4.14 (Chapter 4) shows JB's drawing of her simple synesthesia.

POLYMODAL SYNESTHETES

TP

TP, a 17-year-old dyslexic student, is polymodal. Letters, numbers, and music have color. Food has numbers and falls into "groups," 3 representing heavy foods, and 1 representing thirst and lighter foods. He remembers streets by their color. This trait has been present since childhood. His mother wrote down his color associations when he was a child. He reproduced the list without error 10 years later.

MMo

MMo, a toy designer, is also polymodal. Sounds or specific words evoke flavor, visual shape, and color. Eights are yellow, for example, a square feels like mashed potatoes, and the name Steve is somehow like poached eggs.

CSc

CSc, a doctoral candidate in music, perceives involuntary tastes and smells when she plays the piano or oboe. This occurs only when she herself plays and not when she is listening to others. She first noticed this at puberty. The tastes and smells can be so intense as to interfere with her musical concentration and she has to stop. She is distressed by this interference and its possible disruption of her profession as a performing artist. Taste and smell does not cause music. However, a kiss produces a visual kaleidoscope intermingled with textures that she feels "everywhere."

This subject's experience is reminiscent of the tertiary associations in music cited by Schultze (1912). His subject's colored music was closely associated with gustatory sensations. Instrumental music would produce a sensation first of taste and then of color, as if the stimulus went "from the ear through the mouth to the eye." He would refer to a mouthful of music (*Mund voll musik*) and a perseveration where the taste and color would linger on after the music had ceased. Thus he spoke of digesting the music (*die Musik verdaut*).

Colored Music

MLL

When I listen to music I see colored shapes. If I am tired at the end of the day the shapes seem very near. They are always in color. Shiny white isoceles triangles, like long sharp pieces of broken glass. Blue is a sharper color and has lines and angles, green has curves, soft balls, and discs. It is uncomfortable to sit still. I feel the space above my eyes is a big screen where this scene is playing (9/2/85).

The shapes come, they move, they leave. It lasts for a while and the bad shapes last longer than the pleasant shapes.

Visual Pain and Geometric Hearing

RB

As far back as I can remember I have felt pain in shapes, though it seems to me anyone could do so easily. Often, but not always, I hear voices (particularly singing voices) in shapes; I have felt at times I could draw or paint a song (10/19/84).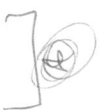

The simple shapes are felt, rather than seen, on the surface of her skin, and are never intricate (Figure 2.4). She does not have a sense of palpation like MW does. The shapes she usually perceives are blobs, grids, crosshatchings, and geometric forms.

That others should express the least surprise at how she perceives is absolutely incredible to RB:

A person who sings with little phrasing or variation in volume has a straight line voice. A baritone has a round shape that I feel. This is so obvious, it's all very logical. I thought everyone felt this way. When people tell me they don't, it's as if they were saying they don't know how to walk or run or breathe (5/6/87).

Colored Orthography that Has Personality

MT

For MT, any graphic representation of numbers and letters stimulates color. Each letter of the alphabet and each digit has a very specific color

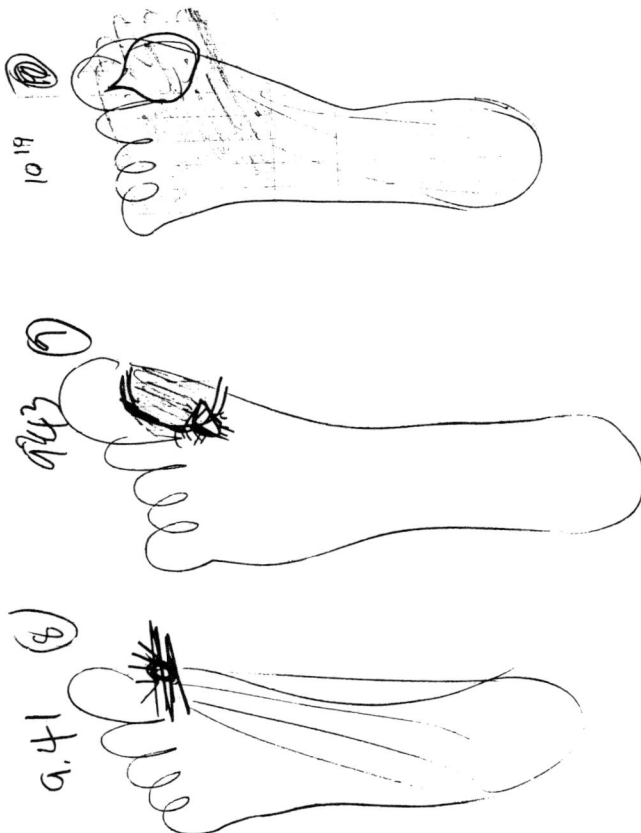

FIGURE 2.4. Drawing by RB of shaped pain following foot surgery. The shape is not constant, but changes with time, just as the experience of the pain is neither constant nor monotonous. Note the simple geometry.

that she sees regardless of the typeface, color of the ink, or language (so long as it uses the Latin alphabet). Roman numerals carry the color of the letters that they use. If a letter is spoken aloud, she first visualizes it, at which instance the color is apparent.

The sensation is not like a hallucination but like "an optical illusion that *never* goes away."

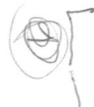

The sensation is unsuppressible, the colors are always present for me and it is very specific. The colors of the letters don't overwhelm my ability to read or function. In fact, they enhance my reading, writing, and spelling. Additionally, the numbers and letters seem to carry personality and gender, the same way they carry color. They are "real characters!" (pun intended).

Dysphoria and Photisms with Foreign Speech

MN

Since about the age of 3, whenever I hear foreign speech (especially French, Spanish and Italian) I immediately see a blinding goldenrod light, feel a tingling sensation up and down my right side, and experience a "wierd" [*sic*] sensation in my ears that I can only describe as similar to the sensation one feels when fingernails are scratched on a blackboard. This permeates my entire body and is most uncomfortable. I cannot keep still or concentrate well.

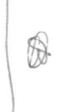

Because I was ridiculed so much about this, told I was spoiled, trying to get attention, etc. (as a child I would put my hands over my ears and squirm until the speaking subsided) I learned to live with it. However, I continue to avoid all foreign films, television shows, etc. (7/7/85).

Colored Hearing in a Swiss Polyglot

JM

We will examine JM in detail because she exhibits many characteristic features of synesthesia.

I had been hoping for a long time to find some information about [synesthesia] or even just a kindred soul. I only became consciously aware of it after reading Vladimir Nabokov's autobiography *Speak, Memory* in which, to my great surprise, he describes exactly the same type of synesthesia as mine: a case of colored hearing, i.e. 'seeing' every letter of the alphabet and every number in a specific color . . . . My colors are not the same as his.

I too never talked about it, not out of shyness but because I always thought that all people were like that. Only after reading Nabokov's description of his synesthesia did I realize that this was rather unusual . . . . I enjoy it very much and would be hard put if these colors would suddenly vanish. I don't think they will; I am 61 now and had it all my life (11/02/86).

JM is facile in learning languages and has varying fluency in Japanese, Italian, French, and Spanish. In all these languages it is the spelling that determines the color. She once studied Russian in preparation for travel and found that the orthography of the Cyrillic alphabet had no color of its own but did when she transliterated it to German. "The words would stick out in color phonetically, the way I would spell them in German. It's simply always there." JM still thinks to herself much of the time in her native Schweitzerdeutsch.

JM wrote down her color list years ago after she read Nabokov, hoping to find someone like her who saw in colors. She never did, but reading Nabokov made her realize that many of her letters are not "definite colors. It is shades." Her color list is reproduced in Table 2.2.

Note that "10" is white, perhaps because its constituents are white. But all the numbers in the 20 series are red, or mainly red, even though "the other colors are there." The 30s, 40s, and 50s are all influenced by

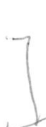

TABLE 2.2. Color list of JM (note desaturation and grays).

a	strong blue, dark
b	brown
c	very yellow, light, almost white
d	light beige
e	also yellow, different
f	yellowishy, but like mustard
g	gray and sometimes with black outline
h	dark gray
i	almost white
j[a]	orange red (with yellow in English; not French or German)
k	pitch black
l	grayish, sometimes a little green
m	brown, different from the "b"
n	red rust
o	white
p	gray
q	grayish white
r	pitch black, even blacker than the "k"
s	bright red, very nice
t	yellow
u	whitish
v	olive green-gray
w	wine red
x	mix of red and brown
y	grayish white
z	orange red
1	white with black outline
2	red, light
3	beige yellow
4	dark green
5	loden green
6	black
7	very violent yellow, like lighting
8	dark red, my favorite number
9	bluish white
10	the combination is white; zero is white

[a]Three days after our interview, JM wrote to tell me that she had forgotten to give me the color for "j" when we met.

the first number. The number 164, for example, is white, black, and green. Large numbers are simply the combination of the colors, although it does not help JM to remember them "unless there's an eight in there because I like it so much."

That a few colors are intense while others are desaturated is a feature that may not be guessed by the frequent reference to "colored" hearing. Even JM remarks that "they're rather dull colors!" This desaturation of chroma is discussed in relation to visual hallucinations and melting of colors off object boundaries in Chapter 9. Desaturation of chroma is also common in achromatopsia (Damasio, 1985; Damasio, Yamada, Damasio, Corbet, & McKee, 1980).

Note the high frequency of pastel or grayish colors in another synesthete, GG, in Table 2.3.

Synesthesia as an Unelaborated Percept

Synesthetes do not perceive complex scenes. They share their perceptions with us only through verbal labels, and perhaps this is how earlier authors, who were psychologists, came to suppose that language was the link in synesthetic perception.

MW

MW, the gustatory synesthete, perceives shape, texture, weight, and temperature whenever he tastes or smells foods. He describes the taste of spearmint as "cool glass columns." Such a description can easily lead others to assume that he is using metaphoric speech or that such a

TABLE 2.3. Color list of GG (note desaturation and grayish colors).

a	bright red	0	white
b	brown	1	black
c	lemon yellow	2	gray-blue
d	yellow-orange	3	bright green
e	gray	4	yellow
f	black	5	orange
g	gray-blue	6	red
h	gray	7	navy blue
i	black, like number 1	8	gray, gray-blue
j	dark gray	9	brown
k	middle gray	10	black & white
l	"	20	gray-blue & white
m	navy blue	30	bright green & white
n	"		etc.
o	white		
p	rose		
q	pale yellow-orange		
r	darker red than "a"		
s	pink		
t	dark, maybe black		
u	pastel yellow		
v	gold		
w	bright green		
x	gold		
y	rich gold		
z	copper color		

description is a product of creative imagination. It is not. It is a verbal interpretation of a sensory experience.

When pressed to describe the tactile qualities that he feels, and pressed to explain how it is that he *knows* it is a glass column, the following occurs: upon inhalation of wintergreen oil, there is a pause of 2 to 3 seconds. His right hand sweeps vertically through the air and he moans pleasurably. He rubs his fingertips together and moves his hand through the air as if palpating an object.

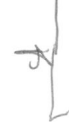

I feel a round shape. There's a curvature behind which I can reach, and it's very, very smooth. So it must be made of marble or glass, because what I'm feeling is this incredible, satiny smoothness. There are no ripples, no little surface indentations, so it must be glass, because if it were marble, I would be able to feel the roughness of the stone or the pits in the surface. It's also very cool so it has to be some sort of glass or stone material because of its temperature. What is so wonderful is the absolute smoothness of it. I can run my hand up and down, but I can't feel where the top ends. I feel that it must go on up forever. So the only thing I can explain this feeling as is that it's like a tall, smooth column made of glass. In fact, with the amyl nitrate [*an adjuvant that intensifies the synesthesia (Chapter 4)*], it's as if there's a whole row of them and I can stick my hand in among the columns and feel the back sides of the curves. There is this funny sort of feeling of being able to reach my hand into this area. It's very, very pleasant.

This is a verbal description of a sensation, comparable to explaining to a blind person what it is like to see by use of analogy. What one has in this example of a sensory perception is the formation of contours in a perceptual process (Osgood, 1956).

DS

Seeing sound/music does not adequately describe the process. There is a spatial presence that incorporates more than just the sensation of "seeing." I think that a better description is perceiving, which also includes the sensation of feeling and denotes integration (3/1/87).

The coloration of the percept is simply that, although it can be associated with shape and movement. Sometimes the color is simply a halo or outline, as in simple synesthesia, or may appear as a wash—a transparent overlay—in which case it is similar to the melting of colors off object boundaries in hallucinations. It can be opaque and block out the real object in the environment. Whether a color is opaque or not is hard for patients to describe since they "fill in the gaps." DS, for example, says that her moving lines block her vision of what is really there even though she "knows" that something is there. This is like filling in the gap in one's physiological blind spot, a process that is automatic and unconscious. Even those who know much about the blind spot and how to find it have difficulty, while viewing the scene in front of them, creating an empty space where the blind spot should be. We can hold our finger up in the temporal field and see that it disappears from our peripheral vision, but when simply viewing the scene in front of us it is hard if not impossible to perceive the blind field that is "really" there.

RP

The synesthetic sense is definitely not "in my mind." It is just sort of there. It is sort of a translucent overlay with depth that I can see through. It is kind of like a heat shimmer, only without the distortion (9/8/87).

Some patients see the colors one at a time, like the flipping down of a number on a digital clock. Others have a panorama that compels the eye to wander. Letters and numbers flash by them like a ticker tape or sequenced electric sign. HC, a 50-year-old painter, has a window in which she views six or seven colors as she counts from 1 to 20. MLP (Chapter 7) feels that some of her letters and numbers have a "spotlight" on them somehow highlighting them with more light when she looks at them.

Validity, Constancy, and Limits to Manipulation of the Parallel Sense

Patients have an unshakable conviction that what they perceive is real and valid. The synesthesiae change little, if at all, over the course of their lifetime and there is little that they can do to intensify or minimize the sense. It is not under volitional control.

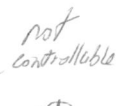

I have never tried to alter the synesthetic perceptions. They are something that I always considered part of normal functioning—like breathing. I have always accepted the sensations, even in the face of skepticism or ridicule. I know what I see and if other don't have the facility I consider it to be their loss.

Concentration will tend to intensify the sensations, while distractions will minimize them (9/17/84).

FKD

FKD is a retired romance language teacher who perceives names, nouns, and verbs "as blobs of color with the printed word lightly superimposed." Sometimes it is so intense that "the printed word will leap out from the page in color."

I was amazed when I realized that other people did not have similar images. The experience comes involuntarily and cannot be altered and is most often the result of *hearing* the word or *thinking* of the person so named (8/7/85).

MN

I experience the synesthetic sense both in my mind and it is also externalized. It is somewhat like an hallucination. It is very real. Once it begins it doesn't stop until the speaker stops (7/7/85).

GH

A consistent stimuli [*sic*] will produce a consistent synesthesia. The shapes and colors will be exactly the same if the sound comes from exactly the same source. For example if you eat a lemon cake baked by one bakery one day and you eat another from a different bakery the next, in both cases you would describe the taste as being that of a lemon cake. But since the cakes are not likely made exactly the same, one would taste somewhat different from the other as described by your taste buds. Now, if a singer sings a song on a record and then live on TV the visual patterns will vary because they're not exactly alike. If I replay a record over and over, however, I will see the same visual pattern.

I usually see geometric shapes of some complexity that is everchanging as does the sound that stimulates it (4/9/84).

JM

Can't stop or start it. I asked my husband "when I talk to you or when you read something, how do *you* see it?" and he says "not at all." Anything—I will read your name or read something, immediately it is in all of its colors.

JM was shown a letterhead that featured the business logo printed in green ink on buff paper. She was asked whether the color of the ink made a difference. "No, here it is light yellow, then it gets a little gray. O is white, L is sort of gray, N is the worst color, so that is very dominant and it dominates the others. R is black, then the rest fades out. Immediately it does that when I look at it."

She was asked about meaning and whether the same word in English (e.g., "color") or German (*Farbe*) was the same. It is not. The determinant is absolutely the spelling.

As soon as I hear words it is spelled in my mind. You know on Times Square how they have the electric band with the news. That it exactly how it is in my head. Any word that comes in flows right through me in color. That's exactly how it is. It goes fast, of course, I mean I haven't got time in a conversation to think of everything—but it's simply there. If I want to I can stop at a certain word and look at it.

Somebody says to me "how is your dog?" First I see the word DOG in color, then I think of my dog. That's how it goes. The color always comes first before I can think of the thing.

DS

I never shift my focus when I see these things. They're always in the same plane—about 6" from my nose. The DEPTH is very important. I get *goosebumps* even talking about it. It's like trying to explain to a blind person what GREEN is. If I hear music that goes UP THERE, beyond what I can see, I just can't listen to it. It's irritating. I can't stand opera because they're always singing up there. I only like what I can see. Too low is the same problem. I've never noticed that music goes off the right or left sides of the screen.

The side borders [*of her screen*] are SHARP. It goes there and it stops. It doesn't go beyond on the sides.

I hate flat lines. Elevator music or Musak [*commercial ambient music*] is like that. And that irritates me as well. I like music that makes the lines move.

Throughout, one notices that the examples are uneven. Those synesthetes who have colored numbers or letters do not necessarily include all the vowels or consonants; some may not have chroma for all digits from 1 to 10 but may assign colors to several higher random numbers. Likewise, some of the months or days of the week may be missing coloration. The same principle responsible for desaturation of color or the presence of grayish tones may be operative here.

MT

As a summary of the sense of validity, consider the explanation of MT:

It is not a hallucination but it is hard for me to describe. As I look at a page, I see the colors there even though I see the color of the REAL ink that's before me. I know it isn't there for real, but I still can't help seeing it. There is still a sensation that the color is there.

I can't remember when I didn't have it. It's not something that I do. It happens all by itself. Letters and colors seems exactly as they are since forever.

Since MT's stimulus is the graphic representation of letters and numbers, no matter what language the text may be in, the obvious questions arise: how does she think, how does she read, and does it not get in the way?

No more than a child learning to read or write and having to look at the letters. After you learn, you take the letters for granted and the individual letters don't get in the way, because you're reading words.

She describes her synesthesia as "an optical illusion that's always there." Her letter states: "I see pages and pages of color." Where does she see it? "On the page, wherever the letters are." So it is not in her mind? "No, it's on the page!"

CORRESPONDENCE OF STIMULI AND RESPONSES

At this point the reader should see general similarities among synesthetes and their perceptions, but perhaps is becoming frustrated at not seeing obvious correspondences among either stimuli or the parallel responses. The search for correspondences is the most common approach to take in trying to bring some order to this subject. It was the assumption taken decades ago, the pursuit of which was fruitless and led to abandonment of the subject.

Even sensory psychologists (L.E. Marks, 1974, 1975) performing sensory differentials could make little order out of it if they assumed that there were similarities either among the stimuli (such as linguistic or phonological components) or the responses (which presumably shared some psychophysical properties). We will show in Chapter 3 that a more fruitful analysis involves the way in which synesthetes map sensory dimensions.

Following are examples of colored hearing in which both subjects have equally distinct but different features that serve as a stimulus. One responds to the *sound* of spoken language; the other is sensitive to the *orthography*. Yet both have word synesthesia.

EWe

Elizabeth Werth (EWe) is a rather well-known subject studied by the linguists Gladys Reichard and Roman Jakobson (Reichard, Jakobson, & Werth, 1949). EWe is a polyglot who learned Serbian and Hungarian as first languages, followed by French, German, English, and Russian. She also reads Latin. The color, shape, and motion synesthesia is essentially the same for sounds in all languages in which EWe can make identifications.

TABLE 2.4. Lack of correlation among speakers of Slavic and Germanic languages.[a]

	Vowels[b]				
Vowel	L(German)	D(German)	S.P.(Czech)	E.W.(Serb)	V.N.(Russian) letters
a	red	red	red	tan	?
æ	pink	—	(orange)	(tan)	?
o	blue	red-brown	red-blue	blue-black	ivory
u	black-brown	black-brown	dark blue	blood red	?
y(ü)	gray	—	(gray)	red base with pinkish spots (Hungarian)	?
ø	light blue	—	(gray-green red)	(dark blue ground with light blurred spots)	?
e	yellow	yellow	bright green	yellow	yellow
i	silver-white	white	canary yellow	white	yellow
w	—	—	—	(steel blue spreading rings)	dull green with violet

Consonants[b]

Sound	S.P.	E.W.	V.N.
p	dust	light brown, tan, or colorless	apple green
b	gray-blue	steel blue	burnt sienna
m	gray-brown	dark tan	fold of pink flannel
f	violet	purple (with dot-circle)	alder leaf
v	matte violet	blue	rose quartz
t	light greenish	no color, but long alternating with sort diagonal lines	pistachio
tj	—	gray with diagonal wavy line	—
d	bright orange	gray or tan	creamy
r	beige	gray	oatmeal
ŋ(ñ)	beige	(green)(French)	—
r	—	(colorless but tufted) (English)	—
k	lead gray (iridescent)	—	huckleberry (for the letter c)
g	dark gray	green	vulcanized rubber
s	"sharply tin color"	gray-white	mother-of-pearl
z	gray-white	steel blue, darker than ʃ	inky
ts	"bright white-blue"	no color but a round group of dots	—
ʃ	blue-silver	gray or colorless	—
θ	tin color	gray	pale rubbery (letter j)
tʃ	"white-blue with some red"	yellow with same form as t	—
dθ	brown-gold	yellow with diagonal lines alternating with one dot	rubbery (English j)
r	bluish black	—	sooty rag
l	watery blue	yellow	limp noodle
lj	—	yellow, soft gum texture	—
θ	—	(steel blue) (English)	—

[a]Reprinted by permission from Reichard, G., Jakobson, R., and Werth, E. (1949). Language and synesthesia. *Word, 5,* 232–233.
[b]L, Langenbeck's (1913) observations on vowels, including his own colored hearing; D, Deichman's observation, cited by Reichard et al.; S.P., Jakobson's (1941) case; E.W., Elizabeth Werth; V.N., Vladimir Nabokov (1949).

To me the numbers 1 to 10 have colors. I can count and reckon only in Serbian. No other language possesses the proper sounds for my mind, the sounds that include the number color.

Characteristically, EWe feels that the synesthesia and method of memorization is "simple" and "natural," but the mental contortions she takes in translating numbers and words into another language and her native colors in order, for example, to remember a telephone number are remarkable!

There is no way for me to remember street or telephone numbers except to translate them into Serbian and arrange them in a sequence, eg a serial of diminishing odd numbers intercepted by even numbers occurring at random as in TR8-9051 where there is in my mind a soft curve of 9, 5, 1 plus the two even numbers that tighten the curve to a zigzag line.

EWe enjoys playing with words, listening to new sound combinations and arranging them in colored patterns. Pronouncing French vowel combinations that she had written out gave her the sensation of "luminous rings;" for others there is texture, sheen, phosphorescence, or sparkling as part of the dynamic of her sounds. The color of a word is dominated by the vowel, which takes on different shades depending on the surrounding consonants. The colors of short English words like jut, jot, lie, and lay "simply run together, obscured by the longer words that stand near them."

EWe makes fine distinctions between shades, and many sounds and sound combinations have shape—dots, rings, horizontal and diagonal zigzags, or wavy lines. Some sounds, such as phonetic *j*, the sound group *ji* (which does not occur in Serbian), and the English *u* (*ju* as in unit), possess form rather than any color at all.

Table 2.4 summarizes a linguistic analysis that Reichard and Jakobson made of Slavic speakers. They concluded that "correspondence is far from regular," as inspection of the table shows. This point is important and will be brought up again in Chapter 6. Suffice it to say here that these eminent linguists and others who have followed them have not found an explanation for synesthetic associations by this method.

DSc

DSc is a left-handed speech pathologist whose letter-color associations seem to be determined by orthographic rather than phonemic features. "In Cathy, Charles and cereal, the k, ch and s sounds, all of which are represented orthographically by 'c,' evoke a golden yellowish color." For DSc, the initial letter tends to dominate the overall color of the word. Vowels are also influenced by the context, whereas in isolation they are white with a black shadow or outline.

COMPETITION OF COLOR

Sometimes there is a very interesting competition between the color of the synesthesia and the actual orthography or semantic meaning of a word. We mentioned the example of one synesthete's frustration in seeing advertisement copy printed in the "wrong" color ink. The color competition can occur in a number of situations.

SO: I recently mistakenly called a new acquaintance "Diane" instead of "Elaine" because she was dark-haired, and "D" is black whereas "E" is red-orange. If a person has a dark, warm coloring, then I can easily recall their name if it is a dark, warm name. Trying to recall a dark name belonging to a light-haired person is hopeless (8/19/87).

MLL: A young woman named Zayas skated to a piece of music that was green and full of squares. Her costume was totally black; her routine started out with curving motions. It became uncomfortable to me to watch such a mismatch, so I just looked at my hands in my lap. She placed last in her category at the end of the evening's judging.

   In the pairs, a girl and boy wearing lovely flowing pinks and grays, skated to music from "Les Miserables," that was a broad river of flowing pink. The judges awarded them 10s. The audience agreed.

RP: My mother says that I have always used colors to describe flavors. Kiwi fruit tastes green, and there is no other way to describe it. Green grapes don't taste green, though, so I know that it does not relate to the fruit's color.

DSc: The word butter is blue.

Rizzo and Esslinger (1988) cited an interesting case of color competition in a 17-year-old synesthetic boy who had perinatal retrolental fibroplasia. His vision was 20/100 OU and he had normal visual- and auditory-evoked responses. The durability of his synesthetic responses to musical notes is shown in Table 2.5, where one sees that he gives exactly the same responses 5 months after the initial stimulus. Table 2.6 shows his

TABLE 2.5. Spontaneous color evokations to notes and durability of synesthetic associations 5 months after the initial testing.[a]

Pitch given	Spontaneous response	Response at 5 months
C	"Bright red"	"Bright red"
$C^{\#}$	"Bright purple"	"Bright purple"
D	"Green"	"Green"
E^{b}	"Sky blue with a little bit of green"	"Sky blue with a little bit of green"
E	"Blue"	"Blue"
F	"Yellow"	"Yellow"
$F^{\#}$	"Dark purple"	"Dark purple"
G	"Dark red"	"Dark red"
A^{b}	"Lavender"	"Lavender"
A	"White"	"White"
B^{b}	"Greenish white"	"Greenish white"
B	"Normal purple"	"Normal purple"

[a]From "Colored hearing synesthesia: Investigation of neural factors in a single subject" by M.R. Rizzo & P.J. Eslinger, 1988, unpublished manuscript. Reprinted by permission.

TABLE 2.6. Color responses to musical chords (note that chords do not contain the colors of the individual notes).[a]

Chords given	Spontaneous response
G Major (G-B-D)	"Pink, blue, and dark red"
A[b] Major (C-E[b]-A[b])	"Lavender, purple, and white mixed with a little blue and green"
C Minor (C-E[b]-G)	"Orange and celery green"
F Augmented (F-A-C[#])	"Black, purple, and yellow"
D Diminished Chord (D-F-A[b])	"Green, purple, and black with some red"
G Minor (B[b]-D-G)	"White, red, and a little purple"
B Major (D[#]-F[#]-B)	"Regular purple, lavender, and white"
A[b] Major (C-E[b]-A[b])	"Lavender, purple, and white"
D Minor (F-A-D)	"Yellow, green, and greenish-yellowish"
C Major (C-E-G)	"Scarlet red and dark red and a little orange and yellow"

[a]From "Colored hearing synesthesia: Investigation of neural factors in a single subject" by M.R. Rizzo & P.J. Eslinger, 1988, unpublished manuscript. Reprinted by permission.

responses to chords. Note that chords do not contain the colors of individual notes. This case is illustrative of absolute versus relative effects of synesthetic responses, as discussed in Chapter 3. The presence of color competition is seen in Table 2.7. He was asked to remember the color of a Munsell color chip that was presented with a musical note stimulus. He was able to learn this in only one trial as compared to controls. The spontaneous response after conflicting color assignment shows that the synesthetic percept is indeed durable and involuntary; the learned association is simply tacked on!

TABLE 2.7. Conflicting color assignment (see text for details).[a]

Pitch given	Original spontaneous response	Conflicting experimental assignment	Spontaneous response after conflicting color assignment
C	"Bright red"	Yellow	"Bright red with a strip of yellow"
D[#]	"Sky blue with a little bit of green"	Red	"Sky blue with a little bit of green and a strip of red"
A[#]	"Greenish-white"	Black	"Greenish-white with a strip of black"
F	"Yellow"	White	"Yellow with a strip of white"
C[#]	"Bright purple"	Green	"Bright purple with a little green"

[a]From "Colored hearing synesthesia: Investigation of neural factors in a single subject" by M.R. Rizzo & P.J. Eslinger, 1988, unpublished manuscript. Reprinted by permission.

Psychological Influence and Stigma

Living in a world of blobs, spirals, moving colors, phosphorescent tastes, and other sensory combinations that the rest of the populace regards as incongruous, to put it mildly, must surely influence the developing personality. Although none of the present cases or any of the historical ones of which I am aware have demonstrated obvious psychopathology, or either mental dullness or genius, there are some trends that can be seen among synesthetes as a group.

The full-blown composite would be the following: a left-handed female, who feels alienated, has a cosmic *Weltanschauung* and a feeling of portentousness, that at any moment something quite special will happen to her. Artistic, creative, and sensitive, she runs the emotional gamut from the highest of the highs to the lowest of the lows. She feels, and is, highly intelligent and intuitive, yet there is an abstruseness that may cause others to perceive her as "dense." The abstruseness may be compounded if the synesthesia is particularly strong and overwhelms thinking (as it did in Luria's patient). In this case, the synesthesia begins to interfere with rational thought. Only a few of the 42 present subjects feel that their synesthesia is ever an interference. At the very least, though, these children grew up shouldering the burden of those who are different.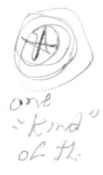

DS

For DS, both pain and pleasure evoke visual and spatial perceptions that are also in color. She was recommended for psychological counseling in high school when she told the assistant principal that "when I kissed my boyfriend I saw orange sherbet foam."

RP

As a child I once mentioned my colors to a teacher, who promptly told my parents I was schizophrenic. That ended my telling anyone about it for quite a while.

I am so used to my colors making me different from others who can't see them. I am both afraid and eager to know what it is like for people who share the trait, to know how different or the same we are. Did the others you studied just shut up about it, and not worry, or did the synesthesia and the difference it created become a part of their definition of themselves?

I know that it was very much a part of my life as a child, a sort of test of friendship, to see how others reacted when I told them. If they didn't believe me, I didn't want to be their friend.

BB

BB, one of the few males with this trait, describes the heightened emotion and portentousness that seeing his color auras create. The stimulus seems to come from people themselves, who have colors around them. "It feels like an emotional bond. The feeling lasts a few seconds. When I realized that others didn't see this, I worried what was wrong with me. I thought it was stress related.''

One particular person comes to mind. There was a very strong feeling and she was surrounded by a dark blue-green aura. It wasn't because she was sexually attractive. I don't know what the emotional feeling was due to because I had only met her twice. But there it was. I think there was some sort of bond or something. I'm not sure which comes first, sometimes I think I see the color and react emotionally; others it may be reversed—I get an emotion and then see this color. I'm not sure. And I don't know what makes it happens (4/2/86).

At times, a scene that is quite ordinary will take on a special perception of clarity, "as if locked in time, looking as a masterful painting, at other times of being part of a motion picture," or a very heightened feeling of merging with the ambient environment while never losing contact with the ongoing stream of consciousness.

DS

DS also has color auras associated with people. An intuitive suspicion that something about a person is not good will produce a "color spike" around them. She feels it is entirely based on her feelings.

My husband was going to hire someone and I had bad feelings, but it turned out I was dead wrong. She's fabulous for the job. Initially, it was that she had lightning bolts—not like grand Zeus—it's zigzag static. I call this my static line. When I meet someone who has this static, small lightning bolts, metallic, silvery, bronzy, I don't like them. I don't see them with this person any more.

MN

Other synesthetes were well aware of the negative consequences that revealing their synesthesia could cause. This is a source of distress.

I tend to describe/analyze in colors, feelings, and sensations, however, I tried not to do this (especially in school) because I wanted good grades and grades were not given out for colors, feelings and sensations. I have always had to make a conscious effort to simplify what I was teaching in my work (former high school teacher) in order to be understood (7/7/85).

MMo

I feel strangely apart from the world. Perhaps this contributes to my incomplete fences separating modes where the to-and-from schloshings form the soup into which inventions are born (9/12/84).

GG

Rarely, the synesthetic sense can interfere with rational thought. This was particularly severe in Luria's patient, S, whose inability to suppress his synesthetic percepts was often so severe as to make it difficult for him to attend to the semantic and meaningful qualities of a discourse. His images would guide his thinking, one association leading to another, rather than thought itself being the dominant element. Such interference is found in only a few of the current patients, where it tends to be mild.

GG, a medical illustrator, describes that while preparing an outline for an article she was to do for a professional publication, she found herself going back over and over every sentence to understand what she was trying to say. In school, short answers on exams were no trouble, whereas she found difficulty with essay answers because

. . . all the colors got mixed up and I didn't have a clear idea. Writing is very slow for me. I read a lot and that seems to go ok, even though the colors are definitely there when I read. But writing is difficult, so the synesthesia can be troublesome for me.

MM

Sometimes speech will dominate perception and I will not be able to understand what someone is saying for the "clutter." This doesn't happen too often, thank goodness. The only real problem is that when I am driving and a very loud sound comes on such as loud music or the Alert Test tone and it is hard to see. The image intensity is directly proportional to the sound level. People laugh when I say "turn that down, I can't see where I'm driving."

JM

JM reads every night and her synesthesia does not interfere with understanding. However, it does influence her feeling toward a person, place, or subject because of the color. For example, her niece was expecting a baby and wrote that they would name it Paul if it was a boy. JM was distraught because

the name Paul is such an ugly color, its [*sic*] gray and ugly. I told her "anything but Paul." And she couldn't understand why and I said "it is such an ugly color, that name Paul." She thought I was out of my mind. At last I thought it really isn't my business and she can do what she likes. The name probably isn't that bad, but in my mind it's very awful. And that influences how I feel about people.

On the other hand, if a name has a color that JM loves very much then the name can be beautiful. She feels that the color of the name has much more influence on her likes and dislikes than the sound of it. For example:

I like blue not that much, but the blue in the A is very nice. So names like Alex and Alexandra—I always call myself Alexandra among my family. I hate the name [*her name*]. My mother was American which is why I have that name. The name Alexandra is such a pretty color and that's why I like it and that's why I always use it.

JM finds it odd that her favorite color, red, appears only once in her whole alphabet, the bright red of the "s." Moreover, all words starting with "s" are not automatically appealing. It all depends on the combinations.

Despite their high intelligence, synesthetes can exhibit lacunae of abstruseness. They can be remarkably dense in some areas, usually a linguistic one, such as dialectic or poetry. Many remark that they have trouble "getting it."

MT: I do sometimes have trouble "getting it" but I think I'm both intuitive and analytical. The difficulty I have in "getting it" arises either from the difficulty of hearing language—"things" often sound like other "things"—or from the way many people string words together sort of needlessly. All I mean is that I have difficulty hearing, but not from a lack of ear power (12/10/86).

DS: I'm always knocking over salt cellars and water glasses because I have to use my hands, not really to talk BUT TO THINK! I need as much support as I can get to think.
  Sometimes I have no idea what people are saying. There is a lot of junk in my mind that makes it hard to pay attention.

What Is Synesthesia Good for?

Synesthesia is a rich way of feeling, highly enjoyable for those who possesses it. To lose it would be a catastrophe, an odious state akin to going blind or not being alive at all. Synesthetes have a well-developed innate memory that is amplified by use of the parallel sense as a mnemonic device.

WORD AND NUMBER MEMORY

DI

For DI, the color of a word is unpredictable from the colors of the individual letters, but once she "sees" a word she thereafter easily remembers the color of it and thus the spelling or the context associated with it.

This may be one reason for my ability to remember things better than most people. I can visualize pages and then *read* what is on them. I use my [*synesthesia*] to remember names and words to the point where I remember actually saying "I don't remember the name but I think it's blue or something."

But note the inconsistency. What kind of memory is this in which the important element—the actual name—is forgotten? Although synesthetes will commonly volunteer that the added sense enhances their memory, *it is more often the memory for the sense itself that is memorable, not the content.*

DI has competition among letters for the overall coloration of the word, prompting her to "wish that this color synesthesia [*sic*] was a little better.

My *feelings* about the word or subject can also 'shade' the overall color of the word.'' An example is given with my name:

R = green   Richard is remembered as green (with white)
 i = white
c = yellow
h = brown
a = red/brown
r = green
d = red
C = yellow   Cytowic is remembered as yellow with black
y = green   because of the influence of the ''w''
 t = darker green
o = white
w = black
 i = white
c = yellow

How this helps her remember my name is not clear, since there must be many green and yellow names. If she subsequently meets me and sees yellow and green how does she know that my first name is green rather than yellow? Unfortunately, this is not an issue I was able to explore. It bears further analysis. A partial explanation may be that when confronted by someone previously met, a color appears. Being associated with a letter or combination of letters thus helps to jog the memory for the actual name.

We see from this and other examples that for those persons with colored letters and words, given elements may determine the predominant color. For some the leading letter is the only determinant; for others it is an amalgamation; in still others the vowels can dramatically alter the coloration of a word.

GG

When asked what good her synesthesia does her, GG responds that it is a boon to her memory, particularly remembering numbers—''they're chromatically arranged. I can recall it much more easily because I'm given a hint. If I knew it before I know it doubly.'' A list of her colors (see Table 2.3) shows that there is not, in fact, a chromatic arrangement for the 10-digit series. ''Isn't that a rainbow arrangement?'' she asks with surprise. Although digits 2 through 6 have a spectral order the notion of chromaticity cannot serve as a method for remembering the 10 digits nor for larger integers.

The spelling of synesthetes is usually good because the word is visualized; the color will tell, for example, whether a word has two ''l''s or an ''e.''

TOPOGRAPHICAL MEMORY

Excellent topographical memory is another common claim of synesthetes. If they want something they can visualize it exactly in a drawer, for example, and go right to that drawer and find it exactly as they have pictured it. This item may be one that they have not used for many months.

HYPERMNESIS

There is also a relationship between hypermnesis and synesthesia. As shown in the example of BB, above, considerable affect may also accompany the reminiscence.

MW

Years after experiments were begun on MW we were discussing feature detection neurons and their sensitivity to highly specific attributes of a visual scene. On learning about feature detection neurons MW volunteered a specific childhood memory about the way the sunlight hit the daffodils at his home. He specifically remembers the "angle" of the sunlight. His profession as lighting designer, requiring knowledge of visual effects related to beam angles of incident light, probably has nothing to do with this childhood memory. The point here is that he has a highly crystallized memory of a perceptual event that occurred on an annual basis. He would observe daily until the luminance was "just so," which it was for a brief period only.

On a specific morning in April, I could plot it year to year, April 7th or 9th I don't recall what day exactly. It was a particular way the sunlight hit on our driveway on the daffodils and it was very vivid and I would look forward to it every year at the same time of the day to be exactly the same way. It was the beginning of Spring for me. I knew it was here. I loved it. It was wonderful. It was beautiful and the beginning of Spring. It was not going to be cold any more. I couldn't wait until that day when the light arrived (12/16/86).

RB

Memory for conversation is excellent, an asset to a court reporter. I can recall dialogue from movies and books.

MLL

My memory is best for things I've seen and pictured; also which side of the page to find a previously seen passage. As a volunteer pot mender for the Smithsonian, I could remember part of a pot assembled one year when I found more pieces the following year. I can remember things from age 3.

MM

The images I see are like really seeing and are stored as regular memory and are therefore available for recall. The things I "see" are therefore just about as real as anything I can remember. I can recall them in sequence at any time.

My memory for faces is very strong. I can remember scenes, and then looking at the memory of it, read a sign on the wall, describe a texture, etc.

OLFACTORY MEMORY

MG, a 24-year-old male, illustrates the memory-like qualities of synesthesia in his visual smell. He smells objects that are seen on TV or in advertisements—cigarettes, bleach, and foods. Thus, although there is a synesthesia between sight and smell, the smell is always specific to the object seen and seems to be qualitatively different, therefore, from the more generic perceptions in other modes—such as visual blobs and lines, smooth or rough textures, elementary tastes, or general somatic sensations. One might speculate that this is because smell is such a low-gestalt sense, or because smell is so intimately related with the anatomic structures serving memory.

Personal experience tells us that smell is particularly apt to evoke memories; but memories and sensations rarely, if ever, evoke the vivid memory of a smell. The smell MG perceives is *not* a memory but a real sensation. His memory is excellent. "I remember sights, sounds and scents from [*age 3*]. Usually I can remember all experiences vividly in its [*sic*] entirety" (11/24/85).

The ability to remember a smell, surely a rare capacity, is found among synesthetes more often than expected by chance. Smell is examined in more detail in Chapter 4, in the analysis of MW (the gustatory and olfactory synesthete), and in Chapter 7, in which smell is intimately related to memory in SdeM, a fact demonstrated by a change in memory following loss of smell as a result of a pituitary tumor.

The memory for scents is not necessarily related to the stimulus for synesthesia, however.

DS: My sense of smell is very important. I cook by taste and smell. I can't follow a recepie [*sic*]. I have to put in what I want to put in. I can remember scents—the smell of a strawberry, or the musty scent of my grandmother's basement. It's not the memory—I remember the smell.

I lost my sense of smell for 2 months while I was sick. And I was miserable. During this time, I seem to recall that the synesthesia was the same.

Familial Cases

Several of the current subjects have first-degree relatives who are also synesthetic (EW, SO, FKD, MT, LH, NM, and SP) [see also Laignel-Lavastine (1901)]. In examining the familial relationships one finds siblings, parents, and children of either sex combination in contiguous generations, all features suggesting an autosomal dominant mode of inheritance. The presence of familial cases serves the argument that synesthesia is a brain-based condition, that is, it is inherited and not learned. It is a sensory function and not a mere psychological association.

Two synesthetes serve as examples. Vladimir Nabokov (VN), although not personally studied by me, is used because he was the first familial case of which I was aware, in addition to the literary merits of his description. EW, whose family has the trait over four generations, is used from the current subjects.

VN

In "Portrait of My Mother" (1949), Nabokov related spontaneous synesthesia as well as

. . . a fine case of colored hearing. Perhaps "hearing" is not quite accurate since the color sensation seems to be produced by the very act of my orally forming a given letter while I imagine its outline.

The "a" of the English alphabet has for me the tint of weathered wood, but the French "a" evokes polished ebony. This black group also includes hard "g"—vulcanized rubber—and "r"—a sooty rag. Oatmeal "n," noodle-limp "l" and the ivory-backed hand mirror of "o" take care of the whites. Passing on to the blue group, there is steely "x," the inky horizon of "z," and huckleberry "k." Since a subtle interaction exists between sound and shape, I see "q" as browner than "k," while "s" is not the light blue of "c" but a curious mother-of-pearl. In the green group, there are alder-leaf "f," the unripe apple of "p," and pistachio "t." Dull green, combined somehow with violet, is the best I can do for "w." The yellows comprise various "e"s and "i"s, creamy "d," bright-golden "y" and "u," whose English alphabetical value I can express only by "brassy with an olive sheen." In the brown group, there are the rich, rubbery tone of soft "g," paler "j," and the drab shoelace of "h."

One can enjoy the metaphoric adjectives attached to Nabokov's colors. "Such confessions must sound tedious and pretentious to those who are protected from similar leakings and drafts by more solid walls than mine are." His mother seemed to find this perfectly natural. As a 7-year-old, he remarked to his mother that the colors were "all wrong" on the alphabet blocks he was using to build a tower. He discovered that she possessed the trait and that "some of her letters had the same tint as mine and that, besides, she was optically affected by musical notes." Unfortunately, Nabokov does not list his mother's colors.

Nabokov also had an unusual aptitude for mathematics as a child, and when sick with a fever "I felt enormous *spheres* and huge numbers swell in my aching brain . . . . Such were the mathematical monsters that thrived on my delerium. . . . Beneath my delerium [*mother*] recognized sensations she had known herself and her understanding would bring my expanding universe back to a Newtonian norm."

EW

EW is a cultural affairs correspondent for a newspaper. She became aware that her synesthesia was unusual when she took a college psychology course. "Professor," she asked "doesn't everybody do that? I thought they did." In his 35 years of teaching, the professor had not encountered a case before her. He urged her to go home and ask her parents if they had it. "My mother didn't know what I was talking about, but my father thought, as I had, that everybody saw things that way."

EW has a "photographic memory" and her number forms, which are also shared by the family, are discussed in Chapter 7, where her pedigree is also shown.

Her son, WW, is a professor of neuropathology. "I suppose I have a somewhat different perspective on the phenomenon than most synesthetes."

Let me say this this is a delightful trait to have, I think. I tend to use it consciously and unconsciously to help me remember correct sequences of numbers, words, phrases, letters, to help me remember names and locations of anatomical structures (especially neuroanatomical structures—you should see the beautiful array of colors in the brain!) and neuropathological classifications.

I have had a long-time fascination with our particular "quirk of the mind" and have kept records from time to time regarding consistency of my "colors," sometimes comparing my colors to my mother's; she did that with her father over some years before his death in about 1950. There are a few other aspects to our synesthesia including certain spatial relationships of series of numbers (which also appear in color, of course). I am quite convinced that "it is in the brain and not in the mind" as I believe the newspaper article stated you seem to think. The apparent transmission of the trait from one generation to another in our family lends support to that idea.

GENETICALLY MEDIATED PSYCHOLOGICAL CHARACTERISTICS OF SENSORY FUNCTIONS

We see that synesthesia runs in families. Some general comments regarding the heritability of sensory functions will conclude this chapter (Fuller & Thompson, 1960). Many people believe that while most physical characteristics are inherited, psychological or behavioral ones are not. In fact, one's genetic endowment (genotype) does indeed drive one to become smart or stupid, or prone to specific talents or personality traits just as it determines whether one is tall or short, or blonde or dark.

As an example of a hereditary sensory talent, the ability to taste phenylthiocarbamide (PTC) as bitter or tasteless is well understood. In most populations taste thresholds (for hydrochloric acid, for example) have Gaussian distributions. But PTC does not follow a normal distribution, the proportion of nontasters ranging from 20% in African populations to 30% in European descendants. The ability to taste PTC as bitter is highly specific in that the substance can be recognized by a "taster" only when it is dissolved in his own saliva. The trait is related neither to overall taste acuity nor to a general ability to taste the bitterness of noncarbamides (such as quinine). Since carbamides are man-made synthetics, it is difficult to fathom what adaptive function this taster gene might serve in human evolution.

Genetic factors are extremely important in both hereditary deafness and many forms of blindness. Little work has been done in the genetic differences in the sense of smell, although scattered reports implicate hereditary factors in selective anosmia [the inability to detect specific odorants (Amoore, 1977)]. Conversely, the presence of "noses" in families of perfumiers and cognac industrialists is legendary.

Personality and intelligence are often said to be reflected by performance on selected visual tasks [e.g., Jaensch's integrated personality (Jaensh, 1931)]. Whatever the validity of such statements, a number of data sets (from twins and other family members) suggest that heritable components mediate susceptibility to selected visual illusions, eidetic or photographic memory, spatial orientation, afterimages, and the ability to detect flicker in a source of light (flicker fusion frequency). Since most studies have involved small samples of people and have done little to control for prior experience, they require cautious interpretation.

One ability that shows a strong tendency to run in families is, of course, musical ability. The pedigree of Johann Sebastian Bach is a prime example, although not a unique illustration. Data gathered from the Julliard School of Music in New York City show a clear degree of heritability in 50 to 75% of parents of opera singers, instrumental virtuosos, and music students. It appears that a significant musical ability emerges early in life and that such aptitude improves steadily among the gifted, even without practice and in a variety of settings. Such data point to a maturation in the gradual unfolding of genotype as a major factor.

This unfolding of the sensory function may be seen in synesthetes' comments that they have had this "as far as I can remember," contrasted with a minority of patients who noted it in their adolescence, around puberty, after which it seemed to develop more strongly. They may attribute this to having paid more attention to it after "discovering" that the trait is unique, a statement that may or may not be valid.

An analogous situation may hold with the familial and genetic aspects of perfect pitch (Profita & Bidder, 1988), which also shows a significant familial incidence, occurs predominantly in females, and is invariably discovered at a very early age. An analogous question can be raised as to whether musical tone sensitivity or perceptiveness is an aptitude that varies continuously between the extremes of the marked insensitivity of the "tone deaf" to the increased sensitivity of those with excellent relative pitch. Profita and Bidder's conclusion is that "perfect pitch is a unique and innate trait which is possessed to a variable degree by a subpopulation of humans."

Perfect pitch is similar to synesthesia in four aspects:

1. It is all or nothing. The talent is either present or it is not.
2. The skill appears naturally without necessity to develop it through the practice that characterizes acquisition of other musical skills.
3. "Most of our subjects with perfect pitch recall their astonishment on learning that *everyone* did not have this capacity."
4. It is recognized at an early age; 25% of Profita and Bidder's 19 subjects recognized their capacity by age 5, 90% by age 10. Pedigrees are compatible with autosomal recessive inheritance, and the fact that 80% are female suggests that the trait is sex-related.

Other studies implicate hereditary musical ability, whether measured by some global score or by instruments with various subtests. For example, Musical Quotients based on tests of musical intelligence have shown identical monozygotic twins to be much more alike than dizygotic fraternal twins. A number of models have been suggested to account for the transmission of musical ability, none of which account completely for the available data (these include single gene action with incomplete dominance, a single or small number of recessive genes, and several major genes with multiple alleles).

In the 19th century Sir Francis Galton, in *Hereditary Genius* (1869), presented the first clear quantitative evidence that genius, as measured by outstanding accomplishment, tends to run in families. Since that time, of course, others have questioned how much education and opportunity (environment) are responsible for the great differences in individual achievement. The consensus is that genius (which Galton distinguished from talent both quantitatively and qualitatively) is a function of both heredity and environmental factors.

Galton himself gave little emphasis to the importance of the environment, although in this century it has been a point of major contention, mostly because of political implications. Numerous studies have shown that within wide limits long exposure to a common environment does not seem to make people more similar in intelligence. In showing this, scores of studies clearly emphasize the role of heredity in intelligence among human beings and other animals. The estimate for the extent of genetic determination in human intelligence is about 80%, and it is unlikely that the genotype contributes less than 50% of the variability.

Thus, both general IQ and specific component ability seem to be heritable, some of the specific talents being more dependent on genotype than others. The precise genetic mode for the transmission of intelligence and its components is incompletely understood. Some theorists favor the notion of multiple genes, some suggesting a major gene pair Nn dominant for average intelligence (IQ range 90–110), with five additional minor pairs of genes acting as modifiers that could push IQ up or down in the absence of the dominant gene N.

The synesthete's ability is inborn and appears early in life, but does not seem to be highly, if at all, modifiable by environmental influences. One possible exception may be in familial cases wherein affected people are encouraged to speak about it openly or at least not feel any need for secrecy, which is the skeptical milieu in which synesthetes usually find themselves.

3
Theories of Synesthesia: A Review and a New Proposal

We have seen in the previous chapter that synesthesia is certainly both odd and interesting. For some, however, the question remains: Is it real? One of the most glaring problems in trying to fathom a mechanism for synesthesia is the lack of agreement among synesthetes about the parallel sense that they perceive. The fact that synesthesia exists is firmly established. What has not been established is how or why synesthesia occurs. Many hypotheses have been proposed, but experiments designed specifically to test these hypotheses are nil. When an explanation is proposed it is consistent only with the case reviewed but lacks empirical support, is a matter of mere speculation on the psychologist's part, and cannot be generalized to all forms of synesthesia.

When individual synesthetes compare associations, they find that agreement is coincidental at best. The expectation for homogeneity among synesthetic perception is a presumption that stems from the consensus we have about the perception of everyday objects. We all agree that roses are red and violets are blue, that a square looks like a square, and that a banana tastes like a banana each time we eat one. We can recognize a piano by its sound and not mistake it for a trumpet or a baby's cry. A look at illusions so common in everyday experience that we take them for granted will illustrate that consistency of perception is not absolute, however.

One such illusion is the perception of a constant color of objects in the varying illumination of daylight. Color constancy and colored shadows are discussed in detail in Chapter 9. For now, it is sufficient just to give the example. Because there is a marked difference in both the brightness and spectrum of daylight from sunrise to sunset, an object viewed in the morning reflects more blue light than the same object seen toward evening, when it should appear redder. Yet we perceive the color of an object as constant, despite changes in both intensity and incident wavelength. The color we attribute to an object is different from what it "really is." It is different from what the physical properties of the incident light lead one to predict and perceive. The question, then, should not be,

"Why don't all synesthetes agree?" but rather, "Why do the rest of us agree so well? Why do we all have common illusions?"

The failure to find universal correspondences among synesthetes may have contributed to the cessation of interest in the subject after the 1920s. A review of papers from the turn of the century shows that "researchers" did little more than make lists of stimuli and synesthetic responses, followed by dismay that agreement was not obvious between individual synesthetes. Moreover, when reading some papers it is hard to know whether the subject is truly synesthetic when we are told only that he was in the habit of "making associations" between two senses. Laurence Weiskrantz (personal communication) says that von Hornbostel's family sat around the dinner table comparing associations—"this soup tastes blue to me," "Oh really, I think it's more round than blue," and so forth. From this anecdote, one gets the sense that they were not synesthetic at all, but rather acting like a caricature of pseudoscientific artistes. One is reminded of the intelligentsia of Paris who flocked to Charcot's evening lectures, seeking a draught sufficiently shallow for them to act fashionably knowledgeable about the new science of neurology (Charcot, 1987). Estimates of the frequency of synesthesia in older literature are very likely overblown. There were never clear inclusion and exclusion criteria for even defining what synesthesia was!

Despite lack of consistency in definition or methodology, there was no lack of theories. Mechanistic theories, in particular, failed. Even Sir Isaac Newton had tried to devise mathematical formulas to "relate" the frequency of sound to an appropriate wavelength of light. We will see below that there *are* generic similarities in the way synesthetes perceive, even though the end result, the actual perception, is unique for a given individual.

Experiential phenomena of temporal lobe epilepsy (TLE) are similar in some ways to synesthetic perception, so we will consider them for a moment. Considerable evidence shows that experiential phenomena are positive effects of limbic seizure discharge or limbic stimulation (Gloor, Olivier, Quesney, et al., 1982). The fact that such experiences can be evoked by stimulation without warning, are not evoked by warning without stimulation, and arise only from highly specific anatomic structures (particularly amygdala) should leave no doubt concerning their cerebral origin. That the phenomena are described in very similar terms further suggests that patients do not embroider their responses, nor are they elaborating a story—that is, verbally elaborating a vague sensation as opposed to describing an experiential fragment.

Yet similar criticism about inconsistency of responses has been leveled at the nature of experiential phenomena, whether they arise naturally as part of a temporal lobe seizure or are deliberately evoked by electrical stimulation of the brain. Halgren, Walter, Cherlow, and Crandall (1978), for example, tried to convince their readers that the responses are "individualized," and that the types of mental phenomena elicited are related more to the patient's personality than to where the limbic stimulation is applied. That is, they argued that "who" is stimulated is more important than "where" the stimulation is applied to the brain. The logical conclusion of such criticism would be to insist that stimulation at point X in all brains must elicit the experience Y. Subjective experiences verbally communicated by the patient cannot be put to the same objective analysis that a finger movement elicited by motor cortex stimulation might be. The variety, vividness, and compelling emotional coloration of these reports might incline the dour to question whether they represent true cerebral responses when compared, for example, to phosphenes or buzzing elicited by stimulation of primary receptive cortices. The same kind of thinking leads to questioning whether synesthetic percepts are of noncerebral origin.

Similar analysis can be applied to the experiential responses of synesthetes. They give similar descriptions of unelaborated sensory perceptions. There is little if any self-referential material woven in as compared to the temporal epileptics. The synesthesiae assume a compelling immediacy similar to reliving past experiences, which the TLE patients liken to actual events. In both sets of patients, however, there is never any doubt that these phenomena are occurring out of context, incongrously superimposed on the ongoing stream of consciousness.

Cumulative data show that stimulation of limbic structures at point X does not produce experience Y in all brains. Rather, it produces a combination of perceptual, mnestic, and emotional components that reflect the functional role of the stimulated area while incorporating elements of the individual brain's past experience. Analogously, a given stimulus is certain to evoke disparate perceptions in different synesthetes. Just as there are consistencies in the mechanism producing experiential responses, there must also be such consistencies in the experience of synesthesia.

The oldest criticism against synesthesia is that it is subjective, a psychophysical phenomenon without external manifestations knowable only through the experiential reports of the subjects themselves. This criticism is an empty one. Many established medical conditions are entirely subjective, such as headache and all pain syndromes, dizzy spells, and TLE. Temporal lobe epilepsy is the better example from these conditions because although TLE patients rarely have convulsions, they do have all sorts of peculiar *subjective* experiences such as disordered time sense, a sense of leaving one's body, and other dissociative states and perceptual distortions; they occasionally have *synesthesia*.

Temporal lobe epilepsy is such a common (1 : 9,600) and well-known entity that a physician can *diagnose* it by the history alone; can *confirm the diagnosis* by prescribing anticonvulsants and causing the symptoms to go away; and, finally, can *prove the diagnosis* by demonstrating characteristic waveforms on the EEG. The word "diagnosis" means "through knowledge," and the diagnosis of synesthesia is made just as is any other diagnosis. Although synesthesia is rare (1 : 300,000 by my estimate), the stories of synesthetes are so similar that it can be diagnosed by the history extracted from the patient; confirmed by meeting five clinical criteria; and proved by objective tests that separate synesthetes from nonsynesthetes.

Diagnostic Criteria for Synesthesia

1. SYNESTHESIA IS INVOLUNTARY BUT ELICITED

Synesthesia is unsuppressable but cannot be conjured up at will. There must be an objective stimulus. It is often said to have been in existence as far back as the patient can remember; sometimes, it is not noted until puberty.

If patients are deeply engaged or distracted, the synesthesia may be attenuated, whereas focused attention in a relaxed state may make it seem more vivid. Otherwise, there is little the subject can do to alter the synesthetic percept. For example, "I find that when working at my computer I am oblivious to everything that goes on around me, and so am not really aware of the colors the clicking of my keyboard makes as I type."

2. SYNESTHESIA IS PROJECTED

The elicited sense if perceived as external and not imagined "in the mind's eye." If visual, the synesthesia is perceived close to the face; in other modes it is in personal space, the space immediately surrounding the body, rather than at a distance.

3. SYNESTHETIC PERCEPTS ARE DURABLE AND DISCRETE

The associations for an individual synesthete are stable over his lifetime. If a sound is blue, it will always be blue; the context of the stimulus does not have a strong influence. This has been affirmed repeatedly by testing individuals without warning up to 46 years apart with the same stimuli.

The synesthetic percepts are generic and restricted. Given choices on a matching task, synesthetes pick only a few, whereas nonsynesthetic controls show a diffuse distribution over the available choices. Their generic nature is demonstrated by the fact that synesthetes never see complex scenes. The percepts are unelaborated: blobs, lines, spirals, and latticed shapes; smooth or rough textures; agreeable or disagreeable tastes such as salty, sweet, or metallic. Replication, with radial or axial symmetry, is also common. Synesthetic percepts never go beyond an elementary level. To do so would be to become a figurative hallucination.

Discrete also refers to signatures of a certain stimuli. We all recognize the distinctive sound of a piano because it sounds like a piano—not a vacuum cleaner or a dentist's drill. As synesthete DS explains, "the shapes are not distinct from hearing—they are part of what hearing *is*. The vibraphone, the musical instrument, makes a round shape. Each note is like a little gold ball falling. That's what the sound *is;* it couldn't possibly be anything else."

4. SYNESTHESIA IS MEMORABLE

Perhaps because of their semantic vacuity, synesthetic percepts are easily and vividly remembered, often in preference to the original stimulus. "She had a green name—I forget, it was either Ethel or Vivian." In this example, the actual names are confused because they are green, but the synesthetic greenness is recalled. There is a strong link between synesthesia and eidetic memory, or at least hypermnesis. Many synesthetes use their synesthesia as a mnemonic aid. The relationship between synesthesia and memory is best depicted in Luria's *The Mind Of A Mnemonist* (1968). His subject's memory, which was limitless and without distortion, was largely so because of the synesthesiae that accompanied every sensation.

5. SYNESTHESIA IS EMOTIONAL

There is an unshakable conviction and sense of validity that what the synesthete perceives is real. There is often a "Eureka" sensation, such as when we have an insight. The universal presence of such strong validity feelings demands investigation of limbic brain contribution to synesthesia. The limbic system subserves emotion and memory, and provides the sense of conviction that people attach to their neocortical ideas and ideals. Moreover, in this primitive part of the brain, which reflects the human's inheritance from early mammals (therapsids), there is the opportunity for the joining of information from the various senses.

These five features define idiopathic synesthesia as discussed in this book and will also serve to distinguish it from acquired synesthesia—such as drug-induced synesthesia, epileptic synesthesia, and synesthesia due to acquired brain lesions, which are discussed in subsequent chapters. Idiopathic synesthesia is diagnosed if the subject meets four of the five criteria above. Subjects who do not possess all five characteristics are usually found to lack projection of the parallel sense. Such patients usually have highly restricted forms such as colored numbers or letters, or a number form in isolation (Chapter 7).

What and Where Is the Link?

All theories of synesthesia assume that there is a "link" between a sensory stimulus and the synesthetic percept. To the extent that one believes that all psychological phenomena have direct physiological correlates, then some type of physiological theory must be correct. Past research has focused on *semantic mediation* as a possible mechanism for synesthesia, a view that simply makes it a subset of the more general phenomenon of cross-modal associations due to shared connotative meaning (D'Andrade & Egan, 1974; L.E. Marks, 1975; Osgood, 1960; Riggs & Karwoski, 1934; Vernon, 1930; Wheeler & Cutsforth, 1922). These studies typically investigate connotative meaning through such devices as the semantic differential (Osgood, Suci, & Tannenbaum, 1957), anthropological measurement of artistic and linguistic emotional expression, and phonetic symbolism. Phonetic symbolism was especially sought by the French symbolist and surrealist poets as a communicative link to the emotional unconscious. An in-depth investigation of these areas is beyond the scope of this book, but the mutual influence of art and synesthesia is undeniable. Such studies show that synesthetic percepts *tend* to follow conventional trends of connotative meaning. In colored hearing, for example, both synesthetes and normals match low pitches with large, dark photisms; high pitches with light, small photisms; and louder sounds with brighter and larger photisms (Karwoski, Odbert, & Osgood, 1942; L.E. Marks, 1974; Ortmann, 1933). The difference is that synesthetes actually report seeing an external photism whereas normals imagine that these "go together" appropriately. This relationship of mapping sensory dimensions explains only a tiny aspect of synesthesia, and only those types in which vision plays a part. Such a restricted view does little to explain other modes of synesthesia or its other constant characteristics. There are surprisingly few direct comparisons between the characteristic perceptual processing of synesthetic and nonsynesthetic subjects. In synesthesia, the precipitating stimulus repeatedly evokes a specific percept, or a narrow range of them at most. Synesthetic percepts are characteristically real, vivid, discrete, and memorable.

In showing only that synesthetic percepts follow some conventional lines of connotative meaning, therefore, these studies do little to clarify the underlying mechanism of synesthesia itself, except to suggest that it is simply a more intense form of normal connotative, cross-modal association. Many aspects of perception that could be entertained as an explanation for synesthesia are amenable to experimental study. Following are some of these brain mechanisms and how experimental data might verify or disprove them. Curiously, this had not previously been done. Rather, existing papers have largely addressed the durability of synesthetic percepts following a retest interval of years (Devereaux, 1966; Gengerelli, 1976; Luria, 1968; Rizzo & Esslinger, 1988), made lists of associations, and seen how synesthesia varies with alterations in stimulus amplitude or interval.

Theories of the Mechanism of Synesthesia

Since much of the research on synesthesia was done decades ago, it should not surprise the reader that most of the references are old. Hardly any beyond the 1920s deal with actual observations of synesthetic patients. The reasons for this are opaque, but surely must go beyond the fact that such patients are rare. Writing about synesthesia without actually having synesthetes to study is like learning to sail by sitting on the beach and reading about sailing. Fundamental problems exist in studying a field in which there are small numbers of patients. This is compounded by geographic dispersement of subjects, and their less than enthusiastic willingness to be queried, poked, and prodded.

Many of the ideas proposed at the turn of the century now seem incredulous. A polarity of thinking is also evident, either purely psychological or mechanistic.

Both ancient and modern thought on the mechanism of synesthesia can be divided into the following categories:

1. Undifferentiated neuronal activity: sensory incontinence analogous to synkinesis in infants.
2. Linkage theories
   a. Neural specificity
   b. Polymodal combination
3. Abstraction theories
   a. Cognitive mediation
   b. Aristotelian common sense

UNDIFFERENTIATED NEURONAL ACTIVITY

The first category comprises undifferentiated theories. Popular in the 19th century, they speculated that the condition was caused by an immature nervous system and likened synesthesia to the normal synkinesis ("joined movements") seen in all infants. An infant reaching for a toy, for example, will experience involuntary overflow movements of the trunk and extremities. Only when the corticospinal and cerebellar pathways have matured and acquired their myelin insulation is a human capable of finely isolated dextrous movements. Labeled the *Degeneracy Theory* (Bleuler & Lehmann, 1881) or the *Compensation Theory* (Downey, 1912; C.A. Myers, 1911), these theories suggest that synesthesia is a form of atavism or sensory incontinence since "there is a level in the development of animals at which no sense differentiation takes place." There is no evidence to support this idea and no one has seriously argued this point in the 20th century.

These theories fail because they predict an impairment of intellect and an indiscriminate perceptual response to a stimulus—characteristics that are quite unlike the actual specificity of synesthesia and contrary to the usual high intelligence of synesthetes.

The gustofacial reflex (Steiner, 1973) bears an apparent similarity to synesthesia. It is a well-differentiated motor reaction of the facial muscles to taste stimuli. Controlled by neural structures of the brainstem, it is a rigidly fixed behavior. Ethologists such as Peiper (1951) and Lorenz (1965) call the gustofacial response an innate behavior, an inherited motor coordination. Characteristic of such innate behaviors is its rigidly fixed appearance, resistance to exhaustion by repetition, and homologous distribution among lower mammals.

In the gustatory facial reflex, different tastes produce fixed facial expressions (sweet = smile; bitter = disgust with tongue protrusion; sour = pursing of the lips). Any resemblance to synesthesia is superficial. The gustafacial reflex is universal with *identical responses produced across individuals*. This is not the case with synesthesia. This fact suggests that the neural mechanism for synesthesia lies above the level of the brainstem.

The neural apparatus of gustation is well developed and functional long before the gestational term. The adult form of the human taste bud is clearly visible in histological preparations of the human embryo in the 5th gestational month.

The striking point of the gustofacial reflex is the ability of the pontomedullary region of the human brain to discriminate between sensory signals and "decide" that some events are welcomed by the organism while other must be rejected as harmful or noxious. People are often inclined to believe that discrimination between good and bad is mainly a cognitive function based on life experience, conditioning, learning, and an emotional attitude. This is not the case.

LINKAGE THEORIES

Linkage theories are based on the assumption that something is "wrong" with the circuitry of the brain. The assumption of crossed wires, short circuits, or cross-talk is the most common intuitive explanation for synesthesia among laymen, but the logical consequences of such an assumption are again contrary to the facts. Linkage theories would especially support universal correspondences, which cannot be found.

The premise of *Neural Specificity* is that inflexible "hard wiring" of neural circuitry mediates between a sensory stimulus and a synesthetic percept. To use colored hearing as a model, for example, the basic hypothesis in all attempts to construct a parallel pitch-color scale is that if

aN, bN, cN . . . represent the vibratory frequencies in a musical scale, then a multiple of aNM, bNM, cNM . . . predicts the spectral wavelength of the synesthetically induced color. Among others (see Ortmann, 1933), Sir Isaac Newton (1730) and Erasmus Darwin (1790) proposed such theories. The elder Darwin, a proponent of colored music, built a *claviere luminere,* a harpsichord-lightbox device in which colored lanterns could shine through a shutter apparatus controlled by the keyboard. The fact that colored-hearing synesthetes have an idiosyncratic relationship between color and pitch predicts this scheme's failure, however.

None of the proposed *Sensory Reflex* theories can be taken seriously today. These theories propose two monosynaptic afferent-afferent limbs instead of the usual afferent-efferent (Donath, 1922; Downey, 1912; Hilbert, 1895; Pierce, 1912).

The synesthesia that occasionally occurs with lysergic acid diethylamide (LSD) and other antiserotonergics is relevant here because the perception of visual hallucinations is facilitated by sensory input from other modalities (i.e., synesthesia). Suppression of neocortical activity with relative activation of deeper structures suggests that emotional meaning might be a relevant "linkage" to synesthetic percepts, a suggestion that is empirically testable. The data on LSD are discussed in detail in Chapter 4.

ABSTRACTION THEORIES

The two main versions of the abstraction theory of synesthesia both involve a filtering out of specific sense elements until one is left with either an abstract *emotional* or abstract *perceptual* residue that serves as a synesthetic mediator.

Those theories lumped under the rubric of *Cognitive Mediation* stress the importance of the secondary and subsidiary meanings. The *Association Theory* (Langfield, 1926; Wheeler & Cutsforth, 1922) explains synesthesia as the operation of chance associations: If A suggests B then A and B have been experienced simultaneously at some previous time. The naiveté of this idea speaks for itself and would seem to have more to do with a psychological notion of imagination than with the actual facts of synesthetic perception.

The *Emotional Tone Theory* (Calkins, 1895; H.L. Smith, 1905) emphasizes intrinsic associations inasmuch as the affective (connotative) component of a stimulus is an integral part of its quality. Its claim that synesthesia and its stimulus have a common emotional background neglects the corollary that synesthesia should be ubiquitous, since emotional coloring is an attribute of all normal sensations and not restricted to any particular sense. One should expect a pleasant color to evoke not only a mellifluous sound but an ambrosian taste, a warm feeling, or the fragrance of a rose. Such a general spread, although logically imagined, it not at all characteristic of the specific response of synesthesia.

Aristotle's *Common Senses* form the second category of polymodal abstraction. Most 20th-century writers have fallen back on Aristotle's common senses to serve as abstract *perceptual* residues that mediate connotative meaning and hence synesthesia. All theories that propose language as a synesthetic mediator also fall back on Aristotelian common sense and suggest that synesthesia is simply a more intense form of the metaphoric speech that everyone uses. The following discussion explains why linguistic theories cannot be correct.

Historically, Democritus taught that all mind events were events of the soul (psyche) and could be predicted by the shape of the soul's atoms. All sensation was therefore reduced to motion. Plato stressed the need to appreciate the *idea* of a sensation as well as its physical attributes. From this, Aristotle (*De Anima,* Books II and III) spoke of the particular and common senses.

By an object peculiar to a particular sense, I mean one that cannot be perceived by any other sense, and in respect of which no deception is possible. Thus color is an object peculiar to sight, sound to hearing, and flavor to taste. . . . Each sense judges the objects peculiar to it and is never deceived as to the existence of the color or sound that it perceives (Wheelwright, 1951, p. 134).

We can be aware of certain aspects of the world around us in more than one way, however. We can see as well as feel the sizes and shapes of bodies, see and hear the motion of bodies from one place to another, and can even tell whether that motion is slow or fast. The common sensibles include movement, number, rest, size, figure, and length. The common senses are not perceived via a special sense organ, but rather indirectly (*kata symbebêkos*) through the particular senses.

Aristotle believed that although the senses come from outside us through different channels of the sense organs, they do not remain separate in our sense experience. The world that our senses gives us is one of bodies of various sizes and shapes, in motion or at rest, and related to one another in space in a variety of ways. Our sense experience of these bodies also includes a wide variety of qualities—the colors bodies have, the sounds they make, the roughness or smoothness of their surfaces, and so forth. We receive passively these sensations through our sense organs but are more active than passive in putting together the seamless fabric of our experience. While sensation comes from the outside, sense experience that arises from our perception of that outside world involves memory and imagination on our part. A unity results from the simultaneous perception of different qualities in one object, "as bile is at once bitter and yellow. This explains why we may mistake a thing, because it happens to be yellow, for bile" (*De Anima,* Book II, ii; Wheelwright, 1951, p. 138).

On discrimination, Aristotle wrote:

Each sense has its own type of sense-object. Residing in its own sense-organ, it discriminates the specific differences of the sense-objects proper to it. Thus sight discriminates between white and black, taste between sweet and bitter, and so on. But we can also discriminate between white and sweet, and in fact between any two sensible qualities. By what means do we perceive generic differences? . . . [*It is not*] possible to discriminate between white and sweet by means of a different sense for each of them; there must be some one sense to which both of the compared qualities are discernably present. Otherwise it would be like trying to establish a difference between two objects on the ground that you perceived one of them and I the other. Objects can be differentiated only where there is a single faculty to discriminate between them. In the case of white and sweet, as they are recognized as distinct, there must be a single faculty to affirm the distinction and hence a single faculty which thinks and perceives them both. We conclude from this that different things cannot be discriminated by a separate organ for each (Wheelwright, 1951, p. 140).

To pursue Aristotle's argument, one is forced to say that the same faculty that *discriminates* white from sweet may also either fail to discriminate them or perceive them as synonymous based on shared qualities—hence synesthesia.

Research in the last century, therefore, focused on shared meanings in language as the link and suggested that synesthesia occurred at the highest levels of abstract processing in the central nervous system (CNS).

Proposal for a Synesthetic Mediator

A variant of the linkage theory, entertained and tested below, may be called *Polymodal Combination*. Heretofore, all recent theories of synesthesia have invoked Aristotelian common sense as a mediator of connotative meaning and therefore as a rudimentary mediator of synesthesia. On reflection, however, an Aristotelian common sensible is not like a synesthetic percept at all (Figure 3.1). An Aristotelian common sensible, such as roundness, cannot be learned by touch alone; it is a concept common to several senses. It is not a cross-modal association or an additive phenomenon but a filtering out of abstract residues, a subtractive attribute that amounts to a superabstraction. By contrast, synesthesia adds elementary percepts (sound and color, for example) to form complex ones without losing the identities of the elementary constituents.

Cross-modal associations per se are familiar enough from everyday life. Even young children can recognize as identical an object seen alone and then palpated in the dark (Ettlinger & Blakemore, 1969; Popper & Eccles, 1977). Cross-modal abstractions are requisite for language, as Geschwind (1964) pointed out:

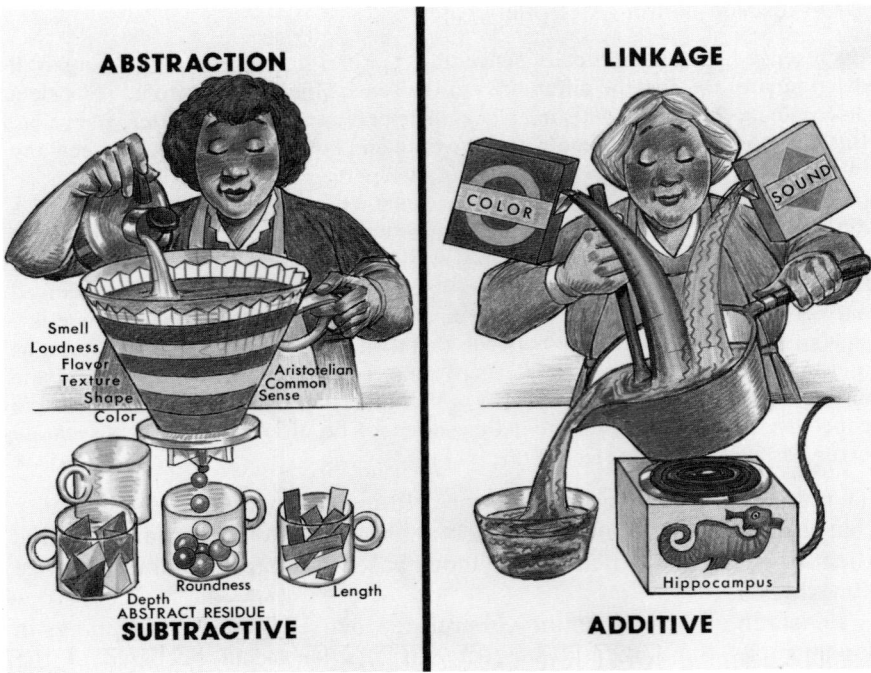

FIGURE 3.1. Theories of abstraction versus combination. In combination, elementary percepts are added into complex ones without losing their individual identities. This is characteristic of synesthesia.

The ability to acquire speech has as a prerequisite the ability to form cross modal associations. In sub-human forms, the only readily established sensory-sensory associations are those between a non-limbic (i.e. visual, tactile or auditory) stimulus and a limbic stimulus. It is only in man that associations between two nonlimbic stimuli are readily formed and it is this ability which underlies the learning of names of objects (p. 155).

At one extreme, for example, the concept of quantity is a polymodal *abstraction* (a nonlimbic to nonlimbic association). The current hypothesis proposes that synesthesia is a polymodal *combination* that is concrete instead of abstract. Based on theory alone, therefore, language should have little to do with synesthesia. This conclusion is supported experimentally by semantic differentials between subjects with colored hearing and the gustatory synesthete MW that show no common meaning between words describing either the stimuli or the synesthetic responses.

Thus, I believe that the place to go fishing in the brain for an explanation for synesthesia is not at the top (in the neocortex where symbolic language resides) but closer to the bottom of the pond, at an earlier stage of neural processing.

Testing the first class of theories, that of primitive loss of differentiation, is infeasible on a priori grounds, but testing the latter two categories—linkage and abstraction—is plausible. Experimental data may distinguish between the two theories in the following way. The proposed model applies to all types of synesthesia.

The solid black dots in Figure 3.2 represent the sensory stimuli and the squares on the right the synesthetically evoked percepts. A high level of semantic mediation implies a broad range and richness to the ultimate perceptual domain: If the associations are mediated through semantically abstract shared meaning, then the precipitating stimulus should engender a cluster of percepts that share the same meaning and the range of synesthetic associations should be as broad as nonsynesthetic controls. On the other hand, a direct one-to-one linkage between two senses would suggest an extremely limited range, which is quite specific as to the particular stimulus-percept combination. If the neuronal-specificity linkage theory is correct, there should be virtually no variability in the stimulus-to-percept associations of a synesthete, unlike normals, who are already documented to mediate via shared connotative meaning. Presumably, there is an intermediate possibility that stresses a small range of associations through a fairly low-level, relatively semantically impoverished mediating structure.

POSSIBLE ASSOCIATIVE ROUTES IN SYNESTHESIA

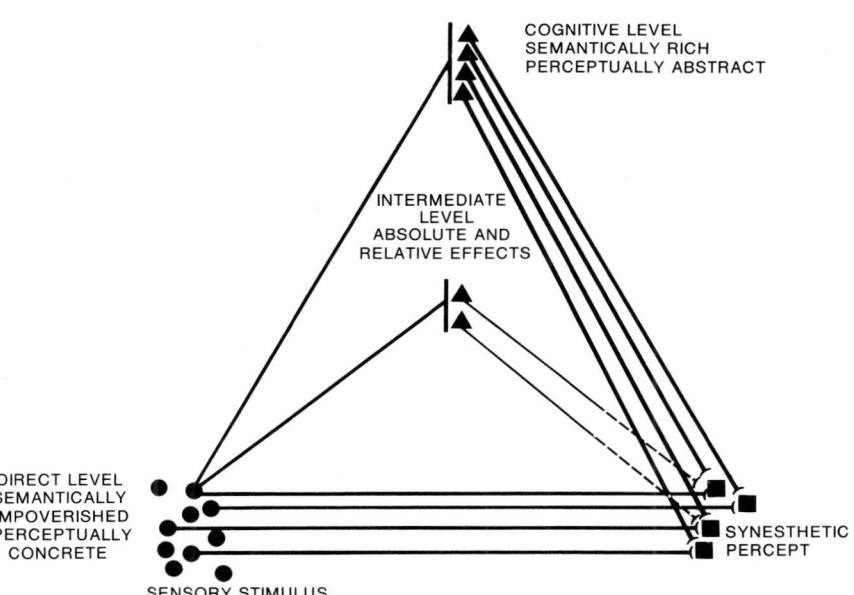

FIGURE 3.2. Possible associative routes in synesthesia. See text for further details. From "Synesthesia I: A review of theories and their brain basis" by R.E. Cytowic & F.B. Wood, 1982, *Brain and Cognition, 1*, p. 29. Copyright 1982 by Academic Press. Reprinted by permission.

In terms of CNS processes, the *semantic mediation hypothesis* would stress that synesthesia flows through the highest levels of neocortical processing, whereas the *neural linkage theory* would stress direct linkages between various sensory channels, at quite low levels of brain integration. An intermediate position might stress a relative attenuation of cortical associative processing with a corresponding enhancement of "lower" associations. *Polymodal combination* would, by definition, invoke a lower level of association than the classical polymodal abstraction theories. Hence, the range of synesthetic responses would be different according to the two theories. Polymodal combination implies a more restricted range than polymodal abstraction.

Within this class of lower level associations, the direct linkage theory can be further distinguished from the intermediate position by a consideration of relative effects in the psychophysical function relating synesthetic perception to the precipitating stimulus. Like the hard-wired knee jerk reflex, the lowest level associations would show no relative effects: a given stimulus would evoke the same percept regardless of the context of the stimulus within a set of recent stimuli. Purely cognitively mediated percepts might be especially sensitive to relational effects. The intermediate position should show a combination of both types of effect.

Operationalizing the Theories of Synesthesia

The alternative theories of synesthesia have been discussed above. Curiously, no direct comparisons of characteristic perceptual processing between synesthetes and nonsynesthetes were made in the past. A number of issues in making such comparisons lend themselves to experimental tests. Briefly, the fundamental question is the level at which the synesthetic association is mediated. A low level of association predicts a restricted range of synesthetic perceptual responses to the same stimulus, whereas a high level of association predicts an extensive range of associations to the eliciting stimulus, all of which are presumably mediated by a shared, high-level cognitive or connotative meaning.

A second experimental issue addresses absolute and relative effects in a psychophysical stimulus-response mapping experiment (Figure 3.2). A very low-level linkage should show no context effects; that is, a given stimulus should always evoke the same percept, just as the knee jerk reflex always produces the same twitch. This is called an absolute effect. For example, if a given stimulus were the highest of a group presented repeatedly to the subject, it would evoke exactly the same response as if it were the lowest of another set of stimuli presented to the subject. A purely relative mechanism, by definition mediated at a higher cognitive level, would predict that the stimulus would elicit quite different percepts, depending on its context within a set of stimuli. In both of these phenomena, range of associations and context effects, there could obviously be an intermediate level, suggesting a corresponding intermediate level of stimulus-response mapping.

The following experiments investigate the psychophysical functions of two synesthetes, each compared to three controls, with specific attention to the question of range and context effects.

EXPERIMENTAL SUBJECTS AND PROCEDURES

Beyond a willing subject who consents to undergo the tedious process of a mapping experiment, one needs a reliable and easily administered stimulus that will consistently produce some synesthetic response. The response should be scorable along a variable dimension and the arrangement of the mapping task should be flexible to permit investigation of absolute and relative effects as discussed above.

Subjects

Two synesthetic subjects, one who perceives vivid geometric shapes and textures in response to tastes and smells (MW) and another with colored hearing (VE), served as the experimental subjects.

MW, the gustatory synesthete with geometric taste, is a lighting designer who feels, rarely sees, and otherwise perceives geometric shapes whenever he tastes or smells foods. His parallel sense is most vivid and sensuous with novel flavors and smells (i.e., those sampled for the first time), although the synesthesia does not fatigue with repeated samplings or familiarization. With repeated inhalations his sense of *smell* will fatigue and the accompanying synesthesia might be absent because "I can't smell anything." But after a pause, when his olfactory neurons have recovered, the synesthesia is present as before. Having discovered that others do not taste shapes, he habitually keeps his synesthetic percepts to himself to avoid ridicule and disbelief, although the percepts themselves are impossible to ignore.

Shapes are felt mainly in the face, hands, and shoulders, in the trigeminal and dermatomal distribution of C2 to T2. There is often a sense of grasping or manipulating the shape, of palpating its texture or temperature. At times, the thumb or middle finger will feel more intensely than the other digits. Years after experimentation with MW began, he was shown a dermatome chart and immediately explained, "So that's why it feels like it's sweeping down my arm into my hand!" Despite the sensation of movement down his arm (spatial and temporal summation), I have never been convinced that he ever perceived in a true segmental distribution. The synesthesiae are almost always pleasurable; rarely, they may be a "slap" or burning" in the face. His obligation to attend to the synesthesia can sometimes be noted by others in his company through his lapse in the conversation, his manual gestures, or his nonverbal behavior that indicates satisfying pleasure. This behavior is nothing like the staring spell or aura of an absence or limbic seizure.

MW has a vivid memory for what he calls "sensory experiences." By this he means an ability to conjure up highly detailed unprojected visual images and to reenact past emotional states. A pilot study showed that he is able, in fact, to form accurate eidetic images after the method of Haber and Haber (1964; Haber, 1969). Of interest is his lack of source memory for a synesthetic percept, although other experiments showed that he can recognize instantly a stimulus he has had before. His hobby of cooking, for example, is guided by a method that I call the "unknown template," in which he has a nonverbal "idea" of what the final dish must "feel" like. Written recipes are not satisfactory to achieve the final desired result. He adjusts seasonings, often by trial and error, to alter the taste's shape, making it "rounder," giving it more "inclination," "sharpening up" corners to give more heft to the vertical component, or giving the overall shape some "points." A "Eureka" conviction of recognition overcomes him when the taste of the actual dish matches his unknown template. "Unknown" here simply means unavailable to semantic expression. This unknown template is just a version of the general instance of knowing what one is looking for only when one finds it.

VE, the auditory synesthete, has routinely, all her life, seen splotches of color whenever she hears music. Occasionally, environmental sounds such as beepers, voices, or clattering machinery will evoke photisms. Her habit is to ignore these percepts except in cases of shrill and loud sounds, where their vividness makes them impossible to neglect. At this level, they may be accompanied by a stabbing pain in the forehead. She is also synesthetic in other modalities, although less regularly so. For example, strychnine smells "pink," the same pink as the taste of her angel food cake. As a young child she had an especially vivid pictorial as well as verbal memory and could easily memorize long passages such as poems and plays.

At the time of these experiments MW was 36 years old and VE 38. The three nonsynesthetic gustatory controls were a 40-year-old chef (control J); a 33-year-old carpenter (control S); and a 43-year-old academic administrator (control W). A fourth gestatory control was eliminated because he insisted that there was no logical way for taste and shape to go together. The three nonsynesthetic auditory controls were a 28-year-old visual artist with strong scientific and mathematical interests (control L); a 24-year-old medical student (control T); and a 54-year-old professional portraiteur and muralist, widely read in the classics and philosophy (control A). All six controls were chosen not so much for rigid age-sex match as for their various experience with and professional response to taste, sound, shape, and color.

Construction of Appropriate Response Domains

For MW, a pilot study determined if certain shapes were appropriate as responses with which he could describe the percepts arising from various tastes. For this purpose, 10 tastes were used in solution: (1) salt, (2) sucrose, (3) anise, (4) critric acid, (5) Campari, (6) menthol, (7) Angostura bitters, (8) vanilla, (9) quinine, and (10) Karo syrup. The responses were developed to permit choices ranging from completely round (spherical) to completely angular (cubic). The response set thus represented a circumplex dimension, and the answer sheet is shown in Figure 3.3.

Stimuli were presented in 10 blocks of 10 trials each arranged in a Latin square counterbalancing sequence. The subject chose one of the shapes on the circle for each of the 100 taste trials and the results showed an orderly distribution of shape choices matched to taste stimuli. In general, simple tastes (such as sweet or sour) elicited a more restricted range of responses than did the complex tastes (such as anise or Angostura bitters), and there was noticeable differentiation in the shape-to-taste mapping.

This pilot experiment also revealed that regular solids radially symmetrical in three dimensions were inadequate as a stimulus set, since the subject often reported percepts that were linear, columnar, or pointed.

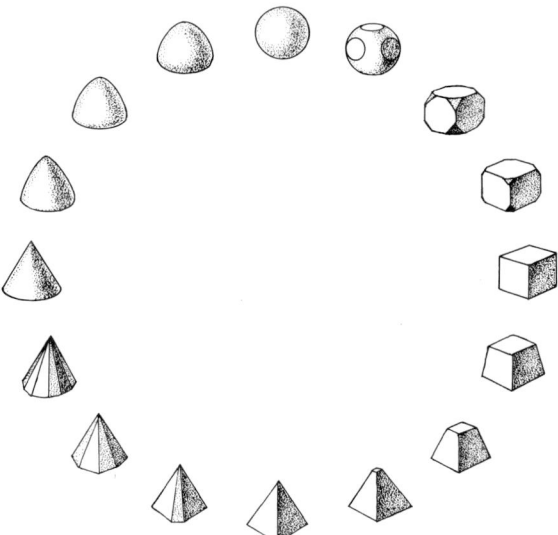

FIGURE 3.3. Circumplex dimension for the gustatory synesthesia pilot study. From "Synesthesia II: Psychophysical relationships in the synesthesia of geometrically shaped taste and colored hearing" by R.E. Cytowic & F.B. Wood, 1982, *Brain and Cognition, 1*. Copyright 1982 by Academic Press. Reprinted by permission.

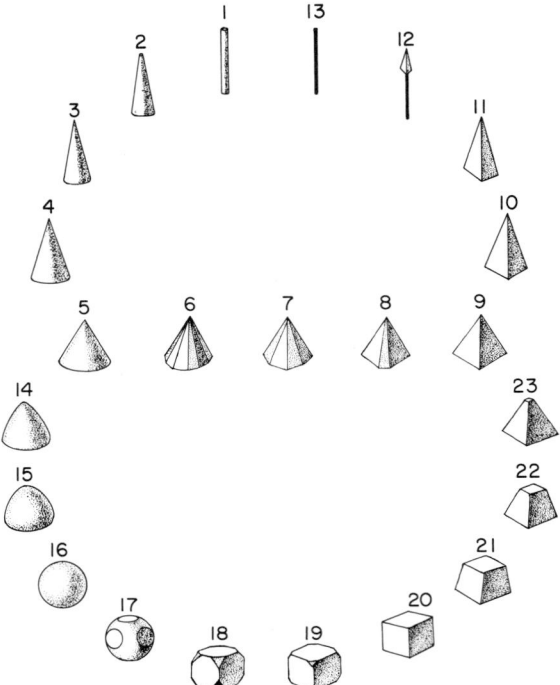

FIGURE 3.4. Revised circumplex for the actual taste-shape matching experiments. See text for further details. From "Synesthesia II: Psychophysical relationships in the synesthesia of geometrically shaped taste and colored hearing" by R.E. Cytowic & F.B. Wood, 1982, *Brain and Cognition, 1.* Copyright 1982 by Academic Press. Reprinted by permission.

Consequently, a revised response sheet was prepared so that it would incorporate some of the reported percepts for those for which the subject was unable to find satisfactory matches on the original response sheet. This revised answer sheet is shown in Figure 3.4. It has an even more complex dimensionality to it, so that shapes can sometimes differ from one another along more than one orderly series of intermediate forms. This figure-eight organization did seem to reflect the response domain as described by the subject: Most members of this figure-eight domain, *in both the upper and lower half,* were included in the subject's description of his percepts in the pilot study.

Pilot studies with VE, the auditory synesthete, demonstrated that verbal labels were quite as satisfactory as actual color chips (see also Williams & Jackson, 1968). An answer sheet was constructed in the following manner. An alphabetized list of color adjectives was printed in

TABLE 3.1. Arrangement of taste and sound stimuli.[a]

	Gustatory synesthesia												
	Sweet							Sour					
Experiment I	1	2	3	4	5	6	7						
Experiment II								7	8	9	10	11	12	13
Experiment III	1		3		5		7		9		11		13

Auditory synesthesia

Specific notes to which histogram numeric scales refer

Tape 1 (A-440)

D♭	D	E♭	E	F	F♯	G	A♭	A	B♭	B	C
1	2	3	4	5	6	7	8	9	10	11	12

Tape 2 (Major thirds)

D♭	F	A-220	D♭	F	A-440	D♭	F	A-880	D♭	F	A-1760
1	2	3	4	5	6	7	8	9	10	11	12

Tape 3 (A-880)

D♭	D	E♭	E	F	F♯	G	A♭	A	B♭	B	C
1	2	3	4	5	6	7	8	9	10	11	12

[a] From "Synesthesia II: Psychophysical relationships in the synesthesia of geometrically shaped taste and colored hearing" by R.E. Cytowic & F.B. Wood, 1982, *Brain and Cognition, 1*, p. 41. Copyright 1982 by Academic Press. Reprinted by permission.

left-to-right order on a single line for each of 144 trials in a given sound-color matching experiment:

BLACK BLUE BROWN GREEN GRAY ORANGE PINK PURPLE RED WHITE YELLOW

Procedure

Table 3.1 summarizes the taste and sound stimuli.

Gustatory Synesthesia

For the shape-taste experiment the stimuli consisted of 13 solutions ranging from pure 0.2 M sucrose for solution 1 to pure 0.2 M citric acid for solution 13. Three different experiments were conducted as follows:

Experiment I utilized solutions 1 (pure sucrose) through 7 (50:50 sucrose/acid), and involved seven sets of the seven tastes arranged in a Latin square counterbalancing table so that each taste occurred in each serial position once and followed every other taste once. After 0.25 ml of solution was squirted by syringe into the subject's mouth, he circled on the answer sheet that shape that best represented the percept, either synesthetic or imagined (for the controls), that resulted from the taste.

Tastes were applied at the rate of one every 20 seconds, with breaks of 10 minutes between experiments.

Experiment II was identical to Experiment I except in using solutions 7 (50 : 50 sucrose/acid) through 13 (pure citric acid).

Experiment III likewise had seven sets of tastes but explored the whole range of available tastes by using odd-numbered solutions only.

Auditory Synesthesia

Sound stimuli for the test of auditory synesthesia consisted of single piano notes recorded on tape. Three different tapes were prepared as follows (refer to Table 3.1).

Tape I consisted of 12 sets of 12 notes, each set containing the half-notes between C-sharp (adjacent to middle C) and C (one octave above middle C). All 12 notes appeared in each set and, across sets, a Latin square counterbalancing table assured that each note followed every other note once and occurred in each serial position once. Sets were ordered randomly, as was the order of tapes. A note was sounded for 5 seconds and followed by a 10-second pause on the tape, during which the subject was instructed to record on the answer sheet the visual percept seen or imagined. A new note sounded at the end of the 10-second pause and the cycle repeated until all 12 notes were played.

Tape II also consisted of 12 sets of 12 notes counterbalanced as in Tape I, except that the 12 notes were not adjacent half-notes but were separated by a major third interval and ranged four and a half octaves, from C-sharp below middle C to A two octaves above middle C.

Tape III was identical to Tape I except for being one octave higher.

The line of color adjectives is described above. Twelve such lines, corresponding to a single set of 12 notes, appeared on a single page. Thus, 12 pages constituted the answer booklet for a single tape. Subjects were instructed to circle the color perceived or imagined as seen in response to the tone on the tape.

Subjects worked at their own speed, taking breaks between sets as needed but no breaks within the set. Each subject completed the three tapes across 5 days of testing. Subjects worked in a quiet room but otherwise had no restrictions on the environment in which they worked.

RESULTS

The results of the mapping experiments show the presence of both absolute and relative effects but are closest to the lower level of linkage. Synesthetes clustered their responses in restricted areas of the response domain while controls spread their choices out over the available options. The synesthetic absolute effect is present in only one part of the stimulus field. Furthermore, there is a prominent relational effect in which the

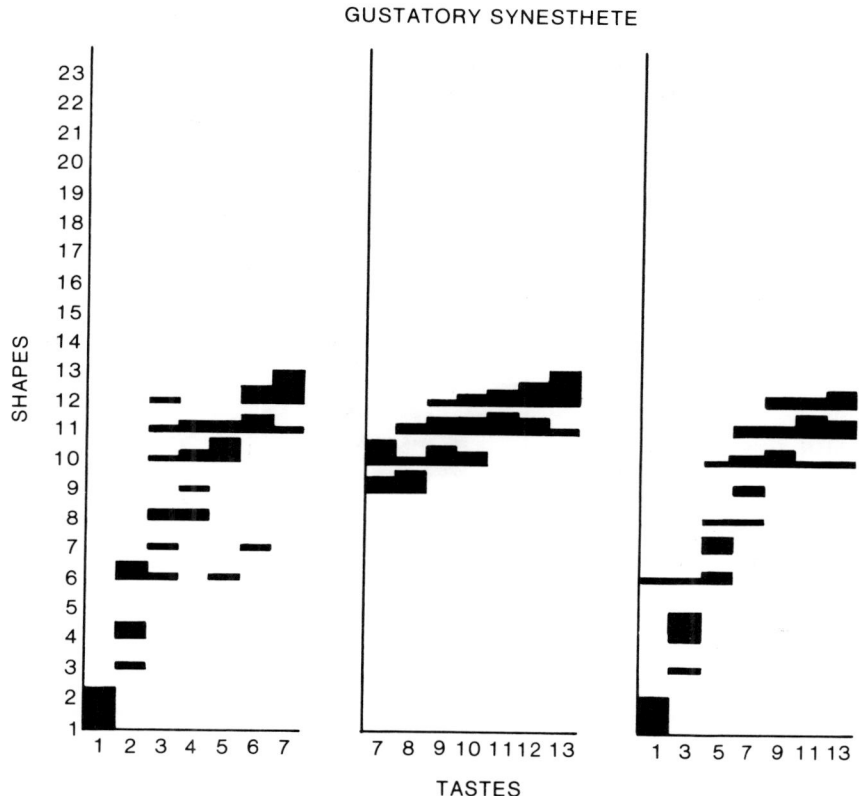

FIGURE 3.5. Distribution of shape choices for MW, the gustatory synesthete. From "Synesthesia II: Psychophysical relationships in the synesthesia of geometrically shaped taste and colored hearing" by R.E. Cytowic & F.B. Wood, 1982, *Brain and Cognition, 1*. Copyright 1982 by Academic Press. Reprinted by permission.

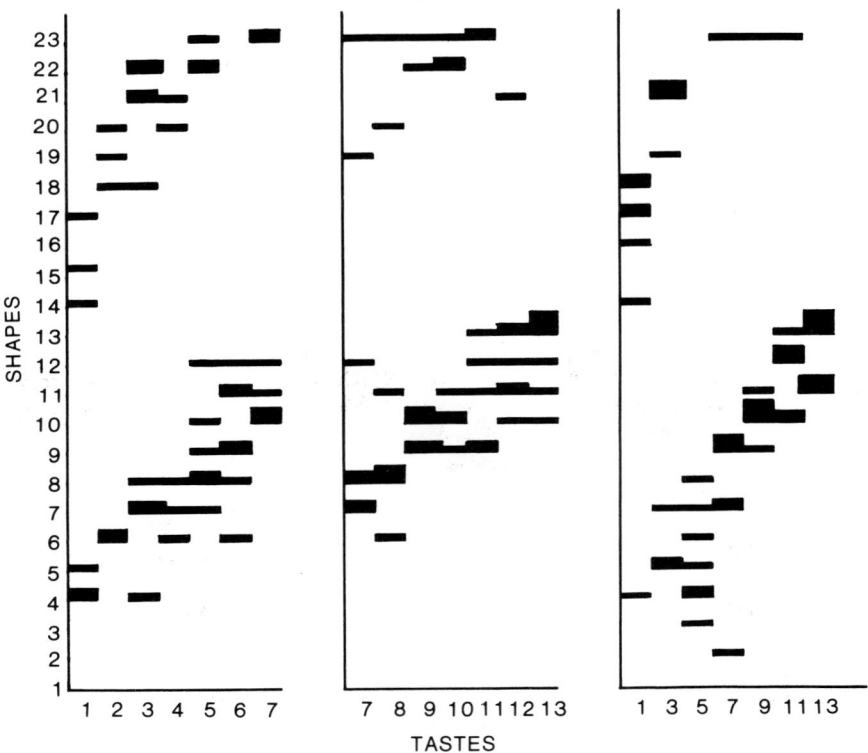

FIGURE 3.6. Distribution of shape choices for control J. From "Synesthesia II: Psychophysical relationships in the synesthesia of geometrically shaped taste and colored hearing" by R.E. Cytowic & F.B. Wood, 1982, *Brain and Cognition, 1*. Copyright 1982 by Academic Press. Reprinted by permission.

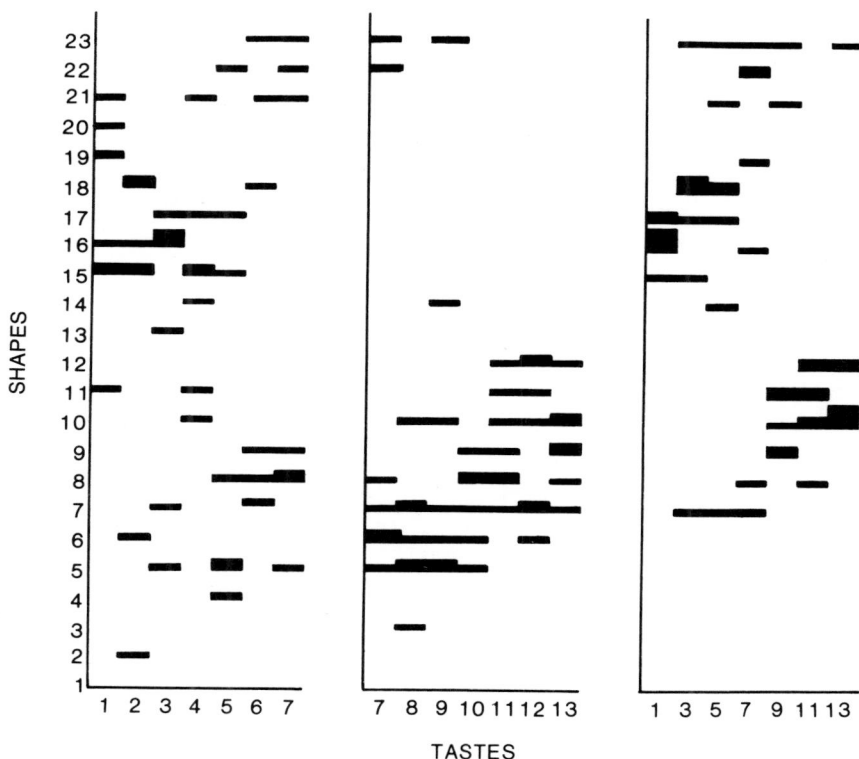

FIGURE 3.7. Distribution of shape choices for control S. From "Synesthesia II: Psychophysical relationships in the synesthesia of geometrically shaped taste and colored hearing" by R.E. Cytowic & F.B. Wood, 1982, *Brain and Cognition, 1*. Copyright 1982 by Academic Press. Reprinted by permission.

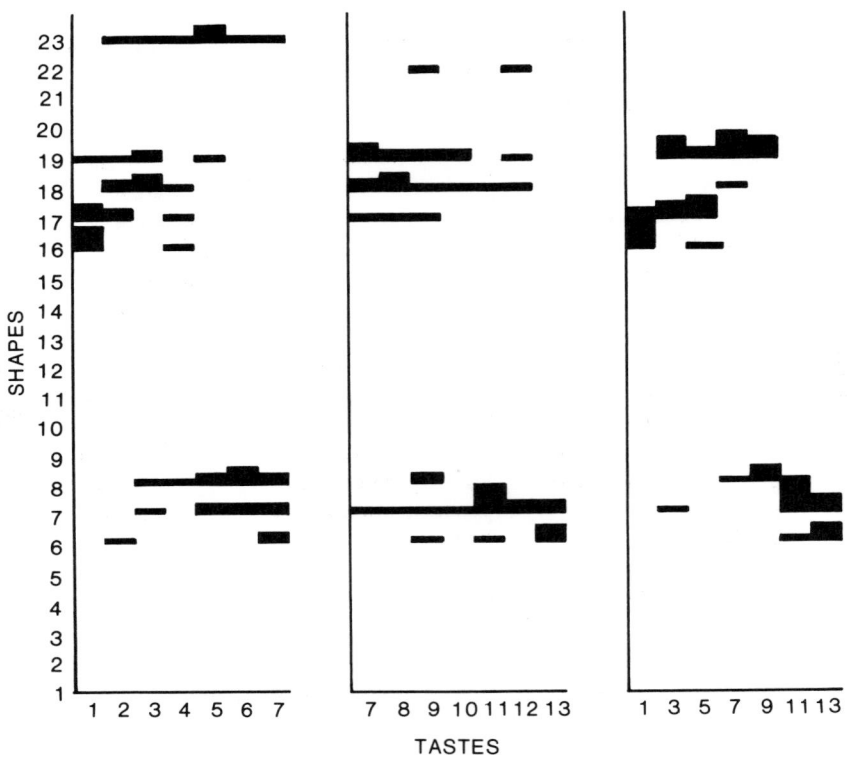

FIGURE 3.8. Distribution of shape choices for control W. From "Synesthesia II: Psychophysical relationships in the synesthesia of geometrically shaped taste and colored hearing" by R.E. Cytowic & F.B. Wood, 1982, *Brain and Cognition, 1*. Copyright 1982 by Academic Press. Reprinted by permission.

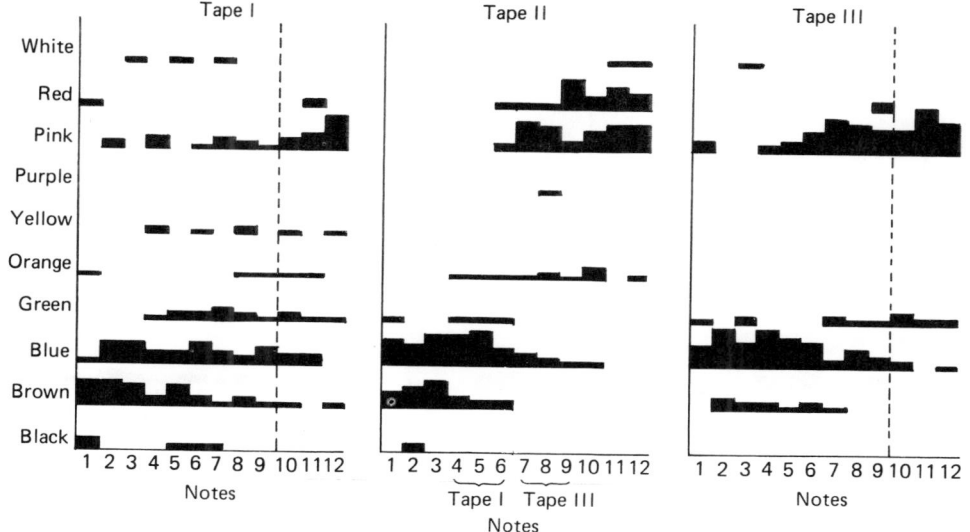

FIGURE 3.9. Frequency distribution of colors for VE, the auditory synesthete. Dotted lines on the low (Tape I) and high (Tape III) octave histograms mark those parts of the stimulus domain that also appear in the extended range (Tape II). From "Synesthesia II: Psychophysical relationships in the synesthesia of geometrically shaped taste and colored hearing" by R.E. Cytowic & F.B. Wood, 1982, *Brain and Cognition, 1.* Copyright 1982 by Academic Press. Reprinted by permission.

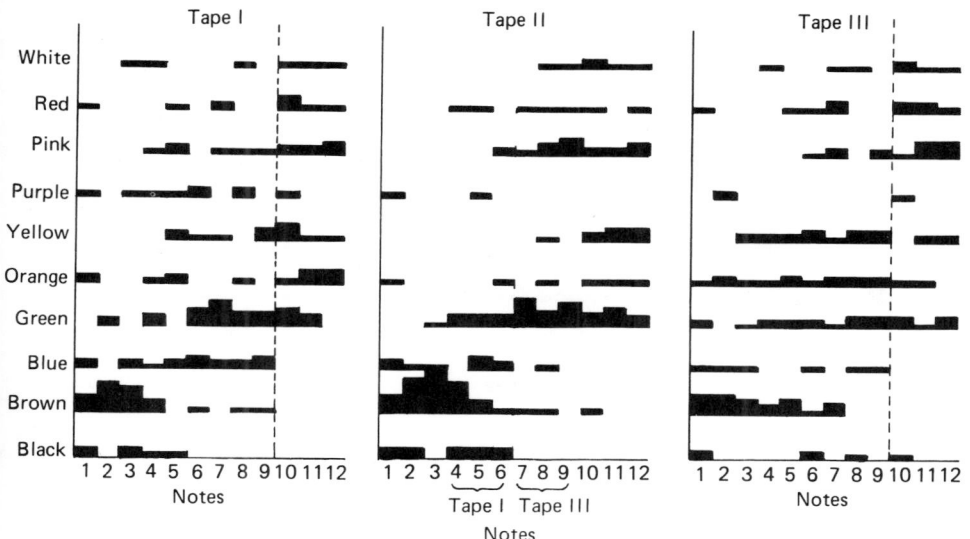

FIGURE 3.10. Distribution of color choices for control L. From "Synesthesia II: Psychophysical relationships in the synesthesia of geometrically shaped taste and colored hearing" by R.E. Cytowic & F.B. Wood, 1982, *Brain and Cognition, 1.* Copyright 1982 by Academic Press. Reprinted by permission.

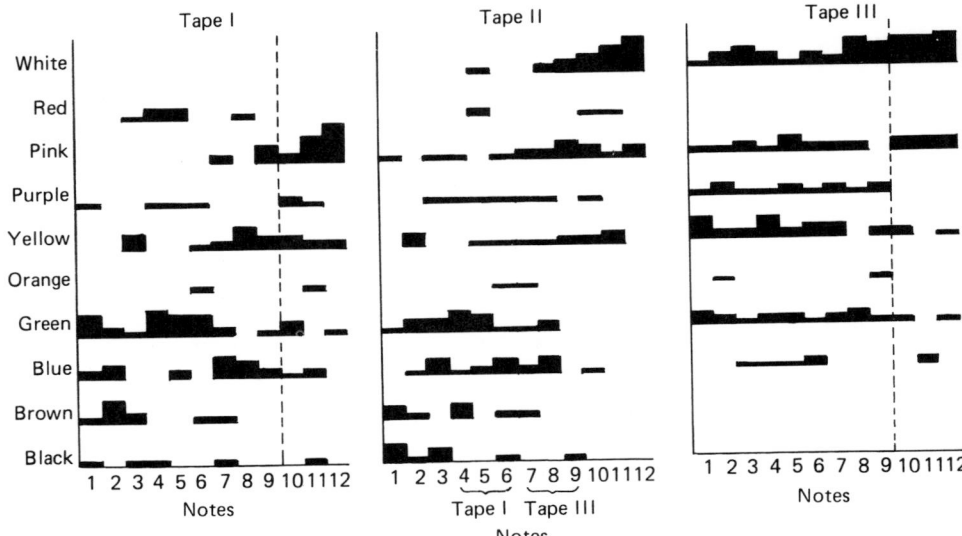

FIGURE 3.11. Distribution of color choices for control T. From "Synesthesia II: Psychophysical relationships in the synesthesia of geometrically shaped taste and colored hearing" by R.E. Cytowic & F.B. Wood, 1982, *Brain and Cognition, 1.* Copyright 1982 by Academic Press. Reprinted by permission.

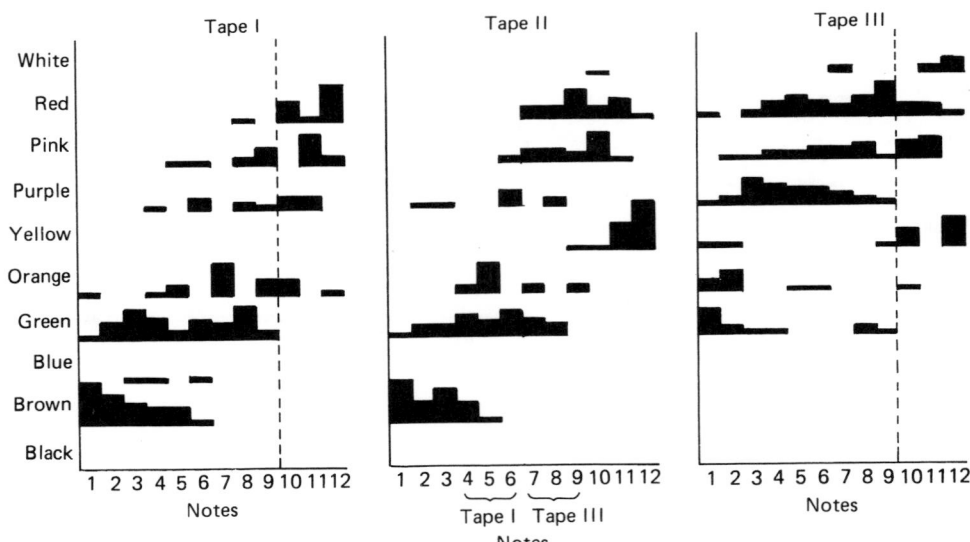

FIGURE 3.12. Distribution of color choices for control A. From "Synesthesia II: Psychophysical relationships in the synesthesia of geometrically shaped taste and colored hearing" by R.E. Cytowic & F.B. Wood, 1982, *Brain and Cognition, 1.* Copyright 1982 by Academic Press. Reprinted by permission.

response mapping of the *entire range* is reproduced in one segment of the stimulus range. These conclusions are examined in greater detail below.

The psychophysical function for MW, the gustatory synesthete, is difficult to describe in view of the circumplex dimensionality (figure-eight form) of the response domain. The results are presented as though the shapes were ordered in a single linear dimension, even though this is to some extent a distortion and oversimplification. The reader should therefore refer often to Figure 3.4 in interpreting this set of results. The frequencies of shape choices for particular taste stimuli for the gustatory synesthete and his three controls are shown in Figures 3.5 through 3.8. Similarly, the color responses to specific tones are shown for VE, the auditory synesthete, and her three controls in Figures 3.9 through 3.12.

The obvious tendency of the synesthetic responses to cluster in restricted areas of the response domain is of special interest. This tendency was tested by a χ^2 analysis, collapsing across stimuli, of the departure from the assumption of uniform distribution of responses across the response domain. This χ^2 was calculated for each set of counterbalanced stimuli for each subject. The relevant χ^2 values were significant at $p < .001$ for all three sets for both synesthetes, beginning at 86.0 (d.f.=10) to 108.0 (d.f.=22). The same was true for two of the controls (W in the gustatory series and A in the color series), where the χ^2 values exceeded $p < .001$ for one set per subject. Reasons for departure from uniformity are discussed below.

On inspection, there are apparent qualitative differences between these particular controls and the synesthetes in respect to the distribution of responses in the different parts of the range. In contrast to the controls, both synesthetes show a unique constriction of the response set at one end of the domain, with a similar and broader range applied both across the whole domain and across the other part of the domain. These tendencies are not subjectable to formal statistical tests, but are considered further in the discussion below.

DISCUSSION

Inspection of the various figures relating synesthetic percepts to eliciting stimuli shows some common features for both synesthetes that are indeed distinct from the nonsynesthetic controls. Compared to controls, the most notable feature of the synesthetic percepts, for both the gustatory and auditory synesthetes, is their greatly restricted response repertoire. The frequency distribution of synesthetic responses in various categories is greatly restricted compared to that of controls.

A second clear feature, shared by both synesthetes but by none of the controls, is a distinct asymmetry of responses in respect to the range of choices that are available in various subsets of the response domain (see Figures 3.13 and 3.14). Both synesthetic subjects use an extremely

GUSTATORY SYNESTHETE

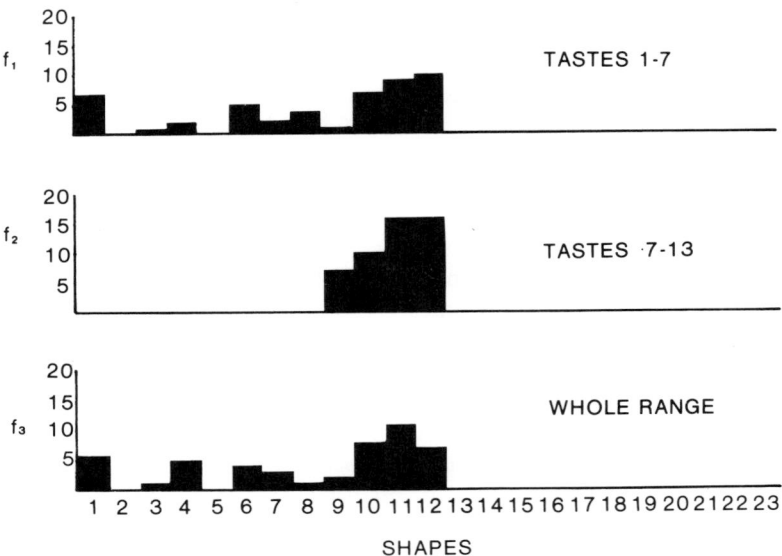

FIGURE 3.13. Collapsed frequency distribution of MW's shape responses for the low (f_1), high (f_2), and extended (f_3) range of taste stimuli. From "Synesthesia II: Psychophysical relationships in the synesthesia of geometrically shaped taste and colored hearing" by R.E. Cytowic & F.B. Wood, 1982, *Brain and Cognition, 1*. Copyright 1982 by Academic Press. Reprinted by permission.

restricted response repertoire in one particular part of the response domain under study. The gustatory synesthete, in responding to various concentrations of sucrose versus citric acid, showed his restriction of responses in the acidic half of the stimulus domain. There were essentially only three shapes that he employed, all some type of pointed and angular shape. These are conceptually close to one another in the response dimension. The auditory synesthete showed the greatest preponderance of blue and pink responses in the high single octave.

In contrast both synesthetes showed a full range of responses in the other half of the stimulus domain, quite similar to that shown when they were responding to the extended range of stimuli between both extremes of the stimulus dimension. Thus, there was a prominent relational effect whereby the response mapping of the entire range was reproduced in one segment of that range; but there was an absolute effect as well, whereby the other end of the stimulus domain elicited a very restricted range of responses.

The six control subjects employed a variety of strategies in their

AUDITORY SYNESTHETE

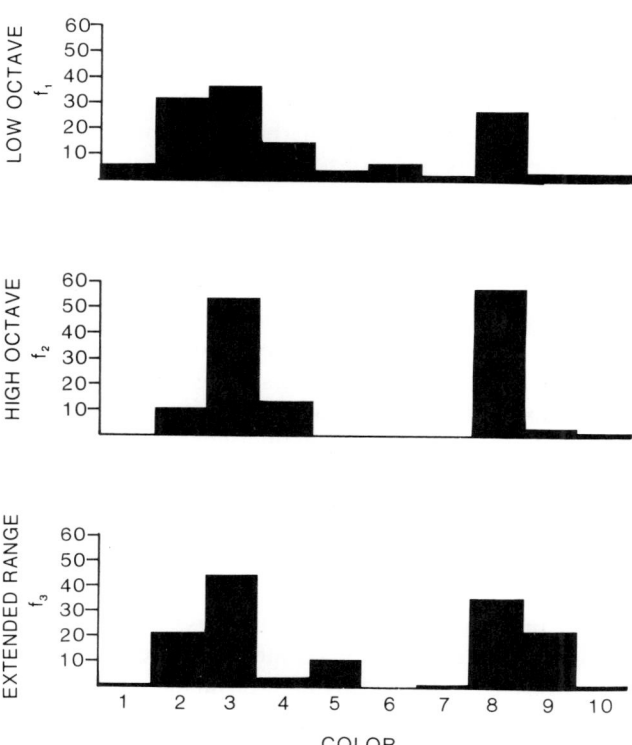

FIGURE 3.14. Collapsed frequency distribution of VE's color responses for the low, high, and extended range of sound stimuli. 1, black; 2, brown; 3, blue; 4, green; 5, orange; 6, yellow; 7, purple; 8, pink; 9, red; 10, white. From "Synesthesia II: Psychophysical relationships in the synesthesia of geometrically shaped taste and colored hearing" by R.E. Cytowic & F.B. Wood, 1982, *Brain and Cognition, 1.* Copyright 1982 by Academic Press. Reprinted by permission.

taste-shape and sound-color matchings. Most of them spread their choices out over the available response domain, giving a very diffuse, although not bell-shaped, and rich set of responses to a stimulus. One control of each in the gustatory series (W, the academic administrator) and the auditory series (A, the professional muralist) showed a restricted and essentially bimodal distribution of choices that was dominated by relational effects and lacking in appreciable absolute effects. This relational effect has been shown previously in nonsynesthetic subjects (Ries, 1969). Control W explained that he *decided* to use shape 17 for sweet tastes, which were "best represented by the concavities of this figure."

Accordingly, his range of most to least sweet encompassed shapes 16 through 19. Those for most to least sour were numbers 7, 8, 9, and 23, the sourness "represented by the complexity of the faceted cone." He apologized during testing: "I hope this isn't boring you because I'm being niggardly in my choices. Basically, if it's sweet I'm choosing these [*round*] shapes, and if it's sour, I pick these [*conical*]." Control A claimed to have no logical scheme for choosing his colors but, like the others, "I just pick whatever comes into my head."

It does not need emphasizing that the controls, even those who show a bimodal distribution, are making conscious choices in their matches and experientially deny having synesthesia.

In relation to the theoretical issues considered earlier in this chapter it appears quite clear that synesthetic percepts show two things: a generally restricted range of responses and a combination of absolute and relative effects. According to the theoretical considerations discussed, therefore, one can conclude that synesthesia is a distinct phenomenon unlike ordinary mediated associations. Its distinctiveness appears to involve an intermediate level of stimulus-response association in which the stimulus-response mapping is neither completely one-on-one nor richly one-on-many. A combination of absolute and relational effects is shown, lending further support to the notion of an intermediate level of stimulus-response mediation.

Regarding the brain basis for a process whose only characteristics are behaviorally described, it is at least possible to indicate that the synesthetic mechanism does seem to occupy an intermediate place in the range of concrete to abstract, one-on-one to one-on-many, and therefore simple to complex brain mechanisms.

The anatomical level of this mechanism is considered in the next chapter, where I propose a disconnection of language areas from limbic structures as a possible explanation for synesthesia. The neural basis for synesthesia will then be taken up in Chapter 5.

4
Overlaps: To What Is Synesthesia Similar?

With a theoretical idea of how synesthesia occurs established, we can ask at what level in the brain it occurs. Bearing in mind the earlier cautions about answering universal questions, our expectation is to make a little progress here and there rather than arrive at any definitive answer.

The mapping experiments and theoretical issues disclosed two fundamentals of synesthesia: (1) a restricted range of responses from the available response domain and (2) a combination of absolute and relative effects. This linkage is neither hard-wired at a one-to-one correspondence nor is it one-to-many as might occur at the highest level of abstract (presumably cortical) processing. It seems to occupy an intermediate place in the range of concrete-to-abstract and simple-to-complex brain mechanisms.

So where is it? It will be argued that synesthesia (1) is in the left hemisphere, (2) is not "cortical" in the conventional sense, and (3) involves temporal lobe–limbic structures.

Phenomena Similar to Synesthesia

In trying to fathom the anatomical and then the functional basis for synesthesia, we can examine those phenomena to which synesthesia is most similar. These include:

Drug-induced synesthesia (LSD and other hallucinogens)
Eidetic imagery and other forms of hypermnesis (Luria's patient S)
Release hallucinations
Simple synesthesiae in deafferented sensory fields
Temporal lobe epilepsy
Electrical stimulation of the brain (Penfield)

Some of the support for the ideas developed will include:

Influence of drugs on synesthesia
Regional cerebral blood flow, cerebral angiography, and magnetic resonance imaging

Neuropsychological assessment
Klüver's form constants

LSD-INDUCED SYNESTHESIA

LSD and other antiserotonergics *sometimes* produce synesthesia. It is not a universal effect of the drug, as many assume from their impressions of the 1960s counterculture. Nor will LSD induce synesthesia every time it is ingested if it has once done so. Much of our contemporary knowledge of LSD is anecdotal, with variation of response unreliable and complicated by factors such as inconsistency of dose, purity, and even chemical identification of illicit street preparations. Such problems will never be resolved; the more reliable scientific work done in both animals and humans will never be repeated. There is no choice but to rely on the information we have.

Synesthetics perform in some ways reminiscent of nonsynesthetic volunteers under the influence of LSD: in their tendency toward concreteness (Fanchamps, 1978; Hollister, 1968; Silverstein & Klee, 1957), decreased productivity (Zialko, 1959), emotional significance (Finkel, 1976), vividness of percepts, and the vivid memory for the hallucinogenic experience (Hollister, 1968; B.L. Jacobs, 1977; Siegel & West, 1975). This vivid memory for dream-like experiences and the marked preservation of detail can be seen in subjects' drawings of their hallucinogenic experiences.

The drug's effect on visual perception and CNS integration is most interesting. The colored visions themselves seem paradoxical in view of increased thresholds for axonal responses beyond thalamic synapses, until one appreciates the facilitating effect of sensory inputs from other modalities on the perception of visual hallucinations (i.e., synesthesia). Almost all measures of color perception are affected in humans given LSD. Particularly noteworthy is the increased elicitation of subjective colors by stimuli that occasionally evoke color percepts (Fechner-Benham flicker fusion) or usually never do (pure tones). The combination of flicker and pure tone stimuli greatly increases visual effects, *both patterns and colors,* over flicker alone (Hartman & Hollister, 1963). The visual image suppresses alpha rhythm (Shirahashi, 1960).

LSD has differential action on central synapses: facilitation of primary evoked responses and inhibition of the recruiting responses (Purpura, 1956a, 1956b, 1957). Purpura has explained this on the basis of anatomical differences in synapses between the two systems. LSD facilitates the primary afferent axosomatic synapses while inhibiting corticocortical association and nonspecific mesodiencephalic axodendritic pathways. This may provide a basis for the intellectual and behavioral disorganization so clearly seen clinically, inasmuch as LSD inhibits human cortical dendritic potentials in a manner similar to that recorded in cats (Purpura, Pool, Ranshoff, et al., 1957).

In both animals and man there are regional differences in EEG activity: desynchronized neocortical activity, suggesting arousal, and synchronized or paroxysmal limbic and sublimbic activity (Bente, Itil, & Schmid, 1957; Ingvar & Soderberg, 1956; Monnier, 1959; Vogt, Gunn, & Sawyer, 1957). In humans (Monroe, Heath, Mickle, et al., 1957), the subcortical activity, which is not reflected in the surface electrodes, correlates with emotional change or perceptual distortion. Perhaps, then, a "stimulated" limbic system in the face of disinhibited neocortical integration results in a subject who cannot discriminate, but who is prepared to respond emotionally (Bridger, 1960). As some of the earlier theories suggested, emotional meaning might be a relevant "linkage" to synesthetic percepts, a suggestion that is empirically testable, although this is difficult to carry out.

The physiological data show that LSD induces a suppression of corticocortical connections with corresponding facilitation of the direct lower level specific afferents (Purpura, 1956a, 1956b, 1957; Purpura et al., 1957). The antiserotonergic action of LSD may be plausibly related to its effect of rendering the cortex less responsive to reinforcement, and thus more responsive to external stimuli (S. Cohen, 1970; Hollister, 1968; Messing, Pettibone, Kaufman, et al., 1978; Weil-Malherbe, 1977). The negative action of increased brain serotonin in interfering with learning, and in disrupting memory consolidation, dream recall, and novel task performance, might be entertained to account for the memorability of the synesthetic percept (Essman, 1977; Fibiger, Lepaine, & Phillips, 1978). Two distinct types of serotonin receptors exist, one excitatory and one inhibitory (Peroutka, Lebovitz, & Snyder, 1981). Inhibition of only the excitatory receptors has been implicated in the serotonin behavioral syndrome. Increased dopamine in the face of decreased serotonin, however, may also be important (B.L. Jacobs, 1977; B.L. Jacobs & Trulson, 1979). These authors suggest a common neurochemical mechanism for the phenomenological similarities between dreams and LSD-induced hallucinations.

Ideas on possible neurotransmitters involved in synesthesia are deductions based on historical and animal work, and are highly speculative. It is premature to take such speculations beyond a level that might suggest a theoretical structure to consider as a mechanism for synesthesia.

As Table 2.1 shows, five of the current subjects have taken LSD in the past. In only 1 (MM) was there intensification of his spontaneous synesthesia while under the influence of the drug. Three subjects had no synesthesia with the drug. Although LSD did not induce synesthesia in a fourth patient (MW), he feels that he was "hypersensitive" to it, experiencing "sensory overload" on one-fourth the dose considered standard (in 1971) among his confreres. He has vivid memories for those three occasions on which he ingested the drug. Compared to his pleasurable synesthesia, the drug made him dysphoric.

HYPERMNESIS

The vividness and memorability of the synesthetic percepts, two of its defining characteristics, also give them some similarity to eidetic imagery and other forms of hypermnesis—that is, mental reminiscences that revive the original percept with hallucinatory clarity. Specifically in this regard, eidetic images, so easily and vividly remembered, are precisely so on account of their semantic vacuity. That is, they carry little semantic or emotional baggage, but rather are reproducible in their original form.

Most of the studies in eideticism are German. Klüver (1928, 1931, 1932, 1965) has been the principle reviewer of this work and Jaensch (1930) systematized its study. Few papers are cited after 1937 until the subject was revived by the Habers (Haber, 1969, 1979; Haber & Haber, 1964). "No serious doubts were raised about the validity of eidetic imagery as a phenomenon, even though the methodology of assessment has been both poorly described and poorly executed. Eidetic imagery just ceased to excite scientists." There was also the behavioristic climate of the time against so introspective a subject.

Luria's Patient, S

An interesting aspect of eidetic imagery is that it has some percept-like qualities and some memory qualities, and yet is qualitatively distinct from both. The relationship between synesthesia and hypermnestic function is, of course, especially familiar in the classic case of S, by Luria (1968). [See also the subject of Reichard et al. (1949), who came to those authors' attention via a class assignment on the topic, "How I Memorize."] S was unavoidably synesthetic for many of the percepts and experiences of daily life. There was no distinct line separating vision from hearing, or hearing from a sense of touch or taste. He could not suppress the translation of sounds into shape, taste, touch, and color.

Presented with a tone pitched at 2,000 cycles per second and having an amplitude of 113 decibels, S said: "It looks something like fireworks tinged with a pink-red hue. The strip of color feels rough and unpleasant, and it has an ugly taste—rather like that of a briny pickle . . . you could hurt your hand on this (Luria, 1968, p. 23).

This same synesthesia enabled him to vividly visualize each word or sound that he heard, whether in his own tongue or a foreign language unintelligible to himself. The thing to be remembered was simply converted into a visual image of such durability that he could remember it many years after the initial event. So specific was his ability that the same stimuli would invariably produce the same synesthetic response, although the synesthetic experience itself was always *secondary* to his recall. There was no limit to the capacity or durability of the traces he retained. As Luria put it, his memory was limitless and without distortion.

. . . I recognize a word not only by the images it evokes, but by a whole complex of feelings that image arouses. It's hard to express . . . it's not a matter of vision or hearing but some over-all sense I get. Usually I experience a word's taste and weight, and I don't have to make an effort to remember it—the word seems to recall itself. But it's difficult to describe. What I sense is something oily slipping through my hand . . . or I'm aware of a slight tickling in my left hand caused by a mass of tiny, lightweight points. When that happens, I simply remember, without having to make the attempt (Luria, 1968, p. 28).

S's inability to suppress these synesthetic percepts was often so severe as to make it difficult for him to attend to the semantic and meaningful qualities of a verbal discourse. An earlier example of synesthesia was of this man, S, seeing a yellow voice with protruding fibers and being so overwhelmed by the perception that he could not understand what was being said to him. He became "trapped" in a synesthetic tangle of evoked percepts, mostly visual, whenever he heard a story. His images would guide his thinking, one picture leading to another, rather than thought itself being the dominant element. Although he could easily manipulate his eidetic images, he was quite inept at abstraction and generalization, at converting encounters with the particular into instances of the general, enabling one to form general concepts even though the particulars are lost.

Perhaps this occurs because the details of a visual experience are essentially unrepeatable, constituting a single episode, whereas the semantic abstractions from a given story are part of the currency of language and can easily be interfered with by subsequent events of daily life and living. Thus it is precisely the concrete level of intellectual processing, a level of encoding conceptually lower but richer sensorily, that appears to facilitate the vivid and long-lasting memory for discrete episodes.

There are sensory memories that can be evoked in hypnogogic reveries (Kubie, 1943; Kubie & Margolin, 1942). These memories merge into the kind of memory mediated by verbal symbols of past events, rather than through vivid sensory images. This is another example of how the semantic abstractions are part of the currency of language. Such memories are necessarily not concrete or vivid because, semantically, they are generalizations. They stand nicely in contrast to the vividness of synesthesia, eidetic memory, and the "recollective hallucinations" of Penfield, what he also calls forced experiential responses to electrical stimulation of the brain.

Luria summarized S's memory as

. . . a striking example of spontaneous recall. Granted that he imparted certain meanings to these images which he could draw upon; he nonetheless continued to *see* the images and experience them synesthetically. He had no need for logical organization, for the associations *his* images produced reconstituted themselves whenever he revived the original situation in which something had been registered in his memory (Luria, 1968, p. 63).

Eidetic Memory

Although eidetikers have excellent recall of visual detail, their performance is not necessarily *discontinuous* from the distribution of control subjects (Furst, Fuld, & Pancoe, 1974). The same might be true of synesthesia.

Like synesthetes, eidetikers describe their images with spontaneity and conviction, giving the impression that they are genuinely *seeing* a stable, externally projected display. Gengerelli (1976) found stability of eidetic images in two subjects after 46 years. An example of verbatim eidetic recall is perhaps the best way to convey this. Pollen and Trachtenberg (1972) studied alpha rhythm and eye movement in Stromeyer and Psotka's (1970) patient. While viewing a print of Chagall's "My Village," no alpha rhythm was present (see Figure 4.1). Alpha rhythm was prominent and convergent eye movements were present when she described details from her eidetic image of the print. "The subject described the painting with a speed that could scarcely have been exceeded had she been looking directly at it." Her description was as follows:

Horse and green man facing each other. Horse or cow. The man has a yellow hat with a red band. The horse is mostly pink and white except he's blue in the neck just above the necklace he's wearing. And under his eye is someone milking a

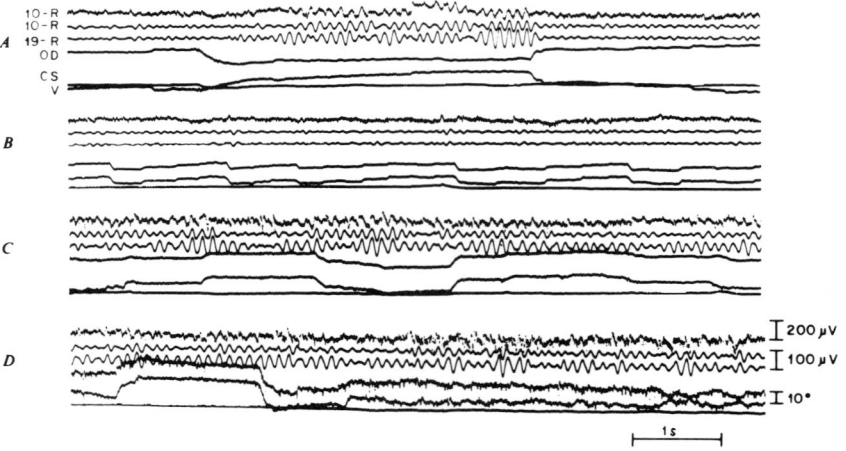

FIGURE 4.1. (A) Absence of alpha rhythm while subject forms an eidetic image of text. (B) Eyes closed, subject reads text from eidetic image built up in A. Posterior alpha rhythm present. (C and D) Describing details from an eidetic image of Chagall's "My Village." High-amplitude alpha rhythm is present. Convergent eye movements seen in D. From "Alpha rhythm and eye movements in eidetic imagery" by D.A. Pollen & M.C. Trachtenberg, 1972. Reprinted by permission from *Nature*, Vol. 237, p. 110. Copyright (c) 1972 Macmillan Magazines Ltd.

cow. Up above this is another sort of sphere like thing. Heading back is a green man carrying a hoe, I think, and a girl standing on her head. Behind them are houses. The one on the left is yellow. It's upright. Then there's a red one upside down, a blue one upside down, a blue one right side up, and then a yellow one right side up. There's a moon over that. The centre of the picture has a red sphere in it. Down in the bottom centre is a tree of some sort in a triangular shape with some little green blobs and a bunch of brown blobs in the branches. And the bottom left hand is mostly reds and pinks. Bottom right there's some yellow and blue. The sky at the top is black. Anything else?

This description was produced in 68 seconds, about the time it takes to read it. The subject made saccades in the direction of objects she described. She had normal alpha rhythm that blocked appropriately to eye opening or tasks requiring visual attentiveness. Of great interest is the presence of large-amplitude posterior alpha rhythm when she scans or reads text from an eidetic image. Pollen and Trachtenberg noted that her speed and detail of recall indicate considerable concentration and mental effort, and cited their own work in noneidetikers showing that alpha blocking occurs with visual tasks that recall resolution or a search for the finest detail rather than the fine detail itself. They suggested that the subject's alpha rhythm during eidetic recall was understandable either if that recall did not require the finest details or if her access to fine detail did not require much searching of the memory.

The reality of eidetic imagery has often been questioned. A few attempts to discriminate eidetic from noneidetic subjects have been remarkable, such as the use of random dot stereograms (Julesz, 1964) that Stromeyer and Psotka (1970) used to test for clarity and duration of eidetic images. The subject must look monocularly in succession at two patterns of dots that superimpose to produce an object or a set of letters (Figure 4.2).

Noneidetic observers are unable to perceive the stereoscopic letters when the two patterns are projected as little as 150 milliseconds apart. Stromeyer and Psotka's eidetic subject could accurately report the figure in depth with an interval between monocular observations of 24 hours. She found the task "ridiculously easy." The patterns are presented monocularly and the two eidetic images are fused to produce the stereoscopic appearance of a third image. Patterns with 10^4 elements were used at intervals up to 3 days, and patterns with 10^6 dots at intervals up to 4 hours, in a double-blind experiment. Reports of binocular rivalry support Stromeyer and Psotka's interpretation that the eidetic image is represented before binocular fusion. Both Jaensch and Klüver found binocular color rivalry in an eidetic image built up from a color chip presented to one eye and a different color chip presented to the other eye.

Stromeyer and Psotka's eidetiker is also cited as being able to halluci-nate "leaves on a barren tree, or a page of poetry in a known foreign language which she can copy from the bottom line to the top line as fast as

1	0	1	0	1	0	0	1	0
1	0	X	A	A	B	B	O	O
O	O	Y	B	A	B	A	1	1
0	1	0	0	1	1	1	0	1
1	1	A	B	A	B	A	O	O
O	O	B	A	B	A	B	1	0
1	1	0	1	0	1	1	0	0
1	0	A	A	B	A	X	O	1
1	1	B	B	A	B	X	1	0
0	1	0	0	0	1	1	1	1

1	0	1	0	1	0	0	1	0
1	0	A	A	B	B	Y	O	O
O	O	B	A	B	A	X	1	1
0	1	0	0	1	1	1	0	1
1	1	B	A	B	A	B	O	O
O	O	A	B	A	B	A	1	0
1	1	0	1	0	1	1	0	0
1	0	Y	A	A	B	A	O	1
1	1	Y	B	B	A	B	1	0
0	1	0	0	0	1	1	1	1

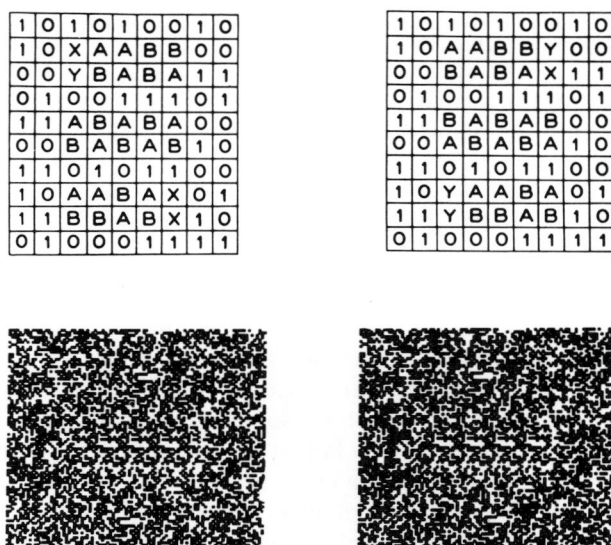

FIGURE 4.2. Example of a dot stereogram. *Top:* Method by which the stereo pair is generated. *Bottom:* When viewed stereoscopically, the sterogram reveals to the viewer an upper rectangle in front of the surround, a lower rectangle behind the surround, and an ambiguous rectangle either in front of or behind the surround. From "Binocular depth perception without familiarity clues" by B. Julesz, 1964, *Science, 145,* p. 357. Copyright 1964 by the AAAS.

her hand can write. These visions can often obscure a real object." There is a report that visual- and auditory-evoked responses are blocked during hallucination, but the methodology is questionable (Schatzman, 1981). One cannot perceive and hallucinate in the same space (see Chapter 9).

Stromeyer and Psotka's subject examined the dot stereogram part by part, "frequently shutting her eyes to see if she has a good image of the part." Luria's patient used the same technique in making eidetic images of numeric tables. What an eidetiker actually does during eidetic recall is not clear. Stromeyer and Psotka's subject recalled the image part by part rather than as a gestalt, some of the stereoscopic images taking up to 10 seconds to construct. *Nor is it necessary for the stimulus images to be in sharp focus,* an observation reminiscent of Land's 2-squares-and-a-happening experiment for edge detection (see Figure 4.3) (Land & McCann, 1971). Also, the lines, streaks, and squiggles that synesthetes see make us pose the question, "What is an edge?"

What makes the Stromeyer-Psotka experiment so appealing is that "hard science" evidence supports the experimental reports of Klüver, Luria, and other neuropsychologists. Similarly, the eye movements

FIGURE 4.3. Land's 2-squares-and-a-happening experiment. Place a pencil over the boundary between the two gray areas. The right-hand paper reflects 80% of the light, the left-hand one 40%. A light at the left of both casts twice as much light on the center of the 40% paper as the center of the 80% paper, producing a linear gradient across the paper. The reflected luminances at corresponding points of the papers are equal. Yet the left 40% paper looks darker than the right 80% one.

When a narrow object, a "happening," obstructs the boundary, the two appear to have the same lightness. The only alteration is the viewer's obscuration of the edge. The change in luminance at the junction between areas both constitutes an edge and leads to a visual difference between the whole two areas. Although the word "edge" suggests a sharp in-focus boundary, boundaries severely out of focus look the same. From "Lightness and retinex theory" by E.H. Land & J.J. McCann, 1971, *Journal of the Optical Society of America, 61,* p. 4. Copyright 1971 by E.H. Land. Reprinted by permission.

recorded by Pollen and Trachtenberg support the observations of others who have noted saccadic movements of subjects reading an eidetic image of text.

Some, like Gray and Gummerman (1975), object that eidetikers simply use more intense imagery than that possessed by the great majority of the population. Haber (1979) reviewed the conflicting interpretations. S. Miller and Peacock's (1982) otherwise good review fails to criticize Gray and Gummerman for using a scaled-down version of the Julesz dot stereogram as an "objective" measure. Eidetikers identified by Haber's method failed this task, which was cited as evidence that eideticism does not exist. Julesz (1964, pp. 357, 360–361) himself cautioned that stereopsis is hard to obtain when superimposing coarse gradient patterns with few pixel elements.

Haber and Haber (1964) established criteria for determining eidetic images. Using colored squares on a neutral background, the examiner demonstrates afterimages so that the subject can distinguish an afterimage (which moves with eye movement) from an eidetic image (which does not). Unlike eidetic images, afterimages fade rapidly, require long fixation to produce, and show negative (complementary) coloration. A type of prolonged afterimage, called the McCullough effect, occurs in workers at video display terminals that have green letters on black backgrounds. The appearance of a pink aura around white letters and objects can last for weeks (Greenwald, Greenwald, Arch, et al., 1983; Walraven, 1985). The Habers' criteria for eidetic images are that an image (1) must be reported, (2) must be positively colored, (3) is projected onto the easel rather than being located in the head, (4) is described in the present tense, and (5) is associated with eye movements appropriate to the location of objects in the scene. A lot of reports on eideticism are in children, and the Habers estimate some degree of eidetic ability in 8% of American elementary school children.

One of the current synesthetes, MW, can form eidetic images after the method of Haber and Haber.

As an interim summary, we see that eidetikers are distinct from a normal population and have variable performance. Like synesthetes, there is a sense of reality and conviction to these externalized images. The link with synesthesia is their hypermnestic quality.

Synesthesia and Memory Function In Current Patients

One of the defining characteristics of synesthesia is that the parallel sense is memorable. Inspection of Table 2.1 shows that 37 of 42 subjects felt that their memory is better than average or excellent. Subjects' comments regarding the utility of synesthesia as a mnemonic device were given in Chapter 3.

Four of the current subjects were studied with the Wechsler Memory Scale, with scores in the superior range (DS, 101; JM, 143; MT, 135; MW, 143). Reasons for the average score of DS are discussed below in her results of neuropsychological testing. An additional subject, MLL, happened to be a normal volunteer in a study of memory performance in aging at the National Institutes of Health. At age 50 years she scored in the superior range on a name-face association task (including delayed recall), recognition of faces (with 40-minute delay), a misplaced objects recall, a news story recall, and a delayed nonmatching task.

Memory of Synesthesia

In Chapter 1, I related the anecdote of how MW's comment that the chicken he had prepared for dinner did not have "enough points" brought his synesthesia to my attention. In December 1986, 7 years after that eventful dinner, MW and I happened to be again dining on roast chicken. I pointed out the irony and misquoted his initial description in saying that there were too many corners on the chicken. MW corrected me, however, and *claimed to remember the original stimulus.*

I corrected you by saying "it was too round, it needs more points" because that's what it *was,* it was round. I was remembering that it was indeed uniformly round and it needed more points. I remember the *shape,* not the anecdote. I remember being disappointed with the chicken because it was too round. I tasted it and I couldn't serve this. I had to fix it. I had to give it points.

It is not the anecdote or a verbal description that MW remembers, "it's the taste, particularly the shape."

RELEASE HALLUCINATIONS

The consideration of release hallucinations is appropriate here. From electrical stimulation of the brain, study of complex partial seizures, and observation of patients with localized cerebral disease, it is conspicuous that the primary receptive cortices play a more limited role in cognitive processes than their name "primary" suggests. Hallucinations arising from these areas are crude and unformed (Penfield & Jasper, 1954); those from association cortex are categorical at best (Lance & McLeod, 1981; Penfield & Perot, 1963). As Lance says, "the hallucinations are not of great complexity, suggesting that the function of the association cortex is to group images into categories of person, animal or thing, leaving the final identification to a further stage involving links with the temporal lobe and limbic system to incorporate knowledge from memory stores." We will consider ictal discharges below (see Figure 4.4).

As Geschwind (1965a) pointed out, the primary receptive areas have no direct links with other cortical areas but establish such connections through the association areas that lie adjacent to them. These in turn project to the temporal lobe and limbic system. These are hard anatomical facts. Stimulation of the association areas or their temporal-limbic projections gives rise to formed hallucinations that are "seen" or otherwise perceived in the external receptive field that is impaired by damage to the primary receptive cortex, as though the association area were "released" from its normal afferent input from the primary sensory cortex (Brust & Behrens, 1977; Cogan, 1973; L. Jacobs, Karpick, Bozian, et al., 1981; Lance, 1976; T.C. Miller & Crosby, 1979). This disconnection is compatible with the electrophysiological data of Purpura and others (MacLean, 1949, 1975). Indeed, such "release" may explain MacLean's "schizophysiology," the discrepancy between what we "feel" and what we "know," and the ability to tell what is real and what is illusory.

The performance of synesthetic subjects may be seen as involving a suppression of rich corticocortical associations, which leaves the more

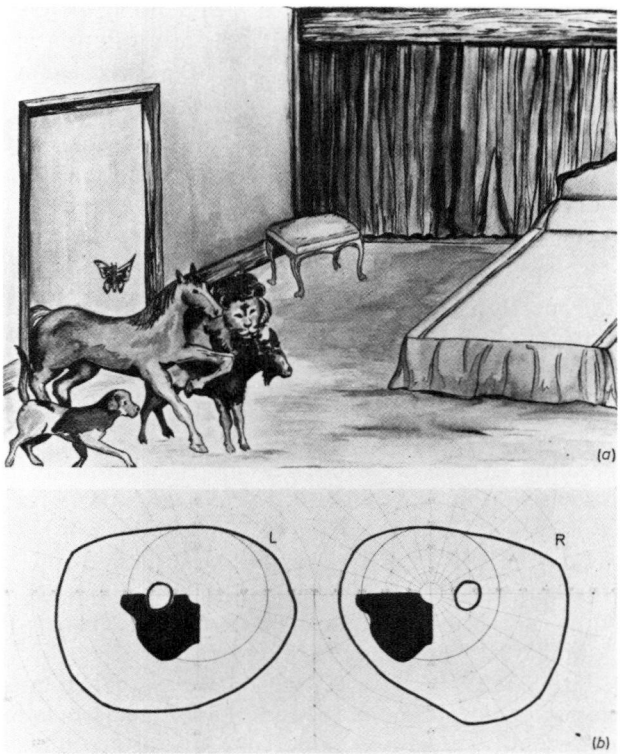

FIGURE 4.4. Categorical release hallucination. Animals appear one at a time in the area of the quadratic field defect. From *A physiological approach to clinical neurology,* 3rd ed. (p. 327) by J.W. Lance & J.G. McLeod, 1981, London: Butterworths. Copyright 1981 by Butterworths. Reprinted by permission.

unelaborated sensory percept (synesthesia, eidetic image, hallucination) to be directly associated at some lower level.

Clinical Examples

Brust and Behrens (1977) reported in detail two patients with release hallucinations in their paracentral scotomas. The first patient's hallucinations persisted for 2 weeks only during the 18 months she was followed. Her field defect remained stable during that time. (Years ago hemianopias were examined more frequently and more closely than they are today. The appearance of a hallucination in or encroaching on the blind field was a strong characteristic distinguishing organic hallucinations from psychiatric ones.) During these 2 weeks, the stimuli that precipitated her hallucinations were quite restricted: watching television or reading a book. They would abruptly disappear whenever she stopped these activities, only to come back when she resumed. She saw "four or five men, variably dressed (two or three in business suits, one in a cowboy's suit and hat, one in a plaid shirt), moving about, not speaking and not relating to one another. She could not make out their faces: "It was as if they were in shadows.'" They were not frightening.

Brust and Behren's second patient, who had a large left homonymous paracentral scotoma that remained fixed, had hallucinations for a year and a half. Computed tomography showed a right posterior temporal lucency. His hallucinations were of three kinds: (1) *simple synesthesia* of perpendicular red and green lines, red and blue spots, and black and white pulsations; (2) *metamorphopsia,* with the lines and spots appearing to move toward him—only the right half of faces would melt and show a yellow or violet color distortion; and (3) *palinopsia,* such as people walking across his scotoma. A palinopsia is a visual perseveration (M.B. Bender, Feldman, & Sobin, 1968). Teuber (1961) described palinopsia in which the image multiplied, and also noted palinopsia after LSD or mescaline ingestion. Other examples of this phenomenon are given by Kinsbourne and Warrington (1963).

A somatic hallucination that bears some resemblance to release hallucinations is the phenomenon of alloaesthesia, a condition in which a noxious sensory stimulus given on one side of the body (where there is a sensory defect) is perceived at the corresponding area on the other side. This has been shown in patients with putaminal lesions as well as anterolateral lesions of the spinal cord. It represents an elementary disturbance of sensory pathways and not a higher cortical dysfunction (Kawamura, Hirayama, Shinohara, et al., 1987).

SIMPLE SYNESTHESIA AND DEAFFERENTATION

Experiments with sensory deprivation show that loss of afferent input leads to psychotic thinking, perceptual distortion, and hallucination. Milder degrees of deafferentation (cataracts, peripheral neuropathy, and hearing loss) lead to less florid results. Normally the brain is constantly bombarded with sensory input, some of which is relevant and most of which is filtered out via "selective attention." At multiple levels throughout the integrated nervous system, recurrent collaterals effect inhibition of competing synapses. This negative feedback is equivalent to raising the signal-to-noise ratio, which sharpens discrimination.

Studies of sensory deprivation (Bexton, Heron, & Scott, 1954; Heron, Doaene, & Scott, 1956) in normal subjects show a progression from mild to severe hallucinations. Visual hallucinations at first are consistent with Klüver's form constants (geometric patterns, mosaics, lines, and rows of dots), later becoming more complex and dream-like, involving bizarre juxtaposition of people and objects. On emerging to a normal environment the subjects continue to have metamorphopsia and perceive an "unnatural brightness of colors." West (in Siegel & West, 1975, chapter 9) suggested that "new information inhibits the emergence and awareness of previously processed information. If the new input is decreased or impaired while awareness remains, stored images may be released and experienced as hallucinations or dreams."

The sensory-deprived brain starts perceiving things that are not there. With a lack of input, the brain starts projecting an external reality of its own. Evarts (1957) was one of the first to note a possible relationship between disruption of information input and the very occurrence of disinhibition phenomenon of the special senses (particularly in the visual system). This condition is not as rare as it might first seem. A very common experience occurs in the shower. When the auditory system is deafferented, sensorily deprived by the white noise of the shower, how often has one hallucinated that the phone was ringing or that someone was calling his name?

L. Jacobs and colleagues (1981) studied 9 patients who had anterior visual loss due to optic nerve or chiasm disorders. All patients had photisms induced by sounds that often startled them. These were usually sounds of daily life and *appeared to come from the ear ipsilateral to the eye in which the photism seemed to be seen.* Sounds included clanking of the radiator, crackling of the walls as they cooled at night, the whoosh of a furnace ignition, a dog's bark, and slamming doors (see Table 4.1 and Figures 4.5 and 4.6).

The photisms ranged from simple flashes of white light to colored forms that looked like a flame, amoebas, oscillating flower petals, a spray of bright dots, or kaleidoscopic effects. All patients' photisms lasted only "a split second, an instant." Some patients had a single stereotyped photism while others experience multiple photisms.

It is of some interest that the photisms were perceived to arise in one eye and to be induced by sounds that were heard only with the ipsilateral ear! This, of course, is contrary to our usual understanding. We are unable to tell which eye is seeing an object unless we cover first one and then the other to determine that only one eye, in fact, can see a certain object (such as when the nose is in the way or when objects are in the nonoverlapping temporal field). Acoustic localization of objects depends on differences in the sound reaching both ears. Yet

. . . the click of an electric blanket thermostat induced a flashbulb photism in the right eye of patient 6 only when the thermostat located to her right clicked; the same clicking from her husband's thermostat located to the left never induced the phenomenon. A petal photism was perceived coming from the right eye of patient 7 when a nurse spoke into his right ear. The photism never occurred when the nurse spoke into his left ear" (L. Jacobs et al., 1981).

The monocular visual-evoked response from the scotomatous eyes showed conduction delays and reduced amplitudes.

TABLE 4.1. Characteristics of photisms and sounds that induce them.[a]

Patient No.	Photism Appearance	Color	Location	Sounds
1	Flame, flashbulb	Red-orange-white, white	In scotoma	Not sure (sharp)
2	Spray, microscope light, kaleidoscope, spot, pollywogs	White, pink, red, black, green	In and out of scotoma	Clap, computerized tomography gantry
3	Flash	White-yellow	In scotoma	Walls crackling, digital clock, pencil striking desk, television scintilllating and crackling
4	Light bulb	White-blue	In scotoma	Not sure (soft)
5	Flash	White	In and out of scotoma	Car or motorcycle engines, others (loud)
6	Flashbulb	White	In scotoma	Electric blanket, digital clock
7	Petal, ameba, goldfish	Pink, white, yellow	In and out of scotoma	Furnace, dog bark, tray crash, voices
8	Plaid	Green	In scotoma	Book or fist slamming desk, others (loud)
9	Flashbulb	Pink	In and out of scotoma	Furnace, door slam, television, radio, voices

[a] From Jacobs, L., Karpick, A., Bozian, D., et al. (1981). Auditory-visual synesthesia: Sound induced photisms. *Archives of Neurology, 38,* 211–216.

We must remember that the task is to investigate and, it is hoped, explain "normal" synesthesia, that is, the synesthesia that spontaneously occurs in various modes in patients who have *no* CNS lesions. What the examples of release hallucinations and simple synesthesia with deafferentation can provide is some help in suggesting a level of the neuraxis at which synesthesia may normally operate. Through these pathological cases one may hope to uncover the structure of a normal process.

The facts that bear on these patients with sound-induced photisms are that they have (1) lesions of the retinal ganglion cells (third-order neurons) resulting in (2) supersensitivity of the lateral geniculate neurons, which are retinotopic. The superior colliculus is also a fourth-order visual neuron and retinotopic and could well become supersensitive too. However, it has no direct cortical projection, at least in the primate (Singer, 1977). Supersensitivity would be greatest in those geniculate cells that are partially deafferented, explaining the occurrence of the photism

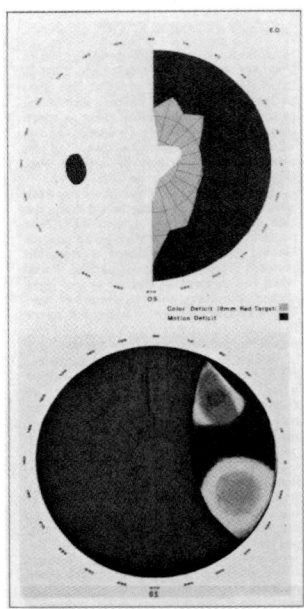

FIGURE 4.5. Visual fields with scotomas indicated in black. *Top:* Nasal defect of left eye visual field. *Bottom:* A flame photism was induced by "sharp" sounds. From "Auditory-visual synesthesia" by L. Jacobs, A. Karpick, D. Bozian, et al., 1981, *Archives of Neurology,* 31, p. 213. Copyright 1981 by American Medical Association. Reprinted by permission.

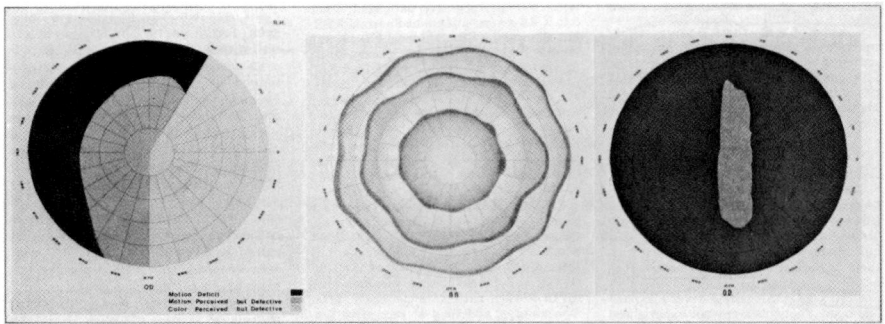

FIGURE 4.6. *Left:* Entire left field is variably defective with anopsia, achromatopsia, and dyschromatopsia. *Center:* "Petal" photism. *Right:* "Amoeba" photism. From "Auditory-visual synesthesia" by L. Jacobs, A. Karpick, D. Bozian, et al., 1981, *Archives of Neurology,* 31, p. 213. Copyright 1981 by American Medical Association. Reprinted by permission.

in the scotoma. The anatomical basis for supersensitivity seems to be axon sprouting and is a well-known feature of partially deafferented postsynaptic fields (Burke & Haylow, 1968; Cunningham, 1972; Echlin & McDonald, 1954; Goodman & Horel, 1966; Merril & Wall, 1978; Sharpless, 1969).

The lateral geniculate normally responds to sound as well as to light, a fact not widely recognized. Cellular recordings in animals from the geniculate will show a response to auditory stimuli (Arden & Soderberg, 1959; Stein & Arigbede, 1972). Paul MacLean (1970, 1975, personal communication) reported the same finding from microelectrode recordings, namely, that what we normally consider a "visual" neuron will in fact respond to a stimulus from another mode, such as a sound or touch. Convergence of afferent impulses on single units are also seen in the reticular formation (Scheibel, Scheibel, Mollica, & Moruzzi, 1955).

Dräger and Hubel (1975) have reviewed the visual, auditory, and somatosensory inputs to superior colliculus in animals. The convergence of multiple sensory modes make it evident that one important function of the superior colliculus is concerned with shift of attention and orienting the head, ears, and eyes toward a stimulus in the environment. Both bimodal and trimodal cells are seen in deeper layers, arranged in clusters rather than segregated into sublayers. They show little habituation to repeated stimulation. That single cells respond to multiple kinds of stimulation, however, is not a sufficient fact to explain synesthesia.

That all 9 of Jacob's patients startled when the photisms occurred is an intriguing observation. It is well known that startle responses will produce pontine-geniculo-occipital (PGO) spikes, that is, brief discharges in the geniculate as well as other portions of the visual system (Bowker & Morrison, 1976; Gogan, 1970; Groves, Wilson, & Boyle, 1974).

What these cases suggest, therefore, concerning an explanation of normal synesthesia is a functional level above third-order neurons (geniculate) but below primary isomodal (e.g., calcarine) cortex. We are presently centered on the level of the brainstem, an intermediate level, in accordance with the theoretical predictions.

T.C. Miller and Crosby (1979) reported on musical and verbal hallucinations in a woman with progressive hearing loss. There was no mental disturbance. The hallucinations were disturbing only in their monotony and persistence. The opinion that such hallucinations are due to deafferentation has not changed in nearly 100 years (Coleman, 1894; Ross, Jossman, Bell, et al., 1975).

Finally, in this group of phenomena one must mention the Charles Bonnett syndrome (Berrios & Brook, 1982; Rolak & Baram, 1987; Rosenbaum, Harati, Rolak, et al.,, in press): formed visual hallucinations with visual loss. Patients are otherwise normal. The syndrome is characterized by the hallucinations being exclusively visual and highly detailed, such as people and scenes. The patient is not psychotic and is quite aware that he is hallucinating. The hallucinations are fairly unemotional and nonthreatening. They are brief and occur in a setting of visual loss: macular degeneration, cataracts, glaucoma, or other acquired causes of poor acuity. The detail of these hallucinations has no relationship to the categorical features of synesthesia or release hallucinations by virtue of their complexity. They are mentioned here because they are sometimes confused. This is a distinct clinical syndrome related to ocular disease.

Simple Synesthesiae With Gross Brainstem Lesions

Vike, Jabbari, and Maitland (1984) reported a patient who had auditory-visual synesthesia that developed ipsilaterally to a large cystic tumor of the left medial temporal lobe and adjacent midbrain. The patient had normal visual function throughout, and the synesthesia resolved after removal of the mass.

This patient is of extreme interest because (1) he had normal vision (acuity, pupillary response, color plate and Farnsworth-Munsell 100 hue discrimination, direct ophthalmoscopy, tangent screen and Goldmann perimetric fields, visual-evoked response, slit-lamp examination with Hruby lens); (2) his synesthesia was stimulus dependent and could be manipulated (increasing click rates at a constant 65 decibels altered the intensity and movement illusion of his photisms); (3) his hearing was normal (audiometry and BER); (4) he believed the photisms to come only from the left eye and only when clicks were presented to the left ear; (5) he had a postchiasmal cystic tumor in the left medial temporal lobe extending to the midbrain; and (6) the synesthesia could not be induced following removal of the tumor.

Cascino and Adams (1986) presented three patients with brainstem auditory hallucinosis who had intact cochleas, cochlear nuclei, and auditory nerves similar to the patient above. These patients had lesions at the level of the pontine tegmentum. Although Cascino and Adams drew an analogy with the brainstem peduncular hallucinosis of Lhermitte (Dunn, Weisberg, & Nadell, 1983), the dream-like quality seen in peduncular hallucinosis was not seen in their patients. In his characteristic style, Raymond Adams summed up an attempt to give a clinicoanatomical explanation to this disorder: "Knowledge of the physiology of ascending and descending auditory centers is too meagre . . ." (Cascino & Adams, 1986).

Nashold (1970) reported the elicitation of phosphenes on stimulating the human superior colliculus. The flashing lights were "white or cold," arranged in straight or wavy lines, off-center, in the contralateral field from stimulation, and superimposed on the visual scene.

Temporal Lobe Epilepsy

Mention was made in the previous chapter of diagnosing medical conditions that are entirely experiential. The peculiar subjective experiences and perceptual distortions caused by temporal lobe epilepsy (TLE) were given as an example. It is important to remember that ictal discharges of TLE can combine the elements of smell, taste, vision, hearing, memory, and emotion (MacLean, 1949; Penfield, 1958).

The phenomena of TLE are well known. The behavioral aspects of it were more a focus of attention in the 1940s and 1950s, particularly as the understanding of the limbic system and theories of emotion were developing. Papez', Yakovlev's, and MacLean's papers are of interest in this regard (MacLean, 1949, 1973; Papez, 1937; Yakovlev, 1948, 1970). Readers are assumed to be familiar with the current kinds of behavioral manifestations seen in TLE, including the so-called temporal lobe personality and multiple personalities (Bear, 1983; Bear & Fedio, 1977; Spiers, Schomer, Blume, & Mesulam, 1985).

Does anything more need to be said than that synesthesia can be a rare manifestation of TLE? Since all association areas have connections with the temporal lobe it should not be surprising that this area may be responsible for complex hallucinations together with an affective component. More will be said of the temporal lobe and limbic anatomy in Chapter 5 when I discuss the evolution of these brain structures and phylogenesis.

Clinical Examples

Jacome and Gumnit (1979) described an epileptic trimodal synesthesia involving vision, audition, and pain in a trigeminal distribution. The patient would hear the word "five" binaurally and then see "5" on a gray background projected in front of him; or he would hear the word "first" and then see it spelled in front of him. These phenomena were associated with a shooting pain in all three divisions of the trigeminal nerve on the right. His EEG showed slow wave reversals at F3 and F7 (i.e., the left temporal) and anterior temporal spikes.

Ictal pain is exceedingly rare. Pain is sometimes a feature of synesthesia. Dudycha and Dudycha (1935) reported just such a patient with "visual pain and visual audition." Among the current patients VE has a sharp stabbing pain in the forehead in response to high-pitched noises or those that are loud; DS sees a thin metallic line and gets a splitting headache from her children's vociferations (recall the geometric pain of RB, Figure 2.4). In a series of 205 outpatients with closed-head injury (Cytowic, Stump, & Larned, 1987) 3 patients (1.4%) had photoalgesic or audioalgesic synesthesia or both. That is, they would have a hemicranial pain associated with seeing painfully bright light or hearing a crashing sound "like gears grinding" or "banging on a pot." Sometimes the pain would radiate into an arm or the trunk, but it always remain unilateral and was never segmental. Never was the head pain in a discrete distribution of the trigeminal or occipital nerves, even though occipital neuritis is extremely common in these patients. Needless to say, these patients were studied in detail and were "normal" in the conventional sense. Electro-physiologic studies were unrevealing. The only perceptual disturbance was found on Goldmann perimetry, in which they had some mild concentric narrowing and a slight nasal step defect.

I am unable to offer any mechanism for this phenomenon in the setting of closed-head injury other than to say that it appears benign and in these three patients resolved within 6 to 9 months (Cytowic et al., 1987).

Various synesthesiae occur in temporal lobe seizures, such as the cases of Gowers (1901), whose patients had elaborate visual and auditory auras. One patient saw "beautiful places, large rooms" and heard at the same time "beautiful music."

Olfactory hallucinations are supposed to be especially suggestive of TLE. Other than Luria's subject, S, who sometimes had all five senses synesthetically engaged, I know of no instance in which smell is the parallel sense in synesthesia. In MW, olfaction can be the trigger for synesthesia and, as we have seen, some of the current patients (MW, above; SdeM, Chapter 7) can remember smells, an ability that certainly does not reflect common experience. For want of a better place I will mention here that high levels of carbon dioxide produce a pungent olfactory sensation reminiscent of gunpowder or rotten eggs. The phenomenon is termed "olfactory hallucination" but may affect senses other than smell (White, Humm, Armstrong, et al., 1952). Such a phenomenon was seen in the degassing of Lake Nyos in Cameroon, a natural disaster occuring in 1986. Survivors also reported feeling a sensation of warmth (Kling, Clark, Compton, et al., 1987), which the authors considered hallucinatory.

Gustatory and olfactory epileptic manifestations are usually grouped together and their rarity makes them difficult to study. Hausser-Hauw and Bancaud (1987) found gustatory hallucinations in 4% of 718 patients with seizures. In their series, there was a clear perisylvian distribution of the epileptic activity and frequent involvement of the amygdala and hippocampus. Tastes are usually not described in detail but in more general terms, such as "bitter," "unpleasant," or "a taste," unless seizures involved the temporal lobe and suprasylvian regions at the same time. Then, the taste was often more specific ("rusty iron," "oysters," "artichoke").

The role of the temporal lobe in the genesis of a gustatory sensation seems difficult to explain from an anatomical standpoint. First-order taste neurons from the taste buds travel in the chorda tympani (a branch of the facial nerve) for the anterior two-thirds of the tongue; the lingual branch of the glossopharyngeal serve for the posterior third of the tongue; the greater superficial petrosal nerve for palatal taste buds; and the superior laryngeal nerve (a branch of the vagus) for taste buds on the pharynx, larynx, and epiglottis. They synapse in the nucleus of the solitary tract in the medulla and ascend to the medial parvocellular part of the posteromedial ventral nucleus of the thalamus. Other projections are to the pontine parabrachial nuclei, lateral hypothalamus, central nucleus of the amygdala and bed nucleus of the stria terminalis. The parvocellular part of the ventral posteromedial nucleus of the thalamus is the synaptic relay of the ascending pathways to the cortical taste area (CTA). Most species have two cortical taste areas as determined by the evoked potential method (Yamamoto, 1984). One is near the somatosensory tongue projection in the parietal operculum and the other in the frontal operculum or limen insulae. In humans, the CTA appears to be in the parietal lobe (Broadmann area 43) encompassing the inferior pre- and postcentral gyri and extending into the parietal operculum. Once considered candidates, the temporal lobe and anterior insula are no longer considered locations for the CTA. Responses of single cortical taste neurons show that more than half the neurons respond to tactile and thermal stimuli as well taste (M.J.Cohen, Landgren, Strom, & Zotterman, 1957; Landgren, 1957). Numerous anatomical reports show corticofugal connections to subcortical structures, yet few electrophysiological studies have been done and little is known of the functional corticofugal pathways. They do feed back to somatosensory, visual, and auditory systems and may be important to taste discrimination (Monnier, 1975; Towe, 1973; Wiesendanger, 1969). Further evidence contributing to the paradox of the temporal lobe in the genesis of gustatory sensation is the fact that only extensive removal of the entire anterior sylvian cortex (including parietal operculum) produced marked and prolonged ageusia (Bagshaw & Pribram, 1953; Hausser-Hauw & Bancaud, 1987).

After a careful analysis of spontaneous and electrically induced seizures, Hausser-Hauw and Bancaud found that isolated gustatory hallucinations in man are related to the disorganization of the rolandic and/or parietal opercula. Seizures originating from the temporal lobe, they found, were intermixed with many other subjective symptoms, a finding that again implicates the anterior temporal neocortex and underlying limbic structures in synesthetic experiences. Following are some examples of epileptic synesthesia involving gustation.

Anderson (1886) cited a 23-year-old male who had a "sensation in his mouth, a rough, bitter sensation" combined with a "peculiar sensation passing down the right arm into the hand, then up the spine from the level of the shoulders to the head, finally spreading over the back of the skull as a cold sensation." He would often shiver during the seizure, and usually see the same scene from his childhood. He was found to have a large pituitary tumor that undermined the posterior three-fourths of the temporal lobe.

The following epileptic synesthesiae are from Hausser-Hauw and Bancaud's (1987) cases:

Case 21. A taste of bile, dysesthesia of the left wrist, abduction of the left
    corner of the mouth and clonic contractions of the left side of the body.
Case 24. Epigastric pain, shivers, a bitter taste, nausea.

Case 25. A lump in the throat, oral movements, phosphenes in the right upper fields, a bitter taste.

Case 28. An intense heat that ascends from the stomach to the mouth accompanied by a disagreeable taste.

Case 30. Bitter taste, hypersalivation, swallowing, spitting (sometimes vomiting), angry outbursts accompanied by shouting.

These are, I think, remarkable examples. One of their patients experienced gustatory hallucinations, similar to his spontaneous ones, 30 to 50 seconds after ingesting food or water. This is, of course, what is known as reflex or sensory epilepsy (Bencze, Troupin, & Prockop, 1988; Forster, 1977; Herskowitz, Rosman, & Geschwind, 1984; Micheloyannakis & Ionnidou, 1986; Reder & Wright, 1982; Wishaw, 1987). For a long time it has been known that seizures could be evoked in certain epileptic individuals by a physiological or psychological stimulus of one of five types: visual (flashing light), auditory (unexpected noise, specific musical themes or voices), somatosensory, reading, and eating.

Electrical Stimulation of the Brain

The work of Penfield and Jasper (1954) is well known; experiential responses were produced *only* from stimulating the temporal lobe. Most responses came from stimulating the lateral and superior surfaces of the first temporal convolution. None were obtained from Heschl's gyrus. Like synesthetes, those patients who have their cortex stimulated are able to appreciate "both worlds." These patients have a strong conviction that the experience they are reliving is real without losing sight of the fact that they are on an operating table in Montreal. Like synesthesia, the elementary percepts, the components of the experience, combine without losing their own identity. As their patient G. Le. put it, "I see the people in this world and in that world too, at the same time" (Penfield & Perot, 1963, p. 635).

Penfield showed that electrical stimulation could make patients relive the past as though it were the present. This was Proust on the operating table, an electrical *recherche aux temps perdu,* yet obviously not *perdu.* Patients were startled to relive an experience.

The recollection produced when the electrode is applied to cortex is not static. It proceeds in a normal time frame. It changes as it did when it was originally seen, according to the patient's point of view, altering when he had perhaps changed his gaze or as a conversation unfolded. "The recollection of a song produced by cortical stimulation progresses slowly from one phrase to another and from verse to chorus. The thread of continuity in evoked recollections seems to be time" (Penfield & Perot, 1963).

The evoked memory is more than an ordinary memory. It is a full somatic participation of the original experience. There are distinctive differences between the characteristics of evoked memory and those that are mediated by verbal symbols of generalizations. Electrical stimulation of the brain (ESB) was thought by Kubie (1943), in particular, to be a shortcut to psychoanalytic technique in recapturing "unconscious memories in the pursuit of insight." But to explore this would take us too far afield.

Penfield's work was the first to suggest that memory was stored in different ways, although he did not fully recognize this. First, memory is stored in patterns of verbal representation as nonspecific generalizations from discrete experiences that are predominantly intellectual and unemotional in content. At the same time, it is possible to reproduce the original episode with all of its vivid sensory and emotional connotations.

Olfaction and Evoked Memories

The experience of the gustatory synesthete MW makes us particularly interested in taste and smell. (CSc, MG, MN, RP, and TP also have taste and smell among their synesthesiae.) It is curious, given the intimate relationship between olfaction and gustation, that tastes and smells did not figure prominently in the evoked experience. Stimulation of the olfactory cortex resulted in simple perceptions just as is the case in somasthetic motor or primary isomodal cortex stimulation (e.g., agreeable or disagreeable odors, metallic tastes).

Penfield did stimulate the uncus and hippocampus almost as frequently as the convexity of the temporal lobe, because epileptogenic foci often arise in the uncus and run back to the temporal incisura. Yet he found no patient whose stimulation caused him to remember a smell. Common experience tells us that a familiar odor can bring back a memory quite vividly, although not as vividly as the recollections discussed in synesthesia, eidetic memory, or ESB. A change in memory in SdeM following postoperative loss of olfaction is discussed later in Chapter 7. In real life, an odor may indeed bring back an elaborate memory, but the memory of an odor is rarely, if ever, brought back.

Weaknesses of Penfield's Method

1. All patients were being operated on for epilepsy and usually had abnormal seizure foci in the temporal lobe. This is a fundamental difficulty of all ESB work. Even later work by Ojemann and others used epileptics. It is unlikely that the ethical constraints of stimulating a "normal" brain can be surmounted.
2. Psychological testing was not undertaken in Penfield's patients. This probably reflects the climate of neuropsychology rather than poor methodology.

3. Inasmuch as the extraction of an evoked memory stimulated such interest among psychoanalysts, a preoperative psychoanalytical analysis would have been helpful to compare to a content analysis of the utterances during operation. So would comparison of operative utterances to what we call conventional memory or those produced by other techniques.
4. It is wrong and probably simplistic to say that the memory resides at the point of stimulation. There is a possible spread of electrical activity, perhaps by callosal pathways. Although Penfield and later investigators reasonably convinced themselves, and others, that the electrical spread was physically not wide, some still question if the memory resides under the locus of stimulation. Increasing the strength of stimulation would produced a seizure, but could never force out a memory if the cortex was "not ready to give it." Excision of the epileptic focus did not destroy the postoperative memory that could be elicited from the excised area (Penfield & Perot, 1963, pp. 620, 677, 689). This is consonant with my earlier comments about two different kinds of memory: the verbal generalizations as opposed to the discrete episode.

Summary

What all these phenomena that we have studied above have in common is a disruption, inhibition, or suppression of higher cognitive activity, with a dimunition or absence of primary afferents or the primary receptive field (sensory deprivation, simple synesthesia, release hallucinations), or the cortex itself (TLE, electrical stimulation of the brain), or both (LSD-induced synesthesia). The electrophysiological data that are available from animal and human experimentation show desynchronization of neocortical activity and inhibition of cortical axodendritic potentials with paroxysmal limbic and sublimbic activity.

The range of anatomical levels suggested by these phenomena are between brainstem and association cortex (either isomodal or heteromodal). The heightened emotional and mnestic qualities as well as the remarkable case of Vike et al. (1984), discussed in the section on simple synesthesia, point strongly to temporal lobe and limbic structures as the neuroanatomical locus of synesthesia.

These cases also show a range of synesthetic performance. As a clarification of nomenclature we will call photisms *simple synesthesiae* if they arise spontaneously; those that are stimulus induced after patients acquire CNS lesions (such as a clanking radiator causing a flame photism in a scotoma) will be called *induced synesthesiae*. This term can also apply to the synesthesia arising from LSD, which we have called *drug induced*. Spontaneous synesthesia occurring as a lifelong characteristic in patients without demonstrable CNS pathology is what we refer to as *synesthesia* throughout this book.

Supporting Evidence for Anatomical Localization

Keep in mind that Vike et al.'s patient had a cystic tumor in the left medial temporal lobe. Unfortunately, neuropsychological assessment was not performed to see whether he had any higher cortical deficits attributable to dysfunction of the left hemisphere. Jacome and Gumnit's (1979) patient with trimodal epileptic synesthesia had an EEG focus in the left temporal region. He showed poor performance on Porteus mazes but no other disturbance on neuropsychological assessment. We have not considered until now that synesthesia could be asymmetrically represented in the brain. We will examine data below that show that this may indeed be so.

Concerning the *what* and the *where* of synesthesia, our hypothesis is that the *what*, that is, the link, is below the level of the cortex and the *where* is the limbic system-temporal lobe. It proposes that synesthesia involves suppression of cortical activity with a relative enhancement of limbic-emotional processing.

Unless otherwise stated, the studies reported below were all performed on the gustatory synesthete with geometric taste, MW. In this subject both taste and smell induce tactile perceptions of shape, texture, temperature, weight, and movement.

DRUG STUDIES IN MW

The fact that the mapping experiments showed that there is some regularity to synesthetic perception led naturally to pharmacology and the question of whether there are any drugs that can modulate synesthetic performance. There would be too many variables in repeating mapping experiments under a drug's influence. Rather, the strategy was to find substances that altered the *experiential response,* that is, substances that would augment or broaden the synesthetic perceptions and those that might abolish it.

Questioning MW about the various settings in which he experienced synesthesia first suggested a diurnal response that, on closer examination, was perhaps related to caffeine and ethanol ingestion. He thought that he had fewer synesthesiae in the morning compared to later in the day, and especially in the evening, when they seemed more intense and vivid. He supposed this might be due to being "more relaxed" in the evening and more able to appreciate his synesthesia without the distractions of work competing for his attention.

This turned out not to be the explanation, however. The "relaxation" he perceived was induced by fairly large quantities of ethanol, as we shall discuss below, and a diary that he was instructed to keep showed that he was in fact experiencing synesthesiae in the morning and all throughout the day. The synesthesiae in the morning and throughout the early afternoon were only attenuated in their development. "It's not as intense." "I just get brief flashes." "There are little things at my fingertips and I don't grab onto them." "The shapes are smaller and further away from me. I have to reach into the distance."

MW's standard breakfast was cigarettes and coffee (5 mugs by noon), and he drank ethanol regularly in the evening. This suggested that conventional stimulants might attenuate synesthesia while depressants could enhance it, an idea that was tested. A third substance, amyl nitrate, markedly enhanced the synesthetic percept and will be discussed below on the section on regional cerebral blood flow where amyl nitrate is shown to decrease cortical metabolism.

Table 4.2 gives a summary of drug effects on synesthesia.

Dextroamphetamine

MW was not naive to dextroamphetamine but had not ingested any in at least 4 years preceding this experiment. Originally blinded, he deduced the drug's identity during the experiment. The stimulus was an inhalation of spearmint essence. This was previously shown on multiple occasions to produce a stable synesthesia that did not fatigue. The characteristic perception of spearmint was of smooth, cold, glass columns that MW could palpate. He could run his hand along the back curvature and up and down the cylinder's length. This synesthesia was reasonably constant and MW was instructed to report any differences in the tactile qualities that he felt. Strawberry essence, as a backup, produced a sensation of round spheres.

Table 4.3 tabulates MW's pulse and blood pressure during the experiment, which were measured to ensure that the amphetamine caused a physiological response. The following comments correspond to the data to the table.

1. Time 0 : 0

Baseline pulse and blood pressure obtained. Five milligrams of dextroamphetamine ingested.

2. Time 0 : 01

No change in vital signs. Amyl nitrate was used as an adjuvant. The "standard method" was to inhale a volatile essence followed by a 2-second inhalation of amyl nitrate. During the synesthesia, in which there was a replication of the columns that was intensified to the point that

TABLE 4.2. Drug effects on synesthesia.

Drug	Cortical Effect	Effect on Synesthesia
Amphetamine	Stimulates	Blocks
Ethanol	Depresses	Enhances
Amyl Nitrate	Ischemia	Enhances

TABLE 4.3. Effect of amphetamine on synesthesia.

	Time	Pulse	BP[a]	Comments
1.	0:00	88	128/80	Baseline
2.	0:01	84	128/80	AN[b] → pulse 132, BP 162/110
3.	0:10	84	128/90	Recovery from amyl nitrate
4.	1:10	100	156/100	"Speeding"
5.	1:15	100	156/100	AN → pulse 118, BP 156/120. "Not as much"
6.	2:30	88	150/98	Still speeding; AN → pulse 120, BP 156/98

[a] BP, blood pressure.
[b] AN, amyl nitrate.

he was "in among the columns, touching and feeling their surfaces," there was a marked rise in pulse and blood pressure *due to the amyl nitrate alone.*

3. Time 0:10

Recovery from the amyl nitrate.

4. Time 1:10

Physiological response. MW acknowledged that he was "speeding." Inhalation of the mint gave an attenuated synesthesia. He described a "small field of perception" with one or perhaps two columns far in the distance, very difficult to touch. "This is quite different. The feeling comes faster than before but they are much smaller. They are still as vivid as a miniature would be compared to a large oil painting. The emotion is less intense but it is still pleasurable. The whole thing is just more distant." He explicated further: "I'm not sure how I can explain it. It's like slipping out of my hands." Inhalation of strawberry essence caused him to feel round spheres but on a smaller scale than that to which he was accustomed.

5. Time 1:15

Positive physiological response from amphetamine continues. Inhalation of mint followed by amyl nitrate adjuvant. Compared to the intensification that MW experienced with amyl nitrate on previous occasions and again in this experiment at time 0:01, the adjuvant effect while stimulated with amphetamine was diminished. "This is not as visceral as an hour ago. Instead of feeling it intensely in my hands, my back, neck and arms, it is more centered on the fingertips and my face. Instead of having a shape which is there all the time on which I can concentrate, it has become a series of small flashes of sensory things, only at the fingertips. I can't feel the quality of the column, the tactile quality is smaller. It is like a scale model, somehow, or a miniature. The whole thing is just incredibly different. What have you done to me?"

6. *Time 2 :30*

Recovery of pulse rate, but still physiological response from dextroamphetamine. Subjectively "still speeding, and pleasurably so." Inhalation of spearmint and strawberry were "pleasurable" but there was no bona fide synesthesia. Additional trials of almond, banana, methyl salicylate, and camphor also could not induce synesthesia. At the most, MW felt lines, dots, and *nongeometric* shapes (quite unusual for him) and most of these were "always receding from my grasp." (Various foods consumed after this experiment were also unsuccessful in producing synesthesia.)

An attempt was made to induce synesthesia with the amyl nitrate adjuvant. Despite a subjective and physiological response to the amyl nitrate, it was not successful. "This is not sustained. It's pulses of a sensation, a sort of cinematic frame-by-frame sensation rather than being a one long shape that I can concentrate on. The poppers [*amyl nitrate*] somehow make the feeling more intense but the small scale and the distance is still the same. With the speed I stay outside of the columns and can't get in, even with the poppers."

Ethanol

A similar experiment was performed with 1.5 ounces of absolute ethanol. This produced a standard physiological response of tachycardia and peripheral vasodilation. The details need not be given, but the magnitude and intensity of MW's synesthesia was increased by the ethanol compared to the synesthesia he experienced at midday (during which time he had not been permitted to consume caffeine) and 5 hours later before the ingestion of any ethanol.

A "natural experiment" then occurred. When I first discovered MW's synesthesia (in 1979) his average ethanol consumption was 8 oz daily. His ethanol consumption began to escalate in 1983 until, when he stopped drinking on April 7, 1985, he consumed almost a fifth daily. For 2 to 3 months after total cessation his synesthesia was attenuated, presumably as a result of supersensitivity and rebound following removal of this classical cortical suppressant to which he had been chronically exposed.[1]

---

[1] Those unfamiliar with alcoholism might think that 3 months is far too long for a rebound stimulant effect to endure, erroneously assuming that all physiological and behavioral effects should be nil following metabolism of the last dose of ethanol by alcohol dehydrogenase, which is on the order of hours. Alcoholics who have maintained long-term sobriety relate similar experiences: subtle withdrawal symptoms pervade all hours of the first few months. The rule of thumb from Alcoholics Anonymous is that it takes 1 month for every year of drinking to "detoxify." The anonymity of AA, numbering 67,000 groups in 114 countries as of 1986, discourages outside researchers and the bulk of practical, experiential knowledge never finds its way into peer-reviewed scientific literature. Information for the medical profession can be had from Alcoholics Anonymous, Box 459, Grand Central Station, New York, NY 10163.

This is in keeping with known effects of alcohol: following withdrawal, there is an enhancement of cortical actvity, sometimes manifested by seizures, and an increased autonomic activity, insomnia, rebound REM sleep, and motor hyperactivity.

He was horrified and distraught that his synesthesia was leaving him. Life was just not the same. Of course, he made no association between the "fading away" of his synesthesia and his cessation of alcohol. Predictably, it returned. At 20 months sober (in December 1986) his synesthesia has resumed its previous intensity and proportion with the noticeable exception of diminution in the morning, congruent with his usual breakfast of caffeine and nicotine, both cortical stimulants. Coffee consumption, previously at 10 cups per day, is now at 3 cups daily.

Amyl Nitrate

Observations indicated that amyl nitrate could intensify the synesthetic experience. Some of its results are noted above. It is important to realize that amyl nitrate in itself does not induce synesthesia. MW's experience with the drug is quite consonant with wider social use of the substance as a recreational drug.

The drug, which peaked in popularity in 1975–1980, was commonly used at discos and during sex. It relaxes smooth muscle throughout the body and because of this its major effect is vasodilation. Its original use for angina pectoris has been supplanted by nitroglycerine. For those not familiar with its effects, they include a withdrawal into the self, slowing of time sense such that music may seem more distant or slower, metamorphopsia, disinhibition, and heightening of emotions so that one appreciated the tribal aspects of the rhythmic throng at a disco. Physiological correlates were a rushing sensation to the head, flushing in the face and chest, and reflex tachycardia secondary to the vasodilation. During sex there is a sense of heightened and prolonged orgasm, an oceanic state of oneness with the sexual partner, a sense of rhythmicity and mouthing, and an abandonment of judgment such that more is not enough. It is nearly universal for users to acknowledge sexual acts performed under the influence of amyl nitrate that they otherwise would be unable or unwilling to do. The whole physiological effect, by the way, is brief, lasting only minutes. Through its use one can dance "like crazy" at the disco and act "wild" in bed. We can readily see that this pharmaceutical briefly turns one into a limbic preparation.

The drug has all the properties of a cortical solvent and that this is so is apparent on examination of the blood flow data. "Solvent" in this context refers to the hierarchical dissolution of higher cortical functions, such as judgment, social inhibition, and reasoning. Ethanol, too, is a well-known cortical solvent that depresses inhibitions and makes one loquacious. Used in increasing amounts one starts to associate with all types of people and exercise poor judgment.

CEREBRAL BLOOD FLOW

The brain is wonderful. Scientists think so, and the public must too if one is to judge by the books, audiotapes, and public television series devoted to its operation, which is usually couched in terms of "mysteries." What they wax rhapsodic over, however, is just the cerebral neocortex, which is hardly the whole brain. This is synecdoche in action, reminiscent of a gorgeous wedding cake that might be on display as a tribute to the confectioner's art. We ooh and ah over the rosettes, the garlands, and the anaglyph in sugar. But there is a catch: there is no cake. Underneath the icing is only cardboard and aluminum foil, nothing that one can sink his teeth into.

The human brain is not like this. The brain is not just neocortex held up by inert filler. To pursue a too-cute metaphor, the grey matter "icing" varies considerably from one cortical area to another, but is *only 2mm thick* on average, only a fraction of the total cerebral volume of 1350 ml. There is, however, plenty of cake underneath. Subcortical aggregates of nervous tissue do a lot of biochemical work. They are not there just to hold the surface up. One can observe extensive behavior in animals that do not have any cortex to speak of (such as birds). Suction removal of large expanses of cortex from monkeys results in animals that can hardly be distinguished from their cagemates, suggesting that the cortex only provides a finer grain of discrimination, better calculation to inform the limbic brain, which is the final arbiter of behavior.

Instead of assuming that synesthesia would be "localized" to some cortical area—such as the angular gyrus, which would be the most logical choice—one could try to prove the opposite: that the cortex was not "working" during synesthesia.

It is well known that in all tissues doing work, there is more energy metabolism taking place than in those tissues that are not working. Skeletal muscle does physical work lifting weight against gravity, and its metabolism correlates very well with the amount of work done. The heart does work by pumping blood out against a pressure head. The same applies to the kidney as it does chemical-osmotic work in concentrating substances against a gradient.

In all cases, the amount of work done correlates well with the degree of oxidative metabolism. Although it is not always clear what is the nature of the physical work that is going on in nervous tissue, the measurement of energy metabolism can serve as a marker for how much work a given part of the nervous system is doing in any functional state. The important thing is to localize this measurement to specific regions of the nervous system, preferably one that can look at all regions simultaneously but independently.

The measurement of regional cerebral blood flow (rCBF) does nicely, because rCBF and cerebral metabolism (as measured by glucose utilization) correlate well (Sokoloff, 1981). Cerebral blood flow also provides the strongest evidence for reduced cortical activity during synesthesia.

Reduced Cortical Blood Flow During Geometrically Shaped Taste Synesthesia

Xenon-133 inhalation rCBF measurements were made for MW in baseline, synesthetic, and adjuvant-intensified states (Cytowic & Stump, 1985). For those not familiar with this technology I recommend the relatively nontechnical explanation of Stump and Williams (1980). The xenon-133 method is able to measure blood flow in multiple discrete cortical regions simultaneously but independently. A fast component flow for the gray matter and a slower component representing white matter are measured in milliliters per 100 grams of tissue per minute. The general procedure is for the patient to lie on a couch with his head in a helmet in which radiation detectors are mounted to measure clearance of the tracer. Each lab establishes that its probes are mounted over the desired anatomical points to be studied. Radioactive xenon-133 is inert in the physiological sense and rapidly diffuses across the blood-brain barrier, and its concentration in the blood can be rapidly and accurately measured. The xenon can be inhaled or injected into an artery or vein. Each route of administration has its own advantages and disadvantages.

For technical reasons, the saturation uptake of xenon is not measured. Rather, the desaturation clearance is measured for 10 minutes after tissues are fully saturated (which happens during a 1-minute administration of the gas). The concentrations of carbon dioxide, oxygen, and xenon-133 are measured in the expired air simultaneously (to permit later correction for recirculation artifact) as counts are obtained for each probe. The radioactivity counts for each probe and for the xenon in expired air are compared. Mathematical analysis of all this permits one to follow blood flow through the brain at each region of interest simultaneously from moment to moment and see which regions on which sides are most active during the behavioral task under study. The data are stored on magnetic medium and are available for comparison with later studies in the same or similar subjects.

Normally, the pattern of blood flow, called a landscape, is obtained during a resting baseline state as well as one or more states of activation, and these different states are compared. The activation state may be either a motor, sensory, or cognitive task, and depending on the nature of the task one expects different brain regions to ''light up'' or be more active than others that are not believed to participate in the specific task. Generally, one expects at least a 10% increase in those regions that participate in the activation task. For example, Ginsburg, Chang, Kelly, et al. (1988) simultaneously measured regional cerebral glucose utilization as well as rCBF in 10 normal subjects performing a somatosensory-motor task: palpation and sorting of mah-jongg tiles by their engraved design. As expected, this somatosensory stimulus elevated the regional cerebral glucose utilization by $16.9 \pm 3.5\%$ and the rCBF by $26.5 \pm 5.1\%$ in the contralateral sensorimotor cortical region.

Method

In the gas delivery system for the inhalation method of measuring rCBF, the subject is attached to the system via a tight-fitting face mask and short hose. A valve is in line to switch from breathing ambient room air to breathing the xenon mixture. It is easier to introduce volatile odorants at the room air intake than to use liquid flavorants sucked through flexible straw tubing passing under the face mask. The latter technique is prone to air leaks around the mask and was subsequently discarded in favor of the inhalation of odorants. From experience, both tastes and smells were sufficient to induce stable, nonfatiguing synesthesiae as outlined in the section on drug studies above.

MW breathed a xenon mixture of 7 microcuries per liter of air for 1 minute and then was switched to room air. Desaturation was measured for the next 10 minutes of clearance. During this time either the stimulus odorant or an odorant followed by amyl nitrate adjuvant was introduced into the face mask and inhaled by the subject. This produced a synesthesia of up to 1 minute in duration. MW was instructed to maintain as near a constant state of synesthesia as possible and to signal for additional stimulation by moving only his left index finger. Eyes were closed, the room darkened, and the ambient environment filled with a steady white noise.

Probe Locations

Scintillation detector probes are placed radially in a helmet with neuro-anatomical references based on a modified 10–20 electrode placement system. Using bony landmarks, probe sites are marked on a cadaver head and holes drilled into the brain. By this method site verification is within 5 millimeters of any desired cortical region. In the left hemisphere probe F3 is in the frontal eye fields of Forester; F2, inferior frontal gyrus (Broca's area); F4, hand region of the precentral gyrus; P1, hand area of the postcentral gyrus; T2, lateral convexity of Heschl's gyrus; P2, inferior parietal lobule, primarily angular and supramarginal gyrii; T0, the anastomotic area between the middle cerebral artery (MCA) and the posterior communicating artery (PCA) circulation; and O1, occipital pole (Figure 4.7, *top*). Probes are similarly placed over the right hemisphere.

Baseline rCBF

Mean flow Gray (Fg) levels in the left hemisphere are reduced for a person of MW's age (56.3 ml/100 g/min), and his resting hemispheric landscape is

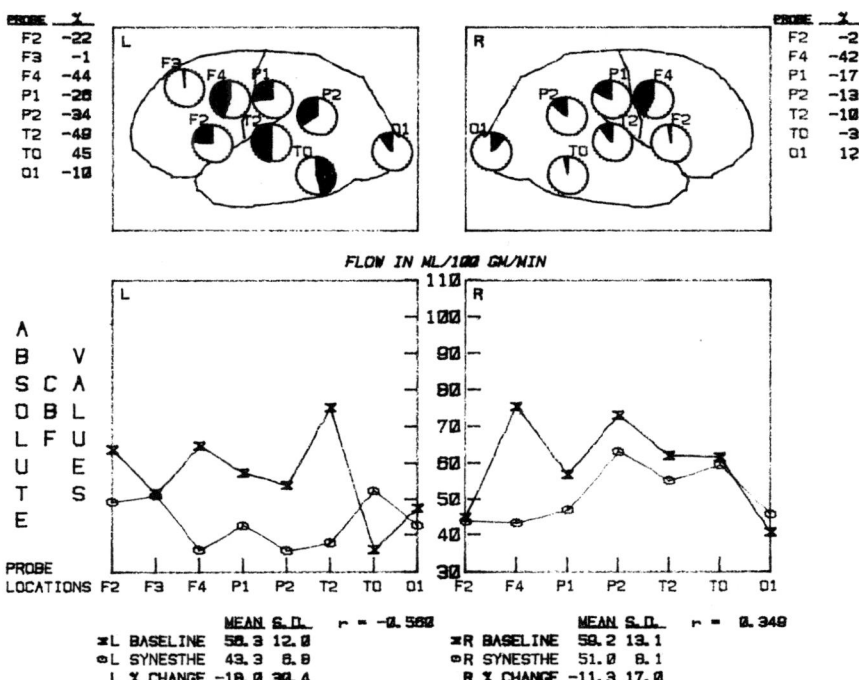

FIGURE 4.7. *Top:* Scintillation detector probe placements for rCBF study. Percentage change from baseline to synesthesia represented by black areas on clocks (those moving clockwise, percentage increase; those moving counterclockwise, percentage decrease). *Bottom:* Absolute blood flow values (in ml/100 g/min) for MW for baseline (X) and synesthesia (○) studies for the probe locations shown at top. Data Display Program by permission, D.A. Stump & L. Hinschelwood.

unusually variable (standard deviation = 12.0) (Figure 4.7, *bottom*). The average person in our lab has a mean flow of 65 ± 4. Inferior temporal and occipital flows (probes T0 and O1) are pathologically low and approaching the floor limits of the apparatus to detect any flow at all. The right hemisphere shows near-ischemic flows in the right inferior frontal and occipital areas (probes F2 and O1), and also has high variability (standard deviation = 13).

The remarkable feature of MW's resting blood flow is its inhomogeneity and areas of ischemia. However, his neurological exam shows no focal deficits nor has there ever been any history of transient ischemic attack.

During Synesthesia

The average left hemispheric flow drops to 43.3 ml/100 g/min, which is close to 3 standard deviations below acceptable limits—a level of flow at which we have never seen a patient in our laboratory who was not symptomatic at the time of study (Figure 4.7, *bottom*). The central MCA territory drops to flow levels in the 30s, which is usually consistent with chronic ischemia or passive flow secondary to stroke (probes F4, P1, P2, and T2).

MW's mean left hemisphere flow drops 18% during synesthesia, an occurrence rarely—if ever—seen in a normal study. Even with 100% oxygen inhalation or aminophylline, which act as potent vasoconstrictors, one sees only a 10% to 15% decrease. This reduction in blood flow seen during the synesthetic experience would be difficult to obtain with a drug in a normal person.

The 11% decrease in the right hemisphere is largely a reflection of the high precentral flow (probe F4) during baseline, possibly due to index finger movement during signaling. Prorating probe F4, the mean decrease in hemispheric flow in the right hemisphere during synesthesia would be 5%, which is within the normal variability.

Hemispheric Symmetry

Hemispheric symmetry (comparing left to right hemisphere) is quite poor for both baseline and synesthesia. Normally, the correlation (r) is .5 to .9 for a younger normal person. The synesthete has asymmetrical hemispheric flow to begin with in the baseline ($r = .164$), which becomes worse during synesthesia ($r = -.05$) (Figure 4.8). Looking only at the MCA territory (probes F2 to T2), one sees a good correlation except that the left hemisphere is about 10% lower than the right, which is inconsistent with what is normally seen. The left anterior temporal and parietal areas are significantly lower than the homologous right hemisphere areas and below the lower limits of normal.

Therefore, there is an unusual dissociation between anterior and posterior circulations during MW's synesthetic experience.

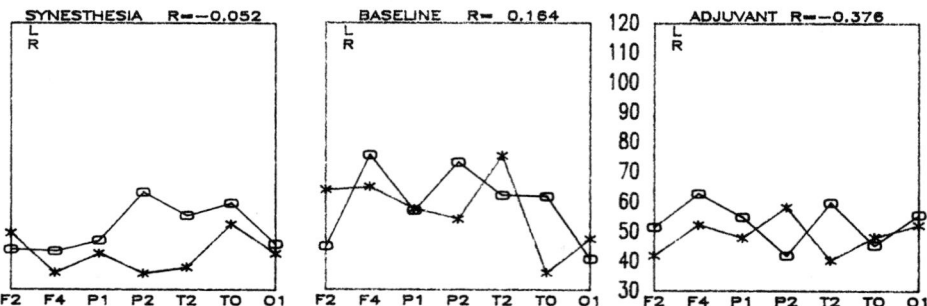

FIGURE 4.8. Cerebral blood flow hemispheric symmetry. *Left:* Flow during synesthesia. *Center:* Baseline flow. *Right:* Flow during adjuvant-activated synesthesia. ×, left hemisphere flow; ○, right hemisphere flow. Data Display Program by permission, D.A. Stump & L. Hinschelwood.

rCBF During Amyl Nitrate Activation

There are no data on the effect of amyl nitrate on rCBF in normal brains. It is known to increase intracranial pressure in animals (Malkinson, Cooper, & Veale, 1985). Some argue that rCBF increases because of increased cardiac output while others argue that it decreases because of vasodilitation. Goodman and Gillman (1975, pp. 727–735) suggested that adverse effects of lightheadedness, dizziness, and telecusis are in fact due to cerebral ischemia and the data here support that idea. Figures 4.9 and 4.10 compare flow during synesthesia to flow during adjuvant. Inhalation of amyl nitrate, which intensifies synesthetic perception (see above), causes a massive redistribution of flow, particularly in the left hemisphere. Areas of the MCA territory dip below the lower acceptable limits of normal while the previously ischemic areas in the posterior circulation now elevate into the normal range. There is an interesting dissociation between flow in the MCA and PCA territories (probes T2, T0, and O1) on the left side. The major difference between plain

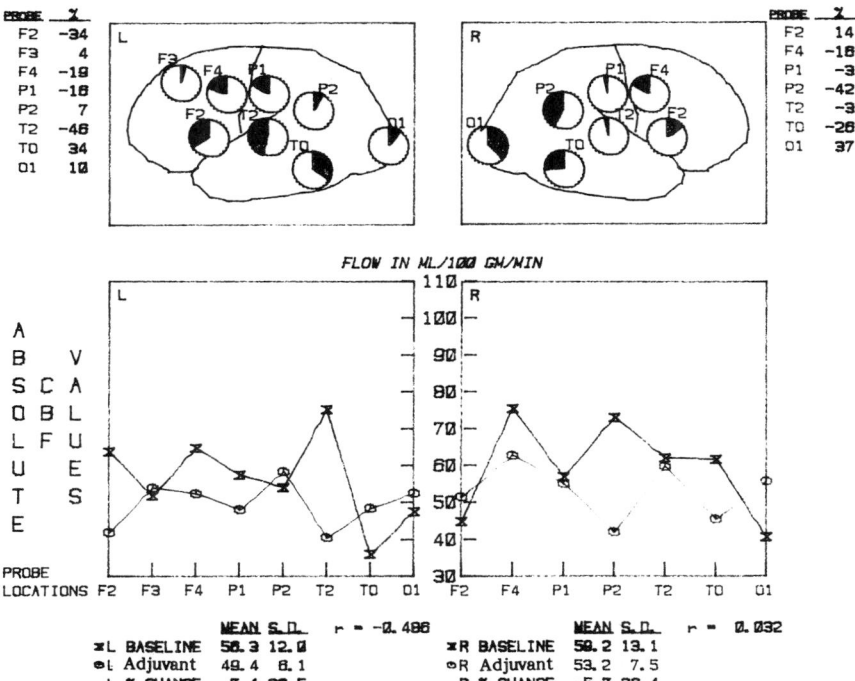

FIGURE 4.9. *Top:* Probe placements for rCBF measurement and percentage change from baseline to adjuvant-activated synesthesia (as described for Figure 4.7, *top*). *Bottom:* Absolute blood flow values for baseline (×) and adjuvant-activated synesthesia (○), measured as described for Figure 4.7 (*bottom*). Data Display Program by permission, D.A. Stump & L. Hinschelwood.

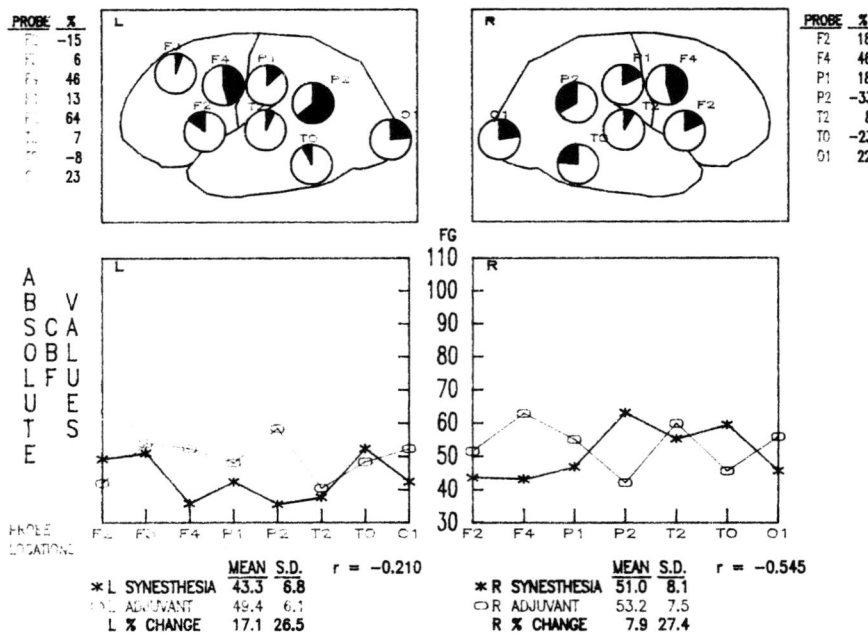

FIGURE 4.10. *Top:* Probe placements for rCBF measurement and percentage change from synesthesia to adjuvant-activated synesthesia (as described for Figure 4.7, *top*). *Bottom:* Absolute blood flow values for synesthesia (*) and adjuvant (○) studies, measured as described for Figure 4.7 (*bottom*). Data Display Program by permission, D.A. Stump & L. Hinschelwood.

synesthesia and synesthesia with adjuvant administration is a higher flow to the posterior parietal cortex (probe P2) and motor hand region (probe F4).

Even though mean hemispheric flows with amyl nitrate are higher than the mean flows during plain synesthesia, the adjuvant flows are still *below* the baseline (−8.0% left, −9.8% right)—well within the range one expects to see with bona fide activation. What is extremely unusual, however, is that MW's flows *decrease* rather than increase with an activation procedure. Normally, with any activation, whether it is hand movement, a cognitive task, or drug administration, one anticipates a 5% to 10% increase in rCBF.

The major effect during this episode of synesthesia is almost exclusively in the MCA territory of the left hemisphere, with a "flip-flop" between the MCA and PCA territories. Baseline posterior flow is low, while the flow during synesthesia decreases dramatically in the MCA of the left hemisphere as if there were a steal in the posterior circulation. MW's rCBF looks, in fact, like those of patients with arteriovenous malformations or subclavian steal, or transient global amnesia patients who also have migraine headaches (Crowell, Stump, Biller, McHenry, & Toole, 1984).

For those not familiar with rCBF measurement, it should be emphasized that the data analysis of the inhalation procedure is mathematically complex. Factors that contribute to this complexity are inhalation of the tracer, recirculation, and extracerebral contamination from saturated muscles of the scalp, bone, air sinuses, and nasopharynx. Xenon concentrations in blood and noncerebral tissue contribute gamma counts to the detectors. That is, the concentration curves of the two contributing sources are intertwined or convoluted. Various equations and computer programs exist to deconvolute these curves. A rough characterization of the deconvolution procedure is dividing the air curve into the head curve, a procedure that provides adequate resolution for the recirculation factor. Other methods are used to account for extracerebral contamination. Numerous parameters, some more obscure than others, are currently in use in various laboratories. In a system with 16 probes, the use of the 12 most common parameters yields 192 separate calculated values. This is a rather large data set.

Because of the highly unusual blood flow patterns both in baseline and during synesthesia and adjuvant activation in MW, both an actuarial approach—that is, a pattern analysis, manipulation of parameters, and the use of indices that separate particular patient populations—and the basic science approach, involving analysis of the clearance curve, the ultimate and primary source of information in this technique, were used. Every effort was made to identify possible sources of artifact. Raw, fitted, and derived curves, as well as Z scores for nine different parameters, were analyzed. The data are an accurate reflection of the actual cerebral blood flow.

The rCBF results support the theoretical hypothesis and are compatible with the experimental data that synesthesia is not a semantically mediated cross-modal association, but a physically based phenomenon that involves a relative suppression of cortical activity.

CEREBRAL ANGIOGRAPHY

Because of the striking abnormality found on rCBF it was medically necessary to investigate MW for a vascular lesion in the left hemisphere. *A left carotid and vertebral angiogram showed absence of the left PCA at the circle of Willis.* There was no disease of the carotid bifurcation and there was excellent supratentorial filling. The vessels reached the inner table uniformly without displacement. There were no occluded vessels, aneurysms, or early-draining veins. The left vertebral injection showed normal visualization of the posterior cerebral vasculature.

Thus, without an anatomical vascular lesion, the blood flow abnormalities both in baseline and during synesthesia become all the more intriguing. The absence of the PCA on the left could explain the flip-flop seen between the MCA and PCA territories but cannot fully explain the unusual ischemia at probe TO, which lies over the anastomotic area between MCA and PCA territories. Why flow should increase in this cortical region during synesthesia, however, is not clear. Nor is baseline ischemic flow on both occipital lobes easily explained. The selective vertebral injection showed excellent filling of these vessels. Although the absent PCA may explain *some* of the results of the rCBF, it is hardly sufficient to explain the unusual landscape of regional flow and its reactivity to ordinary stimuli.

The results surprised us but we were even more flabbergasted by what happened during the injection of contrast material itself. Normal patients experience a flush of heat for the few seconds that the contrast replaces blood in their cerebral arteries. Other than this they manifest no symptoms while the vascular lumen contains nonoxygenating contrast material. In marked contrast to the usual reaction, MW experienced visual, auditory, and tactile sensations during the time that his blood was replaced by nonoxygenating contrast! *This suggests that we are dealing with a cortex that is precariously balanced in its energy metabolism, and becomes pathologically ischemic during the psychophysical state of synesthesia.*

Left Carotid Injection

Visual perception was apparent to MW with eyes closed, but was almost absent with eyes open. "I sense it on the left side. An intense pink and the blackest black I've ever seen. It flashes like lightning and grows in intensity. The pink is mainly on the left side. Everything else is pitch black." He saw this inside his head and not projected outward.

What could account for this visual perception? One hardly expects a carotid injection to affect striate cortex and in fact this injection could not because his PCA is missing. Besides, it would have to involve the right striate cortex since MW is clear that the pink is perceived "on the left." Since his left hemispheric MCA territory flows are already in the low range such visual perception may be due to (1) further ischemia in the inferior parietal lobule (probe area P2) or temporal cortex (the peripheral retina is represented in the lingula of the temporal lobe); or (2) a temporary disconnection of callosal projections to the right hemisphere. If such a disconnection involved the speech regions, the right hemisphere might "confabulate" in the left visual hemifield.

Vertebral Injection

Several sensations occurred during the vertebral injection. There was a ringing in the left ear, a "high pitched whine, higher than a siren. Very, very high beyond 20 kHz."

MW had excruciating pain "bone pain, like a tooth ache" in his neck and occiput and at the vertex. Patients sometimes experience pain in their neck if there are anastomoses between skeletal muscle arteries and intracranial arteries of the vertebral circulation; however, no such anastomoses were present in MW. The angiographer had not seen such an intensely painful reaction in over 20 years' experience. An anatomical mechanism is difficult to propose, but involves the segmental levels C2 to C4 or the spinal nucleus of the trigeminal nerve. Spinothalamic tract disruption is difficult to conceive of without a fuller hemisensory disturbance.

With the small test dose of contrast injected to localize the catheter tip in the vertebral artery osteum, MW saw an intense red spot centrally, "like the fixation point on the perimeter." It obscured real objects in his field. This persisted for 40 seconds. One might assume this to be an ischemic symptom of the occipital pole, which subserves macular vision. Probe O1 was ischemic on baseline rCBF. (Replacement of real object space by hallucinated objects is discussed in Chapter 9.)

Visual images consisted of overlapping geometric squares like art deco that rapidly alternated in a black-and-white pattern shift. This attenuated when MW opened his eyes but did block part of his normal field of vision. He received photic stimulation later during an EEG. As the strobe got faster the shapes of black and white patterns became more complex, "growing like crystals." They started like squares, became hexagons, then developed into overlapping shapes similar to those seen during vertebral angiography, "if not the same."

Cerebral hypoxia has been proposed to play a role in hallucinogenic images (Corales, Maull, & Becker, 1980; Stimmel, 1979); phencyclidine, LSD, and mescaline produce in vitro cerebral artery spasms via specific receptors in cerebral arteries (Altura & Altura, 1981).

ELECTROENCEPHALOGRAPHY

The visual shapes seen during photic stimulation are unusual both in the rarity of their occurrence in this setting (Freedman & Marks, 1965; Smythies, 1960) and *in their similarity to the images MW saw during vertebral angiography*. The EEG was performed within an hour of the angiogram. We have not subjected MW to photic stimulation at a separate time. He showed blocking of alpha rhythm only on the left side during inhalation of volatile stimulants. T1, T2, and nasopharyngeal electrodes were used. No paroxysmal or focal disturbances were seen.

MAGNETIC RESONANCE IMAGING

By all accounts MW had a "normal" brain that was behaving quite abnormally. Perhaps magnetic resonance imaging (MRI) could disclose some abnormal signals in this unusual subject. Geschwind and Levitsky (1968) had shattered the dogma that the hemispheres were exactly symmetrical and this new high-resolution anatomical tool could look into that question. Geschwind had proposed on theoretical grounds alone that asymmetry should exist in the brain. He then showed that one did not need microscopes but could measure these asymmetries with rulers.

Technical Data and Images

Proton MRI has soft tissue discrimination 500 times more sensitive than x-ray computed tomography. The basic principles of MRI, perturbation of hydrogen nuclei by specifically tuned radiofrequency bombardment and computer reconstruction of the resultant signals, apply to all systems. The quality of the reconstructed images is dependent on signal-to-noise ratios, which are affected by several variables. The available signal is roughly proportional to the ambient magnetic field, whereas the noise (mainly generated from the patient himself) is linear. Therefore, by simply increasing the field strength from 0.35 Tesla to 1.5 Tesla, one can achieve a fivefold increase in signal strength. This surplus of signal can be used to realize thin slices with a consequent increase in spatial resolution.[2]

The MRI showed no abnormal signals in the gray or white matter of the cerebrum or brainstem. In symmetrical cuts in which there is no more than 1.0 mm of tilt in the horizontal axis there was a simpler lobulation of the cortical ribbon and fingers of white matter on the left anterior temporal lobe compared to the right. On the lateral basal aspect of the temporal lobe there was a single broad gyrus compared to three on the right. Corresponding coronal views showed this flat broad surface compared to the more configured gyration on the right side. This asymmetry in the gross architecture is tantalizing but, it must be emphasized, highly speculative. MRI is too new and this asymmetry may have no significance. There are no data regarding symmetry of lobulation and similarity of gyration in homologous regions. Whether the asymmetry in MW represents a true deviation from normal or whether it would have any functional significance is not known.

---

[2]The device used in our study is a SIGNA system (General Electric Medical Systems, Milwaukee, WI) operated at 1.5 Tesla. Five-millimeter-thick localizing images are generated in the sagittal plane using a repetition time (T_R) of 400 milliseconds and an echo delay (T_E) of 20 milliseconds. Two hundred fifty-six phase-encoded measurements are obtained by a single excitation over a 240-millimeter field of view. This yields a pixel size of $240/256 = 0.9$ millimeter and a voxel size of $0.9 \times 0.9 \times 5$ millimeters. Total imaging time is under 2 minutes.

A cursor is placed at the foramen magnum and then at the vertex, and a prescription for a multislice acquisition in the axial plane is established. Fifteen to twenty 5-millimeter-thick locations are imaged using a 240-millimeter field of view, a 256×256 matrix, a single excitation, T_R of 2250 milliseconds, and T_Es of 20 and 80 milliseconds. This protocol yields two images per location; the 2250/20 or proton density image and a relatively T_2-weighted study at 2250/80.

Neuropsychological Assessment

Tests Administered

Weschsler Adult Intelligence Test (Revised)
Weschsler Memory Scale (Form I)
Halstead-Reitan Aphasia Screening Test
Drawings on Command
Tapping Test and Grip Dynamometry
Form Board
Reitan-Kløve Sensory Perceptual Examination
Trail Making A and B
Whittaker Acalculia Battery
Minnesota Multiphasic Personality Inventory
Fargo Map Test and New Map Learning

Results of these tests are summarized in Table 4.4.

TABLE 4.4. Summary of neuropsychological testing of MW.[a]

VIQ	128	PIQ	119	MQ >143	
Information	16	Pic Comp	11	Information	6
Digit Span	11	Pic Arr	17	Orientation	5
Vocabulary	18	Block Design	13	Mental Control	9
Arithmetic	11	Object Assem	11	Story Passages	16
Comprehensive	15	Digit Symbol	8	Digit Span	15
Similarities	14			Drawing	14
		FSIQ 129		Ass Learn	20

Form Board	Tapping	Dynamometry
R 3'15"	R 60	R 18 psi
L 2'41"	L 50	L 19 psi

Trails	
A 40"	**Stereognosis:** Normal
B 55"	**Extinctions:** L ear

Finger gnosis	Finger graphesthesia
R Ok	R 5/8 errors
L Hesitant,	L 4/8 errors
3/10 errors	

Acalculia Battery
  Finger agraphesthesia
  Digit to lexical errors
  Lexical misspellings

Fargo Map: Good geography
New Map Learning: Average

[a] VIQ, verbal IQ, PIQ, Performance IQ; FSIQ, full-scale IQ, MQ, memory quotient; psi, pounds per square inch.

Background Information

This 40-year-old right-hander with a B.A. degree in botany was evaluated for synesthesia. No family history of left-handedness or personal history suggesting mixed dominance. Historically, he has difficulty with mathematics and must do calculations on paper, even those pertaining to activities that have great relevance to him in his work as a theater lighting designer (e.g., beam angles involving trigonometry, simple summation of wattages, and calculation of electric loads).

MW has a history of right-left confusion since childhood. He finds it easier to remember "windows" and "bulletin board" instead of "left" and "right," a mnemonic device stemming from the arrangement of his elementary schoolroom.

Behavioral Observations

No behavior is remarkable except for his surprise on encountering difficulty with finger gnosis and fingertip graphesthesia.

Intellectual Functioning

MW's verbal IQ is 128, his performance IQ is 119, and his full-scale IQ is 129. He had difficulty with arithmetical competency as well as a more general use of digits. He had relative difficulty distinguishing essential from nonessential visual details.

Memory Functioning

MW's Memory Quotient is >143.

Language Functioning

MW's drawings were performed like a draftsman; there was no constructional apraxia. Repetition was normal and there was no alexia, aphasia, or agraphia. There was some hesitancy with right-left identification on the examiner. Finger identification on the right was normal, but he had difficulty (3/10 errors) on the left. Speed of answering was much slower and he was uncertain.

Acalculia Battery

Three trials of numerical fingertip writing were performed on the sensory perceptual exam and five trials on the acalculia battery at separate times for a total of eight trials. He made 5/8 errors on the right and 4/8 on the left. An example of errors on the right were calling 8 a 2 or 6; on the left he called 4 a 9, 3 an 8, and 6 either a 0 or an 8. He showed difficulty in digit-to-lexical transcoding and a spelling error in auditory to lexical transcoding. He used the "carry method" in addition and during the task of auditory multiplication, he had a lapse of "forgetting" the multiplication tables.

Sensory-Perceptual Functioning

There was no deficit to unilateral stimulation in the tactile, visual, or auditory modes. MW did show auditory extinction in the left ear with simultaneous stimulation and had errors of fingertip graphesthesia as noted above. Performance on the form board showed appropriate cross-transfer learning. Manual dexterity was appropriate but grip dynamometry showed counterdominance, with the right hand being weaker than the left.

Summary of Neuropsychological Testing

MW shows arithmetical symbolic difficulty, including digit-to-lexical and auditory-to-lexical transcoding. There was a bilateral disturbance of numerical fingertip graphesthesia and finger agnosia on the left. The left ear extinguishes on simultaneous auditory stimulation. Form discrimination is preserved and there is motor dominance for dexterity but weakness of the "dominant" hand on dynamometry.

Results imply an abnormality in the left parietal in the area of the angular gyrus, probably affecting deeper white matter.

Higher Cortical Deficits in Other Subjects

MW is not unique in having mild cognitive difficulties that are suggestive of a left hemispheric dysfunction. Thirty-three of 42 subjects claim to have difficulty with arithmetic, compared to 9 of 42 who felt that their skills were good or better than average.

Subject DS

Tests Administered

Wechsler Memory Scale
Trail Making A and B
Whittaker Acalculia Battery
Reitan-Kløve Sensory Perceptual Examination
Fargo Map Test and New Map Learning
Halstead-Reitan Aphasia Screening Test
Minnesota Multiphasic Personality Inventory

The results of these tests are summarized in Table 4.5.

Background Information

Subject DS has acalculia and a family history of dyslexia. Her son had failure to thrive with stunting of growth. Whether this was a pituitary

TABLE 4.5. Summary of neuropsychological deficits in DS.

MQ = 101	
Trail A 30″	
Trail B 55″	
Aculculia Battery	
Subtraction	
Auditory multiplication	
Lexical-to-digit	
Digits to dictation	
Stereognosis: Ok	**Finger gnosis**
Extinctions: None	RH hesitant
Fingertip graphesthesia	**Right-Left**
LH Ok	Confusion
RH 3/5 errors	
Fargo Map[a]: Low average	
New Map Learning: Failed	

[a] Discussed in Chapter 7.

abnormality was never resolved convincingly. He had trouble reading, learning the alphabet, and learning numbers. Compared to other children he has a noticeable appreciation for rhythm, and "relates to music." He wants to be a ballet dancer despite being clumsy.

"I have severe math difficulties," says DS. She miswrites checks and has to tear them up, adds and subtracts on her hands, and if asked to perform a simple addition or multiplication task in her head will instead draw in the air as she visualizes the calculations. She holds an M.S. degree. Her most difficult course was statistics. "The concepts were not difficult—it was all those numbers."

I didn't want to have anything to do with numbers. I never understood them. If I couldn't visualize a pattern or a relationship with numbers, I couldn't do it. The difficulty started as early as I can remember in grade school. I left Florida and went back up North where I had never heard the expression "naught" for "zero." This made things worse. I felt intimidated. (February 16, 1987).

Acalculia Battery

DS has much difficulty doing subtraction with pencil and paper. She is slow and makes errors that are unexpected for someone with her education. Writing numbers to dictation is particularly difficult. She must vocalize during lexical-to-digit encoding, and even then still makes errors. She gives up during auditory multiplication. "I can't do it. The numbers keep going away. I have to write it down."

Wechsler Memory

Comments regarding DS's memory have been used as examples throughout this book. Although she claims to have an excellent memory, her actual MQ is only 101. She had difficulty in the mental control task of counting by threes and had omissions and transpositions in digits, scoring 7 forward and 5 backward. She drew in the air with her index finger to reorder the numbers in the backward recitation. Learning of paired associates was excellent, but she scored only 5 on visual reproductions. She tended to get the overall gestalt correct but make errors of detail. During story recall she remembered by "visualizing the sentences."

Sensory-Perceptual Examination

There was no loss to single or simultaneous stimulation in the visual, auditory, or tactile modes. DS demonstrated right-left confusion on both herself and the examiner, was hesitant in finger identification in the right hand, and made errors in fingertip graphesthesia on the right index finger (e.g., calling 9 a 0 and 6 either a 2 or a 3). Trails were performed within time limits and without sequence errors.

Geographic Competency

DS's geographic competency is discussed in Chapter 7.

Language

Compared to her disregard for numbers, DS is an avid reader and learned to do so early. "I read in kindergarten [*at 4 years old*]. I wasn't satisfied with the rate the teacher was going. I would get out of bed and sit in the hall by the nightlight reading. My mother yelled at me because she thought I should be asleep."

There was no evidence for an aphasic disturbance, although this was not studied in detail with, for example, the Boston Diagnostic Aphasia Exam. Repetition was normal, as was confrontation naming and fluency of speech. The only suggestion for a disturbance is her comment that during her several hours of daily typing "I find I must continue to look at the keyboard just to make sure I'm hitting the right letters. I often strike more than one key and I substitute locations of keys (I'll be thinking 'F' and hit 'J' instead)." Yet she is good at anagrams and comments "I'm very quick at unscrambling words; usually I can do them in my head. The letters reorganize themselves in different configurations until they make sense. I'm also a good speller."

She expresses a preference for written communication and a need for vocal or subvocal rehearsal.

I am poor at verbal communication and am better able to express myself in writing. I cannot concentrate, organize, or think logically in conversation; but alone, with pen and paper I am more confident. (I am sure this was evident at our meeting.)

Reading is not sufficient if I want to remember. I MUST write down what I want to retain. This is true also with taking directions. In my Tae Kwan Do class I must translate each form [set of prearranged stances involving arm and leg movements] to a written code which I then VISUALLY memorize. I also verbally rehearse constantly when I need to remember, either vocally or subvocally (March 1, 1987).

Thus, although there is no frank aphasic disturbance, there is a certain peculiarity in DS's linguistic performance. She also has elements of Gerstman's syndrome. One gets the impression that there is a visuospatial problem and perhaps an attention problem in addition to the acalculia. Acalculia, of course, does not have to covary with aphasia.

Subject TP

The male patient TP is dyslexic, and still makes reversals and has spelling difficulty at age 24.

Subject DoS

DoS was precocious in math, learning algebra in grade school from her brother, who is 9 years older. The brother is also proficient in mathematics and particularly liked calculus. In contrast to her hypercalculia, DoS has great difficulty learning foreign languages. Attempting Spanish, French, and Hebrew led to termination of study despite her concerted effort. She spoke English early as a child and was voluble.

Subject PO

This 41-year-old left-handed Canadian podiatrist has a colored number form present since childhood (see Chapter 7 for discussion of number forms). His mother is left-handed. "I read the article [*about synesthesia*] in the Toronto paper and almost cried. It struck home. I was so emotionally overwhelmed. I didn't know there was a name for this." He had never told anyone about his synesthesia.

PO had a ruptured right middle cerebral artery aneurysm that did not influence his synesthesia. This lack of change is supportive that synesthesia may depend more heavily on left hemispheric processes.

Summary

The higher cortical dysfunctions in these patients and their first-degree relatives further supports the left hemispheric representation of synesthesia. A few patients have elements of Gerstman's syndrome.

A Disconnection Syndrome for Synesthesia: Analogy to Migraine Theory

I propose that synesthesia can be regarded as a recurrent, stimulus-induced functional disconnection of a language region from other parts of the brain. The only hard experimental evidence for this is the interesting redistribution of rCBF in MW. Careful analysis shows that his rCBF is indeed abnormal rather than a simple reflection of redistribution due to an olfactory stimulus. The logical conclusion from both the hypothesis and the data is that there is a reversible stimulus-induced cortical ischemia during all types of synesthesia. What could be the mechanism for such a spontaneous regional reduction of rCBF?

Such a proposal may seem too speculative, even farfetched, but on reflection it is no more so than the "standard explanation" of migraine, which states that the *clinical syndrome* of migraine parallels cortical blood flow redistribution and an electrical spreading depression (Hachinski, 1987; Oleson, 1987; Skyhøj-Olsen, Friberg, & Lassen, 1987; Welch, 1987). The explanation of cortical ischemia and rebound hyperrhemia has been repeated since the mid-1800s, although no cogent answer to why this occurs in susceptible patients exists. Since this "explanation" appears in countless texts, its lack of cogency seems not to bother us. Because of its appealing simplicity, the hypothesis has easily been grasped by students and even patients. The debate over neurogenic versus vascular causation goes back over 100 years. Abundant data show both the blood flow changes and spreading depression across vascular territories and anatomic boundaries. Although there is contention over hyperrhemia versus ischemia during the aura phase, vascular changes are well documented in migraine and currently accepted as metabolic depression of cerebral blood flow. The spreading depression of Leao (Lauritzen, Balslev Jøgensen, et al., 1982; Leao, 1944) is a surface-negative slow potential that spreads, like a wave in a pond, across anatomical boundaries such as the central sulcus. It is similar to contingent negative variation, an event-related slow cerebral potential modulated by central catecholaminergic systems. Unlike synesthesia, which is evoked, migraine does not even appear to have a stimulus. However, we accept as fact that biochemical and vascular alterations happen in migraine for no apparent reason whatsoever and then resolve.

Like synesthesia, migrane can be influenced by drugs. Noordhout, Timsit-Berthier, Timsit and colleagues (1987) showed normalization of contingent negative variation in migraineurs treated with beta blockade. Their findings support a direct effect of beta blockade on the neural generators of contingent negative variation. A propos of our discussion of temporal lobe and limbic structures in Chapter 5, Reznikoff, Manaker, Rhodes, and colleagues (1986) demonstrated by quantitative autoradiography that beta receptors are highest in all subfields of the human hippocampus. Beta blockade would be a logical manipulation to explore in synesthetes.

There has never been much consensus among headache specialists as to the definition of migraine, let alone its cause. Although changes in cerebral blood flow, both ischemia and hyperrhemia, are well documented, the neurogenic school believes that these changes are secondary to neurotransmitter disturbances. Adrenergic sympathetic systems have been proposed in the medulla, pons, and hypothalamus; others have suggested serotonergic systems in the midbrain raphe. Given that there is so little consensus, I will not draw the analogy to synesthesia further. I have also not discussed migranous photisms in this section on overlaps, but the well-known lines, grids, concentric circles, and zigzag fortification spectrum should be kept in mind during the discussion of Klüver's form constants.

It should not seem farfetched that in synesthesia there is, for an unknown reason, a stimulus-induced ischemia or cortical depression that results in a functional disconnection.

Relation of Synesthetic Perceptions to Klüver's Form Constants

At this point, it is helpful to review the characteristic features of synesthesia. Synesthesia is (1) involuntary but elicited, (2) projected, (3) memorable, (4) emotional, and (5) discrete. It is blocked by cortical stimulants and accompanied by a reduction of cortical blood flow and, therefore, metabolism. The discrete nature of synesthesia, particularly the generic and restricted nature of synesthetic percepts, brings to mind Klüver's "form constants"[3] (Klüver, 1942b, 1966). Synesthetes never see complex dream-like scenes or have otherwise elaborated percepts. They perceive blobs, lines, spirals, lattices, and other geometric shapes. Starting in the 1920s Heinrich Klüver identified four types of consistent hallucinogenic images: gratings and honeycombs, cobwebs, tunnels and cones, and spirals. Variations in color, brightness, symmetry, and replication provided finer gradation of subjective experience. The point is that, given a wide variety of stimulation, the brain seems to respond in finite ways.

Klüver's work was repeated and extended by Siegel (1977; Siegel & West, 1975). Klüver showed that there are a limited number of perceptual frameworks that appear to be built into the machinery of the CNS. They may be part of our genetic endowment.

The analysis . . . has yielded a number of forms and form elements which must be considered typical for mescal visions. No matter how strong the inter- and intra-individual differences may be, the records are remarkably uniform as to the appearance of the above described forms and configurations. We may call them

---

[3] The use of the word "form" by Klüver is unfortunate, since what is really constant is the shape of the percept. Form refers to the larger construct of a work, such as sonata form in music, or the form of composition in a painting. Because of its historical context, however, I will use the term "form constant" to refer to this constancy of shape, which is characteristic of all imagery and hallucinations.

form-constants, implying that a certain number of them appear in almost all mescal visions and that many "atypical" visions are upon close examination nothing but variations of these form-constants (Klüver, 1966, p. 22).

Unaware of Klüver's work, Horowitz (1964, 1975) rediscovered the redundant elements of hallucinations and argued similarly that a "perceptual nidus" resides within the visual system itself. There are "certain constancies" that the visual system itself contributes to illusory and hallucinatory phenomena as well as objective perception.

Similar generic images are seen in sensory deprivation. Brightly colored geometric patterns and cloud formations have been perceived after metrizamide cisternography of the posterior fossa (Bachman, 1984), thought by the author to be from penetration into the temporal lobe; mental and perceptual disturbances are common if metrizamide penetrates cerebral tissue. McKellar (1957) showed that form constants were present in a wide range of states, including drug induced, hypnogogic, psychotic, and feverish delerium. The artist Vladimir Kandinsky (1881) reported such form constants during a feverish delerium: "Pictures, microscopic preparations, or ornamental figures were drawn on the dark ground of the visual field" (pp. 459–460).

Figures 4.11 to 4.15 show that the form constants, often having axial or radial symmetry, can be found in many natural phenomena—from the kinds of medical images we have discussed, to artwork of synesthetics, and even to the craftwork and cave paintings of primitive cultures. For example, the Blanchard Bone and similar Ice Age artifacts carved 20,000 years ago have been studied by Alex Marshack (1975), who made an excellent case that many of the linear and curvaceous notations recorded the monthly lunar cycles, capturing the waxing and waning of the moon. The reason for the configuration can never be known, but its similarity to the form constants is obvious. Marshack also illustrated geometric "symbols" surrounding a Lascaux horse cave painting. They are similar to the simple drawings made by synesthetics of irregular patterns of straight lines.

The form constants seen in the kind of images discussed above are different from the shapes seen with entopic phenomena, such as the ability to see retinal blood vessels, vitreous floaters, and the muscae volitantes. Although retinal vessels and floaters bear some resemblance to cobweb and amorphic form constants, they are fixed in appearance and can be seen or ignored at will. The muscae volitantes are the actual red blood corpuscles coursing through the vessels near the macula. Everyone should be able to see his own, particularly when looking at the sky or at a bright field of snow. The moving objects appears to travel in arcs or lines and then disappear (Scheerer, 1924). Many adults have opacities in the vitreous of the eye whose images may be projected into the environment. Traction of the vitreous or retina may give rise to sensations of light, arch-shaped and achromatic, called phosphenes (Moore, 1935). Some

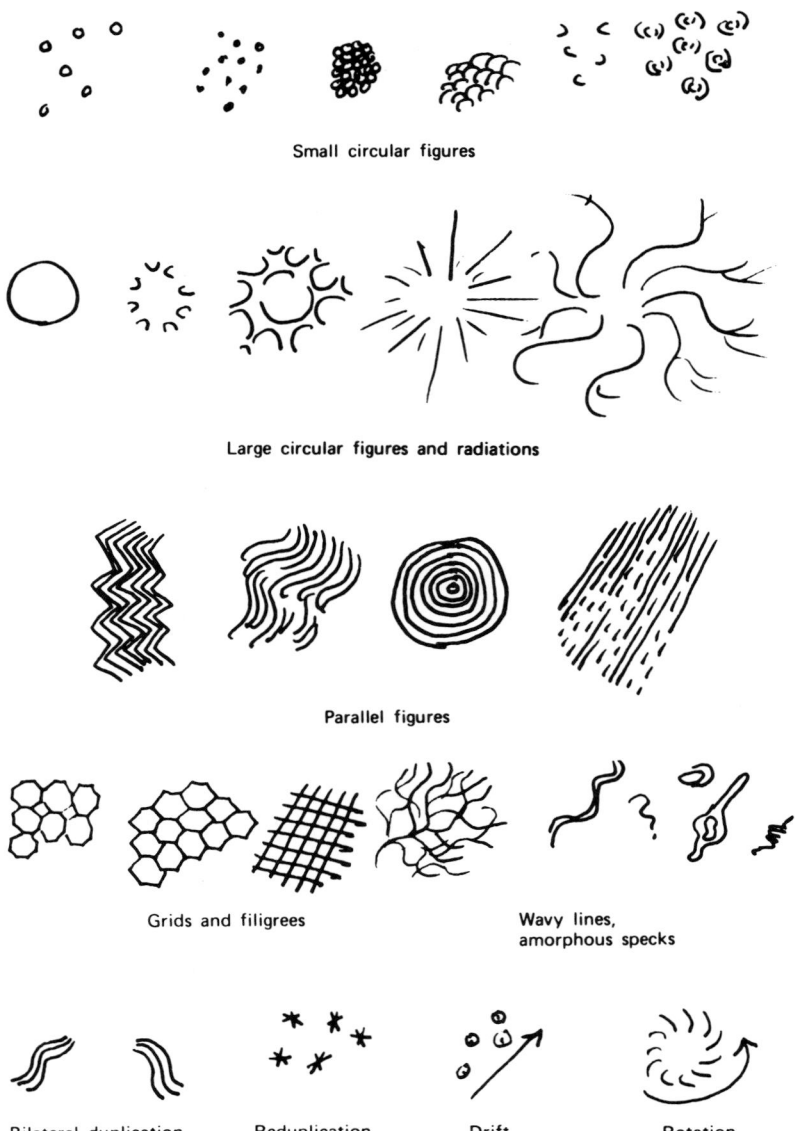

FIGURE 4.11. Generic shapes (Klüver's "form constants") are common to synesthesia, hallucinations, and imagery and can also be seen in primitive art, a finding that has led to speculation about the mind of ice age man. From M.J. Horowitz (1975). In *Hallucinations: Behavior, experience, and theory* (p. 179) edited by R.K. Siegel & L.J. West, 1975. New York: John Wiley & Sons. Copyright 1975 by M.J. Horowitz. Reprinted by permission.

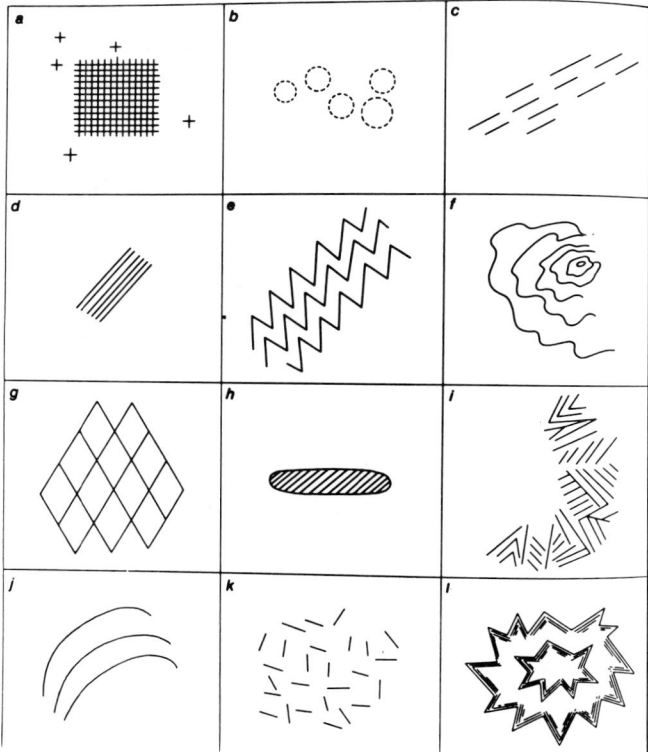

FIGURE 4.12. Eyes-open projected visual images in cocaine-induced hallucinations, showing the typical grid, lattice, and linear configurations featuring axial and radial symmetry. The circular figure in the lower right-hand corner is identical to the "fortification spectrum" seen during the aura phase of migraine. From "Hallucinations" by R.K. Siegel. Copyright © 1977 by Scientific American, Inc. All rights reserved.

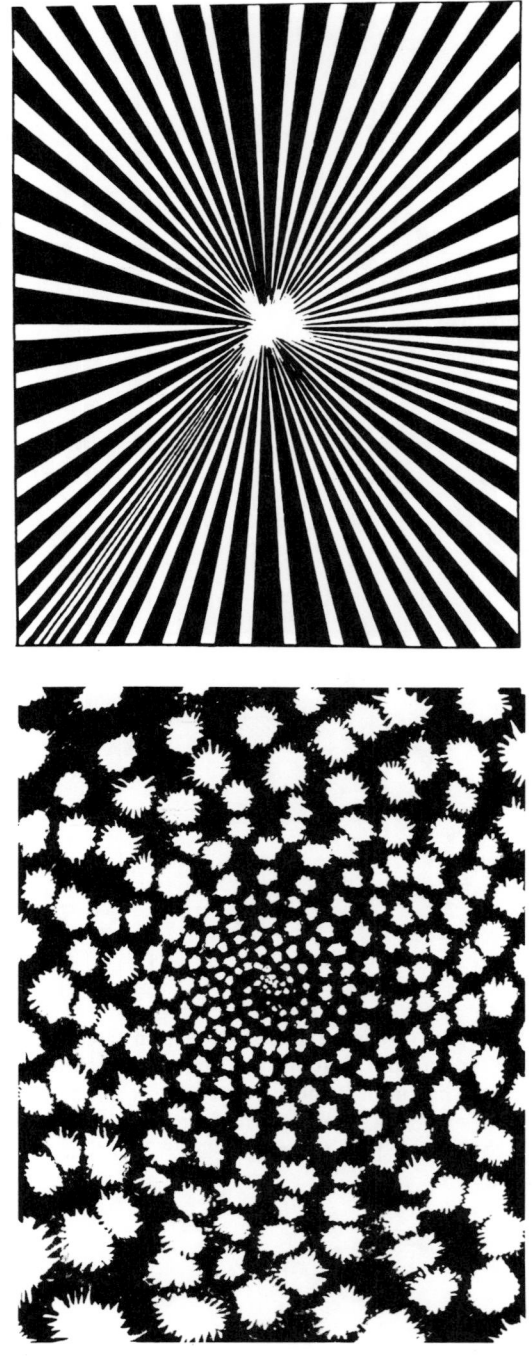

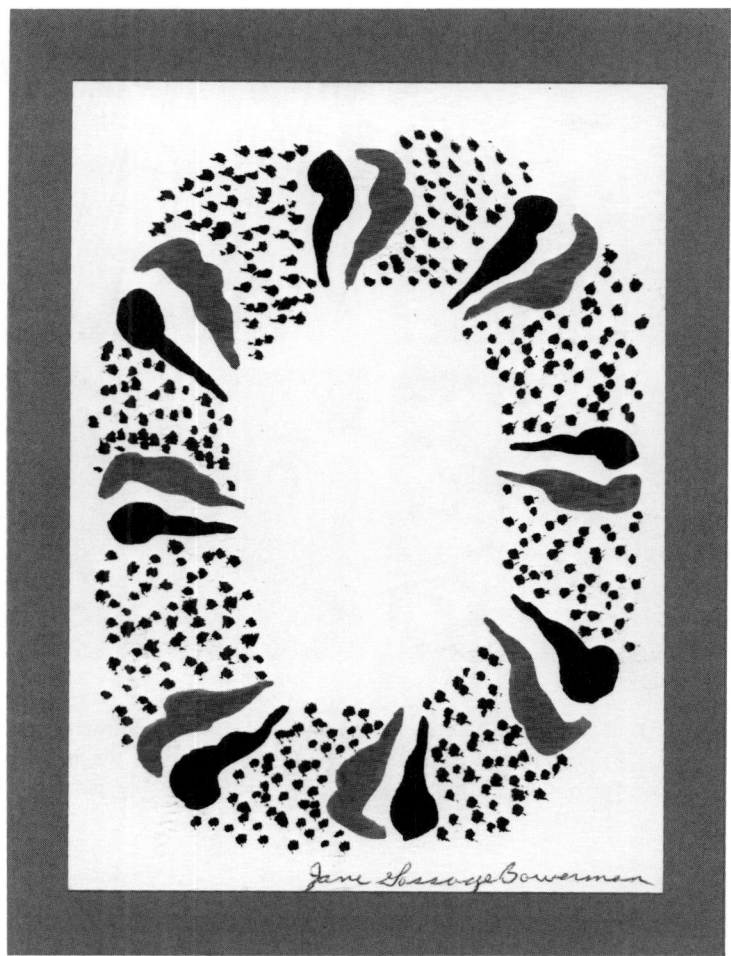

FIGURE 4.14. Christmas card by subject JB. This is a large circular radiation with radial symmetry and replication of amorphous blobs and both colored and black and white elements. Drawn from one of her spontaneous synesthesiae.

FIGURE 4.13. Tunnel form constant. *Top:* "Bright light" with explosion from the center to the periphery. The colors may change. *Bottom:* Spiral tunnel form constant, also with pulsation and rotation. Drawn by the patient from a drug-induced hallucination. From *Hallucinations: Behavior, experience, and theory* (pp. 116–117) by R.K. Siegel & L.J. West, 1975, New York: John Wiley & Sons. Copyright 1975 by R.K. Siegel & L.J. West. Reprinted by permission.

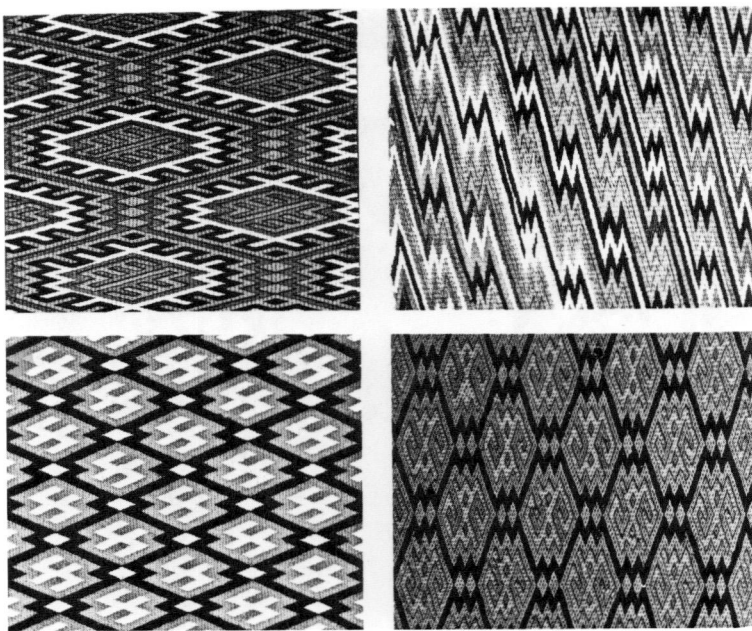

FIGURE 4.15. Four samples of Huichol Indian embroidery, showing geometric lattice forms. Lattice form constants are commonly found in the hallucinatory visions induced by peyote, a hallucinogen that holds a stable place in Indian culture.

individuals have a rare ability to see their retinal vessels and other ocular structures, and to produce a projected image of a cluster of balls or "geode," often in a bluish or purple color. Exactly what they are viewing is not clear, but it may be an elevation of the optic disk (Figure 4.16).

Klüver's analysis was a reaction to the vagueness that others interested in hallucinations and imagery had used for description. Klüver suggested that the novelty of the visions and vivid coloration captured the subject's attention more than the shape did, and that subjects often were overwhelmed by the "indescribable" nature of the vision and simply gave way to cosmic or religious explanations. The notion of form constants gained acceptance. "There are fewer mechanisms than etiologies of hallucinations. There is thus no reason for surprise if different precipitants give wholly or partly similar hallucinatory experiences" (Keeler, 1970). The tendency to attach supernatural meaning is now seen to be attributable to the referential nature of the perception along with its emotional content.

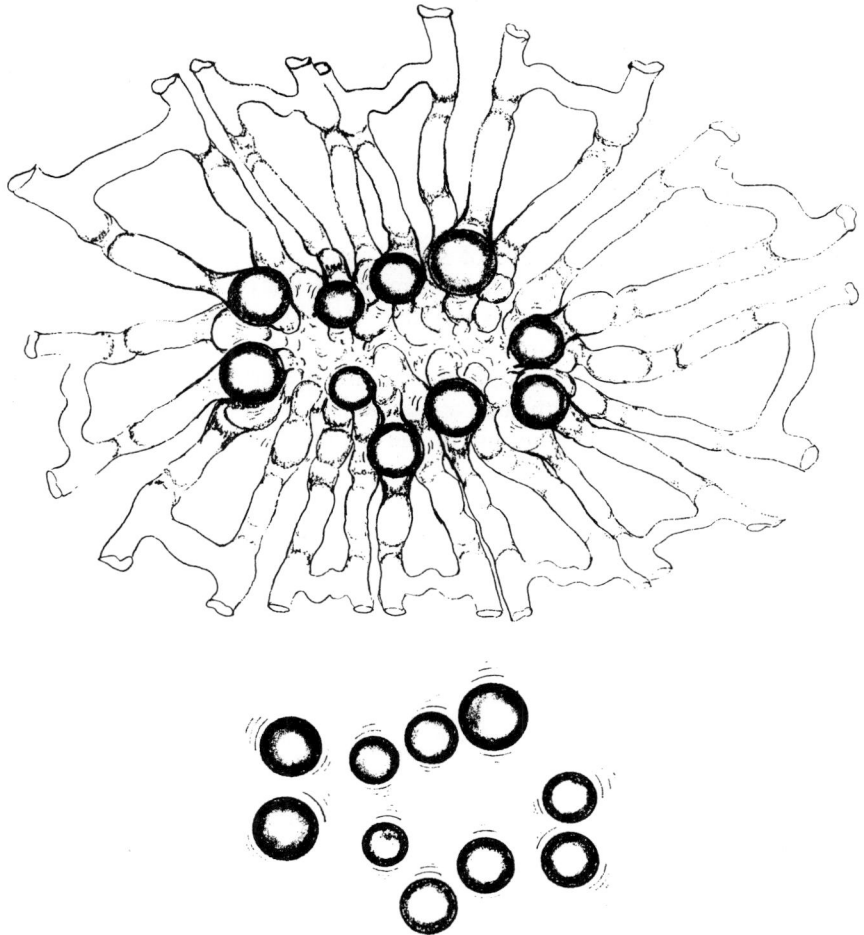

FIGURE 4.16. *Top:* Entopic phenomenon showing idealized retinal vessels with a visual effect of floating balls at the disk, projected externally. *Bottom:* The floating ball effect seen separately. A jiggling or shimmering movement is present. Because this is an entopic phenomenon, the balls move with eye movement, unlike the visual images in synesthesia and hallucination.

For example, Adler (1972) said that "to attach cosmic meaning to these events is a presumption. We are more likely confronting here the projection of affect onto the outside world. The response that one thinks he recognizes is his own projected and reflected image."

Conclusion

The discrete or generic nature of synesthetic percepts should be more understandable now that we have examined various perceptions that overlap with the synesthetic experience. The simplicity of the parallel synesthetic sense is consistent with an intermediate-level neural mechanism. The histories, experiential reports, and experimental data that are available are consistent with such a mechanism. In the next chapter I will look at the evolutionary anatomy of the mammalian brain and suggest a neural basis for synesthesia.

5
The Neural Substrates
of Synesthesia

Conceptualization of Neural Tissue

We progress to smaller systems. Theory and psychophysical mapping suggested a level of central nervous system (CNS) processing for synesthesia. An examination of similar phenomena indicated the anatomical site of the temporal-limbic region. We now consider what the neural basis of synesthesia might be.

Having considered how the senses might combine, we now ask the question in reverse and pose it anatomically. How does the brain physically separate the senses? Since all nervous systems have similar features, we can trace, generically, the phyletic developments in brain architecture by which discrete functions and aspects of sensation emerge out of a less specialized brain.

This chapter emphasizes selective anatomical facts and their functional consequences. At best, comprehending neuroanatomy is difficult; at worst, it is impossible. We will not get bogged down with the minutia of brain circuitry and wiring diagrams, but we will talk in detail about the functional organization of some cognitive functions. We assume that most readers have some understanding of how the brain is wired and have at least a traditional understanding of how it is organized functionally.

REVIEW OF NEUROANATOMY

Some fundamental anatomical facts are worth reviewing. For one thing, it will emphasize the gap that exists *between* what we understand about the anatomical facts (which is a lot) and the psychology of cognition (which is a lot, too). It is one thing to understand the physiology of nerve cells and even nerve networks, and yet another thing altogether to understand how the experience of sensation arises from the apparatus of the brain. The many brain subdivisions each have a characteristic architecture and circuitry and subserve specific functions. Yet the principles of neuronal function are remarkably similar in animals as far apart as the snail and man.

The human brain contains 10^{11} (100 billion) neurons and 10^{14} (100 trillion) synapses, give or take a factor of 10. A typical neuron has a cell body 5 to 100 micrometers in diameter from which emanates one major axon and a number of dendrites. The axon usually branches extensively near its end but may give off branches near its beginning. Generally, the dendrites and cell body receive incoming signals, the cell body averages these signals, and the axon distributes the information to a new set of neurons. Circuitry is not serial but richly cross-linked. Elements operate at low speeds of thousandths of a second.

Neuron processes are intertwined in a dense thicket with adjacent branches separated by fluid films only 0.2 micrometers thick. Virtually all the space is filled with cells and their various processes, a fact that has led to speculation that "cross-talk" or nonsynaptic transmission of information between two cells is possible, an idea that would be relevant to synesthesia. Yet connections are not random, a fact that makes arguments for atavism or "crossed wires" in synesthesia infeasible. Moreover, we do not conceive that a "thought" or "sensation" can occur at the level of only two cells. Rather, 10^4 or more cells probably participate in any unitary cognitive process.

CONCEPTUALIZATIONS OF NERVOUS TISSUE

Our conceptualization of nervous tissue has changed radically many times from that of an amorphous reticulum to a neuronal machine with intrinsic power modules raging a battle of excitation and inhibition. Nowhere is there uncontrolled excitation. Sensory receptors respond to either mechanical (touch, hearing), chemical (taste, smell), or electromagnetic (vision) energy. Regardless of the type of fiber, and whether the process concerned is movement, sensation, or thought, neural signals are virtually identical. There is little in the microstructure of nervous tissue to distinguish one sensory pathway from another. The only variables available to a nerve fiber are to fire or not fire, and the number of impulses per second.

Neurons are connected with a high degree of order and specificity. Conceptualization and "factual" observations of Camillo Golgi's day suggested that nervous tissue was an amorphous net (Golgi, 1883, 1884). Santiago Ramón y Cajal's neuron theory (1911) showed that the neuron was the basic unit of nervous tissue. Their rivalry over conceptualization of nervous tissue was still intense when Golgi and Ramón y Cajal shared the Nobel prize in 1906. Lorente de No (1943) discovered the arrangement of vertical chains of neurons throughout the depth of cortex (which is only 1 to 3 millimeters thick) in addition to the six major layers of horizontal lamination.

Physiological investigations by Mountcastle (1957; Mountcastle & Powell, 1959) and Hubel and Wiesel (1962, 1968, 1972) showed that neurons in tiny columns orthogonal to the cortical surface responded similarly to highly specific afferent inputs. These columns for feature detection are sharply defined, with an average cross-section of 0.1 square millimeter. Szentagothai (1969, 1972, 1974; Szentagothai & Arbib, 1975) showed the structural basis for the "modular" organization of these neuronal columns. The column is a complex organization of specific cell types, and in both structure and function of all cortical areas, the column or module was conceived of as the basic unit. The basic circuit of the module is afferent fiber input; complex interactions within the module; and output channel through the axons of the pyramidal cells. There are major functional differences between the connectivities in laminae I and II and those of laminae III, IV, and V (Szentagothai, 1972).

The modular concept is of well-defined groups of cells (approximately 10,000) with a unitary existence as a result of their mutual connections. They build up power within themselves and inhibit the cells of columns nearby. There are two levels of performance, a powerful one in laminae III, IV, and V involving specific afferents and pyramidal output, and a finer grain of influence in laminae I and II, which is exerted mainly by association and callosal afferent fibers (Szentagothai, 1974). Eccles (Popper & Eccles, 1977) summarized the concept of a module as a power unit:

Its *raison d'etre* is to build up power at the expense of its neighbours. We think the nervous system always works by conflict—in this case by conflicts between each module and the adjacent modules. Each one is trying to overcome the other one by building up its own power by all the vertical connections which Ramon y Cajal and Lorente de No first described and by the projection of inhibition out to the neighboring modules. That functional discriminatory action is really what makes a module. A module is a unit because it has a system of internal power generation and around it is the delimitation secured by its inhibitory action on the adjacent modules (p. 243).

How has conceptualization of neural tissue and the way it functions changed over a single century? The amorphous network yielded to the hierarchical view in which commands from "higher centers" were carried out by less complex brain systems. Parcellation and mapping by cytoarchitectonics followed—the division of all regions of the cortex based on variation of number or type of cell, packing density, or degree and temporal sequence of myelination of the intrinsic or extrinsic connecting nerve fibers. Some scientists believed that each minute and distinct area was a separate cerebral organ that functioned independently of its neighbors, a point not argued seriously for 60 years.

The functional consequence of minute mapping is that each brain region was regarded as functionally unique. It seems that Aristotle was right: the senses were not only philosophically separate, but here was the proof of their physical separateness. This knowledge of multiple specialization was of course not known to those examining synesthesia in the 18th and

19th centuries. This appreciation of neural geography was also not of much use to later investigators, who were psychologists and not neurologists.

It is not easy for the nonspecialist or interested lay person to reconcile changing conceptualizations of nervous tissue. No doubt this is how popular conceptions are so often oversimplified or just plain wrong. Polar thinking led us to assume that one model has to replace another. Yet each contains some amount of truth and one organization is not necessarily mutually exclusive of another. The hierarchical view of the 19th century, which stemmed from Hughlings Jackson and Sherrington, was based on evolutionary theory and held that the brain develops in phylogeny by the successive additions to existing structures. A regulation, if not dominance, of the more primitive and caudal parts is explicit in this view. Dissolution of this hierarchy is revealed by focal disease of the brain in humans or by severing of pathways in animals. This hierarchical view influenced brain research well into the 1950s but is now transcended by conceptualization of the unit module and the distributed system, a concept that sees the brain as a complex of widely and reciprocally interconnected dynamic systems (Mountcastle, 1979).

The Distributed System

The distributed system shows that there is nothing unique about the structure of one region versus another, nothing inherently motor about the motor cortex nor sensory about the sensory cortices. Rather it is the pattern of connections of entities, which can belong to several distributed systems and onto which multiple variables can be mapped, that constitutes the distributed system. This idea of multiple mapping is what we will examine in relationship to synesthesia.

The classical reticular, nuclear, and laminar divisions such as the reticular formation, dorsal horn, basal ganglia, and neocortex are referred to as "entities" and are themselves composed of local circuits that are similar within any given entity (Szentagothai, 1972, 1974). Modules are grouped into entities (e.g., nuclei or cortical regions) by virtue of their specific external connections, by their intermodular interactions, or by cloning a common function over a topographic region. The function of modules is everywhere the same. As we said, there is nothing specifically motor about the motor cortex nor sensory about sensory cortices.

Phylogenetically, the neocortex of primates achieved its enormous size with hardly any change in its vertical organization, one feature that led the vertical minicolumn to be regarded as the basic modular unit. This 30×25-micrometer cylinder is a cord of cells, perpendicular to the brain surface, formed as neurons migrate from the germinal epithelium of the neural tube along the radial glial cells to their destined locations in the cortex (Rakic, 1971, 1972, 1974, 1975, 1978). The nervous system forms from the inside out.

Rockel, Hiorns, and Powell (1974) found an invariant 110 cells in each minicolumn of five different neocortical areas in different species of mammals, except for the striate cortex, where the number is 260. The number of pyramidal and stellate cells, the two main classes of neurons, maintains a constant ratio of 2 : 1 in such diverse cytoarchitectonic and functional areas as motor, somatic, and visual areas of different mammals (Gatter, Winfield, & Powell, 1977; Sloper, 1973; Tömböl, 1974). Mount-castle (1979) thinks that it is unlikely that wholly new cell types that are unique to other brains, including more primitive ones, have appeared at any particular stage of mammalian evolution.

Several hundred minicolumns join to form larger processing units, called cortical columns, onto which several variables can be mapped. The human neocortex contains about 1 million of these larger processing columns.

Several features from the old hierarchical theory as well as the extensive subdivision of the cytoarchitectonists can be incorporated in the present conception of the distributed system. There are distinct cortical areas that can be homologized over a series of mammals, and each region of distinct cytoarchitecture has a unique function (in the conventional sense). Moreover, each neocortical area that has a distinct cytoarchitecture and function also has a unique set of extrinsic connec-tions (that is, its own pattern of thalamic, corticocortical inter-hemispheric, and long descending connections). These three variables of cytoarchitecture, extrinsic connections, and function define a cortical area.

A cortical column is a complex processing and distributing unit that links a number of inputs to *several* outputs. The number of other regions transmitting to and receiving from a traditionally defined cortical area varies from 10 to 30. The cells of origin of different output pathways are sharply separated by cortical layer.

One great advantage of the distributed system is that several variables can be simultaneously mapped onto it while preserving the topology of the area. A large number of variables can be mapped through a given area with preservation of ordered relationships between sets on the source side, those within the area, and those in the target region. Thus, a number of distributed systems can be mapped through a given area of cortex, allowing an integration of their functions with properties of that area determined by some different input to it. Divergent intercolumnar path-ways to different outputs allow selective processing (feature extraction).

The concept of columnar organization does not preclude other systems from working in the cortex in different ways, particularly those that subserve state functions rather than channel functions. The noradrenergic system arising from the locus ceruleus of the pons reaches every cortical region and every cortical layer (Molliver, Grazanna, Morrison, & Coyle, 1977; Moore and Bloom, 1977). Immunohistochemical methods show a fine web of noradrenergic fibers at 30- to 40-micrometer intervals such that any single cell of the locus ceruleus sustains an immense and divergent axonal field. The noradrenergic system is capable of influencing directly every cell of the neocortex.

The functional properties of distributed systems have been elucidated through three sets of discoveries (Mountcastle, 1979). First is the fact that the major structures are constructed by replication of identical multicellular units linked together by complex intermodular connectivity. The basic unit is the vertical minicolumn, which is packed into hundreds of members to form larger processing units called neuronal columns. Second, extrinsic connections between large entities of the brain are far more numerous, selective, and specific than previously supposed. Third, each one of the modules of a large entity does not contain all the connections known for that entity. The large entity is split into subsets of modules, each linked by a particular pattern of connections to similarly segregated subsets in other large entities. The linked sets of modules of the several entities thus define the distributed system.

In contrast with older theories of brain organization, the number of distributed systems in the brain is perhaps several orders of magnitude larger than previously thought. By both definition and observation, the distributed systems are both reentrant pathways and linkages to inflow and outflow channels of the entire nervous systems. Major entities are nodes of more than one distributed system, contributing to each system "a property determined for the entity by those connections common to all of its modular subsets and by the particular quality of their intrinsic processing. Even a single module of such an entity may be a member of several (though not many) distributed systems" (Mountcastle, 1979). The fact of multiple mapping is most relevant to synesthesia, and examples follow below.

Topological Organization

Anatomy underlies but does not itself explain behavior. There are two sides to the equation. If one wants to understand what is happening in synesthesia, one must understand how the brain is organized, not only for sensation but for language, emotion, and other cognitive functions. One must think about organizing the CNS, not just the neocortex, in a way that describes behavior. Various authors have attempted this, and the comments here are naturally highly selective and reflect my personal bias. As we conceptualize different schemes of organization, we can ask, "Where is there an opportunity for derivatives of sensation to join that is compatible with the facts and theory of synesthesia?"

Cognitive "functions" and functional "systems" do not work independently of other "systems" of the brain. No reasonable theory of the activity of any cognitive module or brain system can be developed until a more general understanding of the brain's activities is achieved. Neurobiologists work under the assumption that they can understand the brain, and for the moment they are doing well. But the word "understand" implies a sudden revelation, a moment when all is clear and comprehensible. It is not clear that there can be such a moment nor that we will know it when it comes. Yet the human mind hungers for a theoretical structure to help understand the myriad facts. Because of such a need, hydraulic theories, telephone switchboard theories, hardware-software analogies, parallel distributed processing supercomputation constructs, wavefront theories, and holographic models have all been advocated. The triune brain of Paul MacLean is such a model. All of these are only metaphors taken from other contexts and applied to brain theory. As long as they are not mistaken for fact, metaphors are extremely useful.

One current fashion is to look at patterns in behavioral neuroanatomy. The classic emphasis has been on cytoarchitectonic organization that emphasizes the uniqueness of regions. In all schemes, whether the cytoarchitectonic maps of Brodmann, Exner, or von Economo, some regions are clearly associated with specific functions while others are "silent." Bearing in mind what we have said about modules and distributed systems, topological organization stresses common characteristics of a region. Topology bears the same relationship to topography as geology does to geography. It means a science of place, a qualitative geometry. Functional correlates of topology and architectonics as they relate to synesthesia and other sensory aspects is our concern here. A broad review of the macroscopic and microscopic topology onto which behavior can be mapped is not possible here but can be found in the first chapter of Mesulam (1985) or other standard texts. Some knowledge on the part of the reader is assumed.

The topological approach shows that the cortical mantle can be divided into only five common types that display a progressive increase in structural complexity and differentiation. Figure 5.1 shows this topological schema and Figure 5.2 shows the topological regions mapped onto the conventional Brodmann areas.

As Figure 5.2 graphically shows, the functional topological zones overlap the conventional cytoarchitectonic regions widely. There is no direct interaction between the primary sensory areas for somasthesis, vision, and hearing, yet interaction obviously occurs when, for example, we identify an object felt with an object seen. We conceive that identification must occur in some system to where the primary areas project. The conventional view would hypothesize that synesthesia is localizable to that region of the cortex where somasthesis, audition, and vision come together in a tertiary association area (Brodmann areas 39 and 40). The topological view, as represented by Figure 5.1, takes us away from considering primary sensory- or modality-specific association areas as the neural real estate for synesthesia unless one endorses the

EXTRAPERSONAL   SPACE

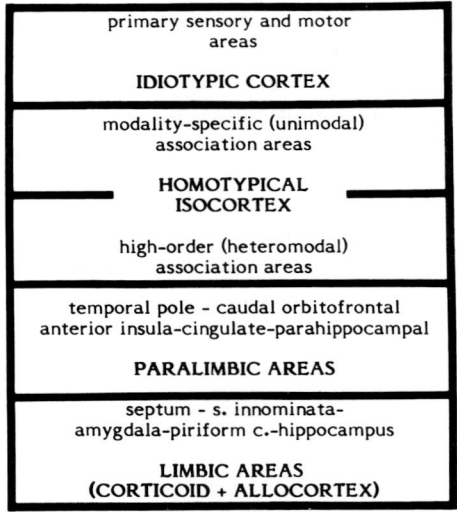

HYPOTHALAMUS
INTERNAL   MILIEU

FIGURE 5.1. Topological cortical regions in the human. See text for further details. From *Principles of behavioral neurology* (p. 8) by M-M. Mesulam, 1985. Philadelphia: F.A. Davis Co. Reprinted by permission.

notion of cross-talk or nonsynaptic transfer of information. Likewise the heteromodal association areas are not likely candidates given the results of regional cerebral blood flow studies and related considerations discussed in Chapter 4. Consider also that the neocortex is not necessary for many forms of auditory, visual, or somasthetic discrimination (e.g., Diamond & Neff, 1957; Weiskrantz, 1980, 1986). The quintessential ability of the neocortex is to efficiently process information that has too many fine details to be easily handled by simpler and evolutionarily earlier brain systems. What the topological scheme does, however, is suggest that the separation of derivative aspects of sensation occurs further downstream and that there is the opportunity for these derivatives— color, directional movement, linearity, shape, texture, temperature—to combine in the paralimbic or limbic areas. Furthermore, it is here that the autonomic responses could join in to give the pleasurable sense that synesthetes experience in their parallel sensation. The limbic system also provides the sense of conviction that they experience is real and occurring outside in the world in limb space.

In Chapter 1 I articulated the romantic notion, which I do not hold with strong commitment, that synesthesia is a fundamentally mammalian characteristic. My ideas are based on structural topology that leads to general principles about the distribution of neural connectivity and the distribution of behavioral specialization throughout the brain. They are also based on an awareness that the brain of man resembles the brain of "lower" animals much more than it differs from them (Sarnat & Netsky, 1981). My metaphor is that synesthesia represents a fundamental quality of sensation. However, this point cannot be argued satisfactorily until synesthesia becomes localized with certainty and neuroanatomists finally agree on a definition of the limbic system. More will be said later when commenting on MacLean's triune brain.

PHYLETIC DEVELOPMENT THEORY

Consider now the point of view of phyletic development from the same basic blueprint from which all vertebrate brains develop. This represents a very traditional view peppered with evolutionary theory that is usually put forth to illustrate fundamental advances in brain function. As one ascends the phylogentic scale there is an increasing separation not only of the senses but of all cognitive functions during the process where discrete functions emerge out of a less specialized brain. In man functions become not only separate but lateralized as well between the hemispheres as the brain develops the capacity for multiple specialization.

In simple organisms, little or no plasticity in behavior is possible. The brains of lower animals tend to react immediately to the stimuli in their environment with a simple, unvarying program of behavior. These are unthinking brains that, because of their small size, have little room for flexible responses or for joining information from several senses.

For example, the hydra or sea anemone (phylum Cnidaria, class Anthozoa) has a largely reticular nervous system. Neuroepithelial cells located at intervals on the body surface make direct connections with underlying muscle cells. If you poke the animal, as a marine aquarist knows, stimulating one cell stimulates all of them and the animal recoils and closes up. This simple reflex arc between sensor-effector has been replaced in higher organisms by a series of interneurons interposed between the sensory and effector cells. More advanced animals such as the crown jellyfish (Ctenophora) or tube worm (Phoronida) retain the reticular nerve net throughout their bodies. It provides undulating movements to direct food to the mouth. Isolated conduction in a separate ring of neurons around the rim of the umbrella causes the synchronous contraction of the marginal lappets by which the jellyfish swims and the tube worm withdraws into its tube. One now finds conduction of a nervous impulse over a distance without interfering with all the neighbor-

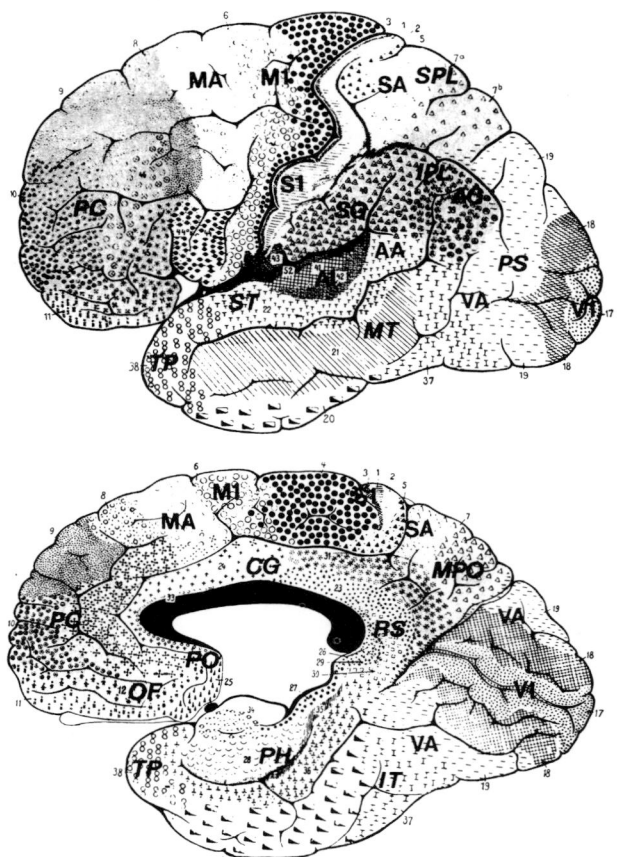

FIGURE 5.2. *Left:* Brodmann's cytoarchitectonic map of the left hemisphere of the human brain in lateral (*top*) and medial (*bottom*) views. Numbers indicate the various areas as originally mapped by Brodmann. Compare with Figure 5.2 *right* (opposite page). From *Principles of behavioral neurology* (p. 9) by M-M. Mesulam, 1985. Philadelphia: F.A. Davis Co.

ing cells (that is, it does not stimulate the reticulum). This separation of the reticular system from the conducting ring system represents a fundamental advance. An analogy could be drawn to the separate human pathways serving channel and state functions. It is in the great proliferation of these intercalated neurons (interneurons) that central nervous systems of higher organisms have evolved and, with their appearance, a corresponding plasticity of behavior.

Flechsig's (1901) principle states that the primary receptive areas have no direct neocortical connections except with adjacent association areas

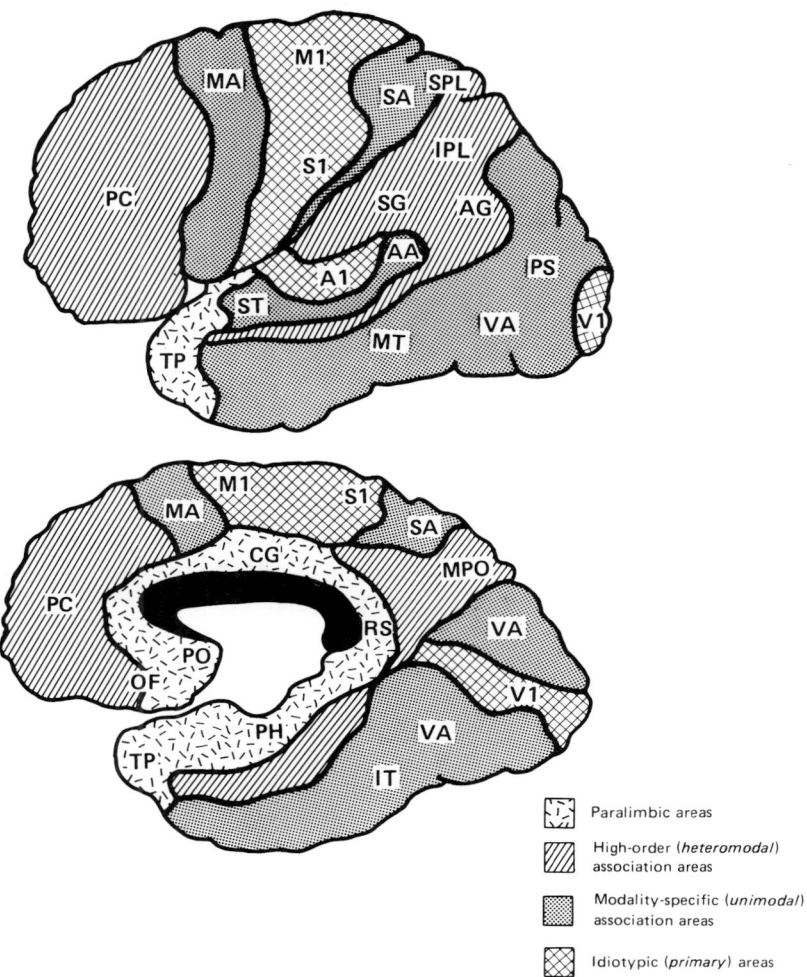

FIGURE 5.2. *Right:* Distribution of topological and functional zones in relation to Brodmann's map. Boundaries are not precise. *Key: AA,* auditory association cortex; *AG,* angular gyrus; *A1,* primary auditory cortex; *CG,* cingulate cortex; *INS,* insula; *IPL,* inferior parietal lobule; *IT,* inferior temporal gyrus; *MA,* motor association cortex; *MPO,* medial parieto-occipital area; *MI,* middle temporal gyrus; *M1,* primary motor area; *OF,* orbitofrontal region; *PC,* prefrontal cortex; *PH,* parahippocampal region; *PO,* parolfactory area; *PS,* peristriate cortex; *RS,* retrosplenial area; *SA,* somatosensory association cortex; *SG,* supra-marginal gyrus; *SPL,* superior parietal lobule; *ST,* superior temporal gyrus; *S1,* ´primary somatosensory area; *TP,* temporopolar cortex; *VA,* visual association cortex; *V1,* primary visual cortex. From *Principles of behavioral neurology* (p. 9) by M-M. Mesulam, 1985. Philadelphia: F.A. Davis Co.

(Bailey & Bonin, 1951; Geschwind, 1965a, 1965b). These primary areas also have no callosal connections nor any significant connections with other parts of neocortex in the same hemisphere (R.E. Myers, 1962). There are indirect and subcortical pathways, however, such as thalamic projections going to specific afferents, and primary receptive areas sending long fibers to subcortical regions, such as collicular projections from striate cortex (Geschwind, 1965a, p. 243; Popper & Eccles, 1977, p. 322; Trevarthen & Sperry, 1973). As we ascend the phylogenetic scale, anatomical evidence indicates that association fibers may arise from primary projections areas. With increasing phylogenetic complexity these connections are probably transferred to newly developed association areas (Geschwind, for one, argues this). That is, they do not appear de novo but are elaborations of parts of the projection cortex. One conclusion, of course, is that some of the more primitive connections that join primordial zones persist in higher forms, and therefore explain some synesthetic perception. On the evolutionary scale, the gradual process of separation of association areas from primary projection areas is probably a later stage of a process in which the primary motor and sensory areas (and also later projection areas) became individuated out of a less specialized brain, such as the sea anemone and jellyfish.

The argument is then developed that as we ascend the phylogenetic scale, the associative activities become separated from the receptive ones and cytoarchitectonic differentiation increases. Patterns of cells and patterns of connectivity become sharply demarcated from one another. Table 5.1 shows such an organization. Figures 5.1 and 5.2 show the ultimate development of this kind of complexity. Topographic relationships among individual cortical types is highly ordered and highly regular. Paralimbic cortex is always flanked by allocortex at one extreme and by isocortex on the other, while unimodal association cortex is always found between primary sensory areas and heteromodal cortex. It is from these constant relationships that one can draw principles about the organization of neural connectivity and the distribution of specialized behavior.

The phyletic point of view leads to an interesting paradox, however, as far a synesthesia is concerned. That paradox involves multiple representation. Ever since Sherrington and Grünbaum (1902) demonstrated in

TABLE 5.1. Theoretical increasing separation of function as one ascends the evolutionary scale (such a concept concludes that synesthesia cannot exist in humans).

Species	Developmental feature
↑ Humans	↑ Separation of primary projection areas
Primates	Development of association cortex
Mammals	Multiple specialization and parcellation of areas
Marsupials	Overlap of primordial zones

anthropoid apes that the central fissure demarcates the "precentral" motor area that lies in front of it, and since Cushing (1909) demonstrated in humans that a "postcentral" sensory area lies behind it, one can demonstrate a dividing line identical to the central fissure in all placental mammals. This dividing line was confirmed with the development of detailed electrical mapping of sensory areas. Woolsey (1952) then showed that the organization of the sensory area behind the central fissure is a mirror image of the motor area in front. The existence of two spatially separate areas, each with its own function, is a basic tenent of neuroscience.

However, there is considerable overlap of motor and sensory areas in marsupials such as the opossum or wallaby (*Thylogale eugenii*, a small member of the kangaroo family) (Lende, 1963). In cats and some primates, one can attach an electrode to what is supposed to be a visual neuron and discover that it also responds to sound or touch (Buser & Imbert, 1961; Horn, 1965; MacLean, 1970, 1975; Murata, Cramer, & Bach-y-Rita, 1965). Multimodal cells are also found in subcortical regions such as the caudate and red nuclei (Fessard, 1961), the cuneate nucleus (Atweh, Banna, Jabbur, & Tómey, 1974), and the trigeminal nucleus (Dubner, 1967). Other examples of multimodal cells are given on page 107. These multimodal cells are like the inverse of a feature detection neuron (a cell that responds only to highly specific features of the environment). Cellular response is not all-or-nothing, however. It is a question of degree that a cell that is interested in color or a particular feature responds robustly to a specific modality and not very much to other kinds of stimulation. That supposedly modality-specific cells will respond to other modalities would seem to be the essence of synesthesia. One could develop the argument and assume that there is a range of performance in humans such that cellular modules that "aren't supposed to respond" to certain things do in fact respond, hence synesthesia. Multiple representation of different senses does exist according to the experience of cell recording. My point is that the lines are not drawn as sharply as dogma says they are, even though the evolutionary trend is clearly for increasing separation of function. This seeming difficulty can be explained by the fact that although cytoarchitectonic differentiation increases the later one travels on the phylogenetic scale, the most important connections of association cortex are with the neocortex of the temporal lobe, which in turn feeds into limbic structures. Connections with any *one* sensory modality and the limbic system tend to be powerful in their arousal of emotional and autonomic responses, whereas nonlimbic sensory-sensory connections are weaker in this regard.

In summary, the phyletic and topographic view leads to the conclusion that there is an increasing separation of function and that synesthesia should therefore not exist in man, who presumably represents the most differentiated species. At the same time, there is the paradox of multiple representation of function. This is best illustrated by the clinical example of achromatopsia, a type of modular processing that has particular relevance since color figures so prominently in synesthesia.

Achromatopsia

Students of classical neurology, psychology, and even physiology labored under the notion that the neural equipment of vision was organized in a series of steps such that the features of vision were extracted in a gradual process. One step led to another, and somehow the different properties of vision that were identified in traditional psychology, such as shape, vision, stereopsis, and motion, were extracted together. Everything was concurrent at the retina, lateral geniculate, and cortex, and somehow features would be successively extracted in a cascade of operations that were sequentially linked. There was supposed to be a togetherness of function.

That idea is no longer tenable. The way the brain extracts these properties is now conceived of as parallel. There are multiple representations of these different properties that we assemble in a beautiful illusion called vision. These representations correspond to different operations at different levels of the brain.

INFERIOR CALCARINE LESIONS AND ACHROMATOPSIA

Occlusion of the posterior cerebral artery causes infarction of the visual cortices on the medial aspect of the occipital pole. This involves primary as well as association cortices (areas 17, 18, and 19). Such a patient (or animal) has a homonymous hemianopia, a completely blind hemifield. In lesions entirely below the horizontal calcarine fissure, area 17 has not been damaged either in the lower or upper lip of the calcarine fissure (Damasio, 1985). The optic radiations are intact, so visual information can arrive undamaged at the primary visual cortex and be available to a variety of other cortices for processing. Such a patient has hemiachromatopsia, an acquired loss of color perception in the contralateral field. Yet such patients can, in the contralateral field, perceive shape perfectly. They can even read.

One finds this remarkable dissociation between the ability to process color and the ability to process shape and a variety of computations that come out of shape such as stereopsis, motion detection, depth, and texture. We know since the time of Holmes (1918, 1919) that the visual field is retinotopically represented in the inferior and superior calcarine cortices. That is, there is a point-to-point correspondence. The inferior field is represented superiorly, the superior field inferiorly, right maps left, and vice versa. Yet we have just described a lesion in association cortex entirely below the calcarine fissure producing a vertical defect in color covering the entire hemifield! The color system is obviously eccentrically distributed!

To such a patient, the world looks like a television picture whose color is turned down. Once an object crosses the vertical meridian, the grayish hues become normally colored (Damasio et al., 1980). Patients do have *some* chroma left but complain that the colors are washed out, dirty, or pale. Compare this to the colors of synesthetes, who, like JM for instance, say that their colors are often pastel or only tints (Chapter 2).

The anatomical lesion causing achromatopsia is inferiorly placed in the occipitotemporal association cortex, involving the fusiform and lingual gyrii (Damasio, 1985; Dejerine, 1892; Verrey, 1888). Visual discrimination for shape is preserved in the colorless field because the superior calcarine cortex and the optic radiations remain intact. Some studies suggest that defects of color perception are more common in the right hemisphere (Assai, Eisert, & Hecaen, 1969; De Renzi & Faglioni, 1967; F. Lhermitte, Chain, Aron, Leblanc, & Jouty, 1969; Scotti & Spinnler, 1970). Damasio (1985) believes this conclusion is not justified. However, the right hemisphere may very well process color differently than the left. Confounding this issue is the fact that unilateral right hemisphere lesions may less often come to clinical attention; patients with left hemisphere or bilateral lesions usually have prosopagnosis, alexia (Damasio & Damasio, 1983), visual agnosia, or blindness for both shape and color in the affected field. Thus, they are more likely to come to medical attention. The point is intriguing since I have suggested that synesthesia resides in the left hemisphere. Unfortunately, no further conclusions can be drawn at this time.

Experience tells us that we are able to perceive minute differences in color. How do we do this?

SUPERIOR CALCARINE LESIONS AND SPATIAL DISORIENTATION

Patients with superior occipital lesions have a different kind of problem than patients with inferior lesions. Patients with superior calcarine lesions have a severe disturbance in their construction of space while retaining normal reading, color, and recognition of shape and faces. What they do see is not properly placed in the three-dimensional Euclidean space that we believe we have around us. Objects appear to be broken, with one part sliding over another or distorted in some way (this is metamorphospia). They may lose the object and have to search for it in the visual field after it disappears on them abruptly. In general, the inferior cortices are in general directed toward object vision, deriving a very fine description of the type that will allow us to interface with previously stored memories. The superior visual cortices are interested in the construction of space around us, and in placing that particular object in space according to given coordinates. The more local level in the construction of the multiple dimensionality of an object (e.g., the multiple dimensions of a face) may be in part dependent on some of these finer appreciations of space. One can say that the lower part of the visual system is interested in *what* is out there and how to describe it, while the superior part of the visual system is interested in *where what is* (Levine, Warach, & Farah, 1985; Rizzo & Hurtig, 1987). It is interested in placement in space. Thus, Euclidian space can be dissociated from object vision as well. Apropos of this, the interesting spatial maps of subject CS are described in Chapter 7.

We can see from these examples of inferior and superior calcarine lesions how information from the retina remains retinotopic until area 17, the primary visual cortex. Segregation begins immediately beyond that, where the job of doing this or that is farmed out to different cortical areas. The job of analyzing whatever it takes to give us the experience of color goes in one direction. The many things that constitute shape and lead to the description of an object, or the description of a space where that object is inserted, will be handled somewhere else.

Thus, there is not only a breakdown of continuity the minute information arrives at area 17 but also a breakdown of the neat arrangement that corresponds to the world as we think it is out there impinging on our retinas. The world becomes multiply mapped in a very peculiar arrangement in the visual system. The cubists, it seems, were right.

I will mention briefly here that the art of aphasics, like that of psychotics, unmasks a cognitive style in which *form is altered* (Arnheim, 1986; Bader & Navratil, 1976; Cocteau, Schmidt, Steck, & Bader, 1961; Prinzhorn, 1919, 1922, 1972). Jason Brown (1977), the proponent of microgenetic theory, has a collection of paintings done by aphasics, and argues that aphasia is a cognitive disorder and not just a linguistic one. The drawing of a conduction aphasic, for example, shows problems with perspective, foreground, and background, and yet shows reasonably intact drawing skills. As one penetrates more deeply into this system, one can appreciate the cognitive style or mood as revealed by the changes in the patient's art.

In creating a visual rendering of the Cowboy story, for example, there is a tendency toward a purely ornamental style with excessive details. This is a quite common feature in the breakdown of art in schizophrenic patients. The elements are all there but the excessive ornamentation gives the drawing a dreamlike rendering.

Brown's point is that aphasias tap levels in cognition and that there is a kind of cognitive aura around every aphasic disorder. There is not just a language module in the back of the brain, but a cognitive module that spills over into level-specific areas of cognition. Aphasia is just the most prominent symptom. The reader should bear this idea in mind when examining the personality of synesthetes in Chapter 7.

ANALYSIS OF COLOR

Color is the psychophysical combination of chroma (hue) saturation (density of chroma), and luminance (brightness). These three dimensions, which can be selectively disassociated, enable us to perceive 10^6 colors. What is it that is disrupted when we lose color perception? The reader may wish to refer to Figure 5.2 during the following discussion.

Rizzo (1988; Rizzo, Kritchevsky, & Damasio, 1986) reported a patient with a right hemisphere lesion below and above the calcarine fissure and a left hemisphere lesion in association cortex (18 and 19) below the calcarine fissure. The patient had a left homonymous hemianopia but a patent right visual field that was achromatopic. In the right hemiachromatopic field his colors were drained out but the patient could read, discriminate shape, and detect motion. (He also had prosopagnosia, a typical combination of such bilateral lesions.) Rizzo studied chroma and luminance and found that in the achromatopic field the patient had normal luminance and normal saturation, but defective chroma (hue). Such patients have a selective disturbance of chroma in the absence of saturation and luminance defects.

There is excellent evidence in animals that the color system is segregated in areas 17 and 18, and continues to be segregated as late as V4 (in the lunate sulcus) (Baizer, Robinson, & Dow, 1977; Van Essen, Maunsell, & Bixby, 1981; Zeki, 1973, 1977). V4 represents the peripheral part of association cortex in monkeys. This may be partly homologous to the most peripheral part of the visual association area in man. Microelectrode recordings show that in V4 there are a large number of cells that respond to color above all other qualities, and the distribution of color-sensitive cells is highly selective. These cell columns consistently respond to certain bands of the spectrum.

Hubel (1982; Livingstone & Hubel, 1984) discovered sets of cells in areas 17 and 18 of the monkey that are unequivocally associated with color processing. They are packed in areas called "the blobs" because of their spatial arrangement. An electrode penetration in the area of the blobs shows them to respond only to color and not to edge, orientation, contrast, or other derivatives. They do not respond to an edge, an angle, or a line orientation, which means that they do not participate in the kinds of detections that would be useful for spatial computation or derivatives of shape. However, the cells in the interblob areas respond strongly to shape and orientation, but little to color. At 17 (V1), corresponding to the calcarine fissure in man, one finds a marked division between the cellular packets that are interested in color and those that are interested in shape. Moreover, the arrangement of those cells is peculiar. The kind of geniculate input that those cells receive is different, as can be traced with horseradish peroxidase. The pattern continues into area 18 (see Figure 5.3).

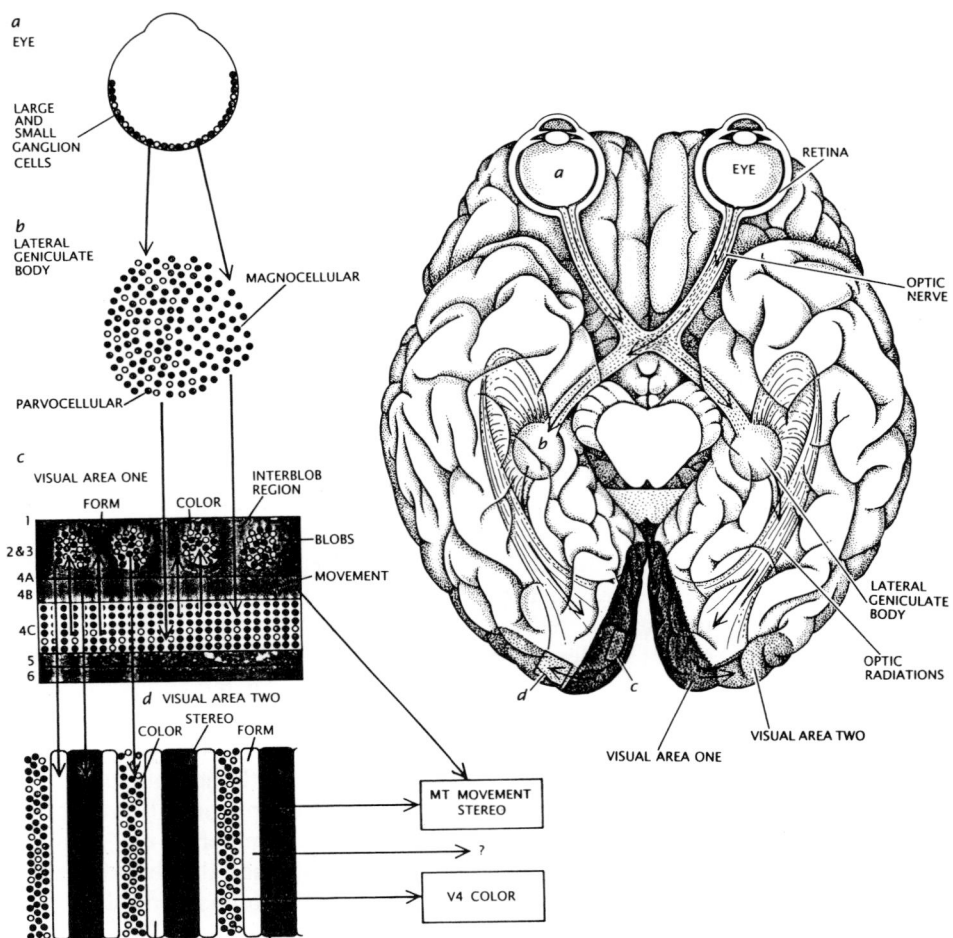

FIGURE 5.3. Separate systems for color contrast, luminance contrast, and movement as explicated in the text. The first separation in information processing occurs in the lateral geniculate bodies (*b*), where the small cells in the parvocellular region carry color contrast information and the large cells of the magnocellular part carry luminance information. The basal view (*right*) shows the proximity of visual machinery to the mesencephalon, suggesting how brainstem lesions such as those discussed in Chapter 4 (page 108) might cause simple synesthesia. Information regarding luminance contrast passes from the magnocellular region of the geniculate to layer 4B of area 17 (visual area 1) and then to the thick stripes of visual area 2 (*bottom*). These signals yield information about motion and depth.

Input from the parvocellular system ascends to the interblobs of visual area 1 and then the pale stripes of visual area 2, where it yields information regarding shape. Input from both the parvo and magno systems is combined in the blobs and processed for color and luminance. It then continues to the pale stripes of visual area 2 and then on to visual area 4. From "Art, illusion and the visual system" by M.S. Livingstone, 1988. Copyright © 1988 by Scientific American, Inc. All rights reserved.

In summary, there is a highly ordered anatomy at the cellular level that leads to the anatomical separation of color and spatial processing. Finally, these color-processing cell packets, or "blobs," stain with cytochrome oxidase, a mitochondrial stain that indicates that they are metabolically very active. Their high metabolism means that they are quite sensitive to ischemia and stroke, which is perhaps why these inferior lesions result in achromatopsia with preserved spatial processing.

These color cells are functionally discrete—as "modular" an example of brain processing as one could wish for. The high metabolic activity and susceptibility to ischemia is particularly interesting in light of the ischemic cerebral blood flow seen in MW (Chapter 4) and subsequent discussion regarding a functional (reversible) disconnection in synesthetes in general.

TWO SPECULATIONS

Before closing this section, I want to make two speculations, one addressing the absolute effects and consistency of the synesthetic psychophysical mapping, and the other addressing the deep emotional feeling that usually accompanies the synesthetic experience. A number of anatomically based modules for these speculations are possible, each with no more hope of being supported or proven wrong than the other. The one that follows is the one I like best.

The first speculation is based upon facts given above that the color-sensitive cells have a specific physical distribution in the occipitotemporal lobe. In the adjacent medial and ventral white matter are the intra- and interhemispheric visual pathways that connect visual association cortex with language areas and fiber systems linking auditory and somasthetic association cortices. Although I have previously eschewed the notion of "cross-talk," now that we know the location of the color cells (which, of course, does not explain how or where we perceive color) there does seem to be the possibility for these cells to be stimulated by recurrent collaterals or other sensory channels that are also coursing in the temporal stem on their way to the hippocampus and limbic system. This may be one anatomical reason why color figures so prominently in the various kinds of synesthesiae. If the blob cells, which are highly active metabolically, or the components to which they project are stimulated in the limbic system, then one could perceive color incongruously.

The topological organization of primary sensory cortex (retinotopical, tonotopical, somatotopical, gustotopical) does project in an orderly way to entorhinal cortex (Brodmann area 28) and the limbic system. It follows that this regular physical arrangement may underlie some of the absolute effects that are seen in synesthetic response mapping. However, this is speculating that proximity of structures infers interconnections, always a risky assumption in brain science. Our knowledge of the auditory association areas in man is also not well understood.

For example, there is a linear tonotopical organization of frequency perception in Heschl's gyrus in the temporal lobe. Highest frequencies are perceived anatomically most medially, and the lowest tones are subserved by more lateral tissue. Thus this tonotopical organization may give some explanation for the relative regularity of the psychophysical stimulus-response mapping as we saw in Chapter 3. In colored hearing, tones that were perceived as high by VE were also perceived as pink, whereas the lower tones were perceived as blue. This is not to imply that the synesthesia occurs at the location of Heschl's gyrus, because it is likely that the projections to and from this isomodal auditory cortex are involved in the appreciation of the parallel synesthetic sense.

The thalamus also maintains an intimate relationship with the limbic system and for all senses except olfaction is the first sensory relay. (Olfaction projects directly to pyriform cortex, which has well-developed hypothalamic, paralimbic, and limbic connections.) There is somatotopical organization of the thalamus, as well as areas that are quite modality specific, while others are heteromodal and paralimbic (see Figure 5.4).

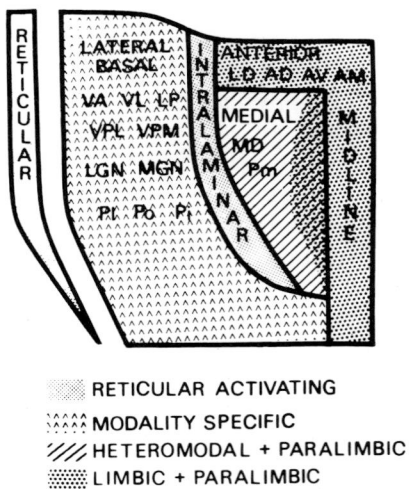

▓ RETICULAR ACTIVATING
ʌʌʌ MODALITY SPECIFIC
/// HETEROMODAL + PARALIMBIC
▓ LIMBIC + PARALIMBIC

FIGURE 5.4. Schematic topology of the four major groups of thalamic nuclei. *Key:* *AD*, anterior dorsal; *AM*, anterior medial; *AV*, anterior ventral; *LD*, laterodorsal; *LGN*, lateral geniculate; *LP*, lateroposterior; *MD*, medialis dorsalis; *MGN*, medial geniculate; *Pi*, inferior pulvinar; *Pl*, lateral pulvinar; *Pm*, medial pulvinar; *Po,*oral pulvinar; *VA*, ventral anterior; *VL*, ventral lateral; *VPL*, ventroposterior lateral; *VPM*, ventroposterior medial. From *Principles of behavioral neurology* (p. 43). by M-M. Mesulam, 1985. Philadelphia: F.A. Davis Co. Copyright 1985 by F.A. Davis Co. Reprinted by permission.

The clinical cases from Chapter 3 showing brainstem lesions are recalled in this regard.

Knowing and the Limbic System

One of the interesting features of synesthesia is the sense of certainty that patients have about it. This sense of validity, which is unexplanable in rational terms, is what MacLean calls the "schizophysiology" of the limbic system—that is, the difference between what we intuitively "feel" with our limbic system and what we "know" with our neocortex (MacLean, 1949, 1975, 1985). It is difficult not to mention MacLean in discussing the limbic system, particularly since, upon handing me a reprint of his 1949 paper years ago, he pointed out to me the hippocampus as a possible neuroanatomical mechanism for synesthesia:

Here [*in hippocampal formation*] the possibility exists for correlating not only olfactory, gustatory, and other visceral sensations, but auditory, visual, somasthetic and, perhaps, sexual sensations as well. . . . It is important to stress that there is an overlapping of the three main fiber systems into the subiculum of the hippocampal gyrus. There are also longitudinal fibers associating the hippocampal formation throughout its entire length. In the light of these observations, there is a possible neuroanatomic mechanism to explain some of the seemingly paradoxical overlapping (*or synesthesia*) of the various qualities contributing to emotional experience (p. 347).

We will review the triune brain and the topic of unconscious knowledge, or subception, in relation to the "knowing" in synesthesia and its hypermnestic quality. The limbic structures and connections in the anterior temporal lobe may provide an anatomical structure for this experience. The structural and functional organization of the mammalian temporal lobe has been a focus of interest for 50 years since the dramatic studies of Klüver and Bucy (1939) revealed its profound importance in social behavior, attention, and learning at a time when conceptualization of a limbic system and the allocortical components of the temporal lobe had not changed since the time of Broca's (1878) original formulation of a limbic lobe.

SUBCEPTION

One of the current areas of neuroscience is cognition that occurs outside of consciousness. This is called subception. There is strong evidence for dissociation between processes that occur at the level of consciousness at which patients can give testimony, and processes that occur below consciousness. Most brain processes obviously occur at a level about which we can have no awareness or sense of the strings being pulled. We still labor under the notion that everything that a patient does reflects some kind of processing that the patient could conceivably be aware of. This simply does not happen.

Patients with superior occipital lesions have such a dissociation. When asked to "touch my finger," such a patient goes immediately to the finger but says he cannot see it. He has enough visual information to inform his motor system to hit the target that he claims he cannot see. There is a full dissociation between his own experience of the visual target and what his motor system can do. This is ocular apraxia, or Balint's psychic gaze paralysis (Damasio, 1985).

Faces are the prime example of a stimulus about which one cannot give a conscious account. Face recognition is a visually triggered episodic memory. Patients with prosopagnosia can look at multiple faces and adamantly insist that they have never seen them before when in fact they knew the faces quite well previously. The patient does recognize the object as a face. It is the identification of a specific member within a generic class that fails him.

Obviously some parts of these patients' brains are quite knowledgeable about what it is that they say they cannot see or recognize. This can be shown by a skin resistance paradigm, showing that they have a signal event. Faces that they do know (target faces) will cause a response, whereas those that they have definitely not seen before will not. Obviously, the patient does not know consciously, but there is something in the neural machinery that responds to the recognition of the target face. The autonomic system betrays that the patient has a variety of intact perceptual processes that are deriving a description of the face in front of him with an outlet to the autonomic nervous system but no outlet to conscious awareness. A forced-choice paradigm will also show the same process. Cognition is not an all-or-nothing system. Most of the knowledge is simply not accessible to consciousness. Synesthesia may be an example of knowledge at a level that is so low it cannot produce a sense of familiarity or allow inferences to decide identities of objects.

ORGANIZATION OF BEHAVIOR

Yakovlev, Papez, and MacLean are three neurologists who divide brain and behavior into three categories. Yakovlev (1948, 1970) organized the brain according to three types of neuronal systems that he claimed were found in all brains and whose operational representations were empirically derived. These systems were the reticular, the nuclear, and the laminar. Yakovlev was one of the early neurologists and neuroanatomists who popularized the idea of behavior as simply movement. As human beings we are bombarded by electromagnetic flux, which we call the physical world around us. The only response that organisms can make to the environment is contraction of skeletal muscle or secretion from glands. That is, we can either squeeze or squirt. This movement of being alive we call "behavior." Yakovlev's "three spheres of motility" were visceration, the expression of internal states (emotion) and effectuation, corresponding to movements of the body within the body (autonomic) for the reticular; movements of the body upon the body (extrapyramidal) for the nuclear; and movements of the body outside the body (pyramidal) for the laminar arrangement of neurons.

MacLean's 1949 paper on the limbic system was influenced by Papez (1937), who also divided the brain into three levels of circuitry: streams of thought, streams of feeling, and streams of movement. Based on evolutionary theory, comparative anatomy, and neurochemistry, Paul Mac-Lean (1970, 1972, 1977, 1978a, 1978b, 1978c, 1980, 1985) believes that neural and behavioral distinctions can be made from three types of systems found in brains of mammals. The usefulness of the triune brain model lies in its description of behavior in terms of the actions and interactions of relatively self-contained anatomical systems. Repeatedly oversimplified, misunderstood, and appropriated by others as a basis for grand social theory, the triune brain is nonetheless an excellent idea that deserves serious consideration as a metaphor for the hierarchical structures of the brain as they relate to behavior. No theory of limbic system function is adequate. The triune brain does offer a broad outline for a scheme of limbic system function.

FEATURES OF THE LIMBIC SYSTEM

French anatomist Paul Broca (1878) emphasized two aspects of what he called the limbic lobe: (1) its strong relationship to the olfactory apparatus and (2) its common presence in the brains of all mammals. The actual structure of the brains of mammalian antecedents can only be guessed at. There is no way to determine the brain structure of creatures now extinct. Theories about their structure must rest on inferences drawn from living species available for study today. Having been subject to natural selection acting over thousands of years of genetic transfer, these existing animals are considerably different from their ancestors. Therefore, it is most surprising to find considerable uniformity in the interconnections among limbic structures of all living vertebrates. It is on this basis that many investigators believe that the study of the brains of lower animals can provide help in understanding the patterns of neural organization of all vertebrates.

Broca used the term "limbic," meaning border or hem, to designate the brain tissue surrounding the brainstem and that lies beneath the neocortical mantle. Grossly, this includes the cingulate and hippocampal gyri, the tissue connecting them, and the various gyri that surround olfactory fiber tracts. Structures are organized into two layers within this inner lobe of the brain. Allocortex tissue, thought to be phylogenetically the oldest, makes up the inner ring, and the outer limbic ring, whose cellular structure resembles neither neocortex nor allocortex, is called transitional cortex. The inner "ring" is actually not a continuous band of tissue but nodes of discrete entities that can be recognized by gross dissection. The structures of the inner portions of the limbic lobe are surrounded by transitional cortical tissue that has different names in different regions. Most of the information known today about the limbic system is about the inner ring structures of the limbic lobe; much less is known about the transitional cortex. Historically, there are heated debates about various anatomic structures of the inner brain that "should be" regarded as belonging to the limbic system. The nervous tissue is not easily distributed into categories.

Douglas and Marcellus (1975), for example, showed that two independent evolutionary trends in "higher brains" are expansion of the neocortical surface and associated subcortical regions, and expansion of the limbic structures. Some species may be high in either one or the other. Monkeys, for example, have a substantial neocortical development but little limbic enlargement; rabbits show the opposite trend of substantial limbic systems and poor neocortical development. Humans are probably unique in having substantial advancement in both limbic and neocortical dimensions.

We tend to conceive that the rapidly and massively expanding neocortex overwhelms and suppresses earlier systems, but limbic pathways do not diminish as the neocortex develops. Although the relative volume of limbic system structures is less in animals with large neocortical development, the number of axons in the fiber tracts is greater both in absolute number and relative to other fiber systems of the brain. In humans, there are five times the number of fibers in the fornix as in the optic tracts! (There are also three times more fibers in the optic tracts than in the auditory system, and both account for 85% of afferent fibers. Perhaps this is why color and visual phenomena are most prominent in synesthesia.)

The limbic system developed from the old olfactory brain and is especially concerned with emotional experience and forming memories. It includes primitive areas of cerebral cortex that are distinct from the great newly developed neocortical areas. It is here in the limbic system of sequential neuronal nodes that conscious experiences are elaborated with emotion. By their projection to the prefrontal lobes, the hypothalamus and other parts of the limbic system modify and color with emotion the conscious perceptions derived from sensory inputs and superimpose on them motivational drives.

There are pathways for complicated circuitry from the various sensory inputs to the limbic system and back to the prefrontal lobe, with further circuits from that lobe to other limbic components and back again. That is, the prefrontal and limbic systems are in reciprocal relationship, a continually looping reentrant circuit.

Hippocampus

The major input to hippocampal formation is the perforant pathway from the entorhinal cortex. Output of hippocampal formation contains large components directed toward association cortices. The transitional cortical areas of the hippocampal formation represent the critical portion of the structure for influencing other cortical regions of the brain.

There is general agreement that the amygdala is one site of convergence of a broad spectrum of sensory volleys. A ceaseless surge of spindling patterns from 25 to 40 Hz are seen in a variety of species (Adey, 1977). Hippocampal EEG rhythm signatures are in the theta range. This spindling EEG rhythm signature in temporal allocortex and amygdala may be related to motivational drive states. These facts may be useful in hypothesizing a relationship between synesthesia and paroxysmal activity in the limbic system.

Papez Circuit

Papez (1937) considered the limbic system to be the anatomical basis of emotions. The mammilary bodies, anterior thalamic nuclei, and cingulate cortex were prominently featured in his theory of a limbic system. Current knowledge has expanded the original circuitry of the Papez circuit (see Figure 5.5). The current version shows that the hippocampal

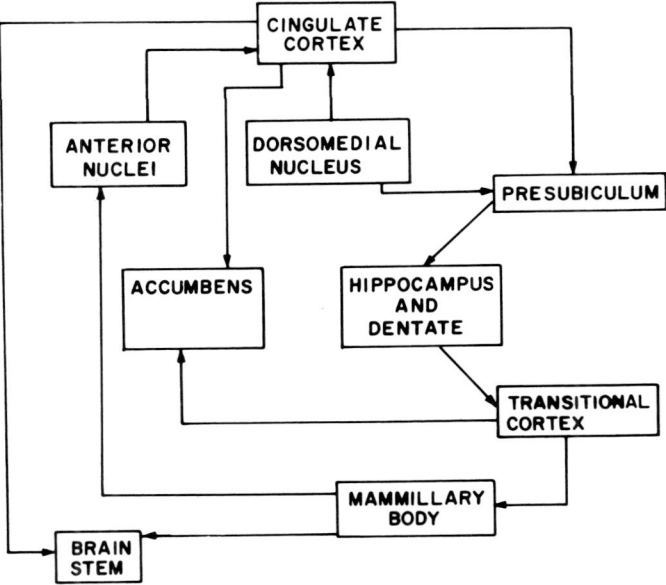

FIGURE 5.5. Modern conceptualization of the Papez circuit. From *The limbic system,* 2nd edition (p. 59) by R.L. Isaacson, 1982. New York: Plenum Press. Copyright 1982 by Plenum Press. Reprinted by permission.

formation influences distant regions primarily by its actions on cells in the subiculum, that the cingulate cortex receives multiple thalamic input, and that an important basal ganglia target for the major cortical areas of the circuit—the hippocampus and cingulum—is the nucleus accumbens. Whether this new version of the Papez circuit is any better than the classical one is not clear, but it does offer a new route for influencing behavior: a link with basal ganglia, particularly nucleus accumbens.

PLEASURABLE REACTIONS

Hypothalamus

All limbic influences converge on the hypothalamus, yet the limbic system's influences on behavior extend far beyond actions directed toward maintenance of homeostasis. They involve many subtle aspects of learning, memory, motivation, and performance. They include cognitive acts, forming strategies, and casting hypothesis.

The view that the hypothalamus is only a regulator of physiological systems was shattered by Olds and Milner's experiment (1954) on pleasurable reactions from electrical self-stimulation. Reports from patients whose brains have been stimulated in "reward" regions have indicated that the experience obtained is, in fact, pleasant (Bishop, Elder, & Heath, 1963). Generally, most limbic regions will support self-stimulation. Catecholamine systems are strongly associated with self-stimulation behavior (Isaacson, 1982).

Synesthesia is almost always pleasurable, and to lose it would be an odious state. Like rats pressing a stimulation lever, synesthetes too have "favorite" music, sounds, names, words, food, and colors that evoke their pleasurable synesthesiae. They never tire of it.

Because of its close ties to the neocortical, basal gangliar, and limbic systems, the hippocampus stands as a neural modulator of activities in many brain regions. It is not surprising that its dysfunction should produce abnormalities of "higher" capacities. The actual disruptions, however, should be thought of as disruptions of many systems and not just due to a faulty hippocampus.

The Triune Brain

MacLean's basic divisions of the brain are a protoreptilian brain, or R-complex, a paleomammalian brain, and a neomammalian brain. He conceives of the R-complex as a fundamental core of the nervous system, consisting of systems in the upper spinal cord, midbrain, diencephalon, and basal ganglia. The paleomammalian division is essentially the limbic system; the neomammalian brain is the neocortical expansion so prominent in primates. What MacLean believes to be the R-complex in existing mammals derives from early mammal-like reptiles (therapsids) that disappeared in the Triassic period. Skeletal remains have been found in southern Africa and evidence of their existence found on all continents. Modern mammals may have developed from these mammal-like reptiles (MacLean, 1977, 1978a, 1978c, 1985). The R-complex structures of mammalian brain are quite different from the neural organization of the brains of living reptiles, which, in their current state of evolution, probably bear the vaguest resemblance to the reptile-like mammals of the Permian and Triassic periods. As emphasized above, the usefulness of the triune brain metaphor lies in its describing behavioral functions in terms of specific anatomic systems.

THE REPTILIAN BRAIN

The protoreptilian brain is responsible for stereotyped behaviors based on "ancestral learning and ancestral memories," playing a crucial role in the establishment of home territory, finding food and shelter, breeding, and social dominance. MacLean considers the paleomammalian brain to be nature's tentative first step toward providing self-awareness, particularly of the internal milieu (by definition, the emotions). It is a "visceral brain" (MacLean, 1949). The elaboration of internal information is necessary, in MacLean's view, for forming significant memories, with the hippocampus being an especially good place to combine "internal information" from the septal area and "external information" from sensory systems projecting to nearby transitional cortical areas (MacLean, 1949, 1972, 1973).

The neocortex is the "mother of invention and father of abstract thought." As opposed to the internal signals that project to the limbic cortex, the neocortex provides a fine-grained analysis of the external world and has a predilection for dividing things into smaller and smaller units. The neocortex affords "a vast neural screen for the portrayal of symbolic language and the associated functions of reading, writing and arithmetic" (MacLean, 1977).

Isaacson (1982) agreed about the functions of "three brains in one," particularly in seeing the limbic system as a strong modulator of the R-complex. How this modulation is achieved is a current topic of neuroscience.

THE PALEOMAMMALIAN BRAIN

The limbic system is an advance in neural tissue, a device for better coping with the environment and integrating the internal and external worlds. Parts of the limbic system are concerned with primal issues of food and sex, others are concerned with emotions and feelings, and still others combine messages from the internal and external worlds. Epileptic disruption of limbic activities produce a host of experiences and feelings, some of the most interesting being associated with knowledge of fundamental truths, feelings of depersonalization, hallucinations, paranoid feelings, and synesthesia (MacLean, 1970, 1977). Mandell (1980) attributed many "other worldly" experiences to deregulation of limbic activity. The hippocampus can be seen as a mechanism that suppresses the activity of the R-complex when the unexpected happens (Isaacson, 1982). Life becomes uncertain when old patterns of responding fail to produce anticipated rewards, when old habits fail to pay off. This suppression prevents the animal from continuing in its old ways of responding and from overreacting in general. The paleomammalian brain can be viewed as a mechanism directed toward the elimination of the stored memories of the protoreptilian brain, that is, influences from the past. Finally, each of the limbic structures, including the hypothalamus itself, is a complex set of subsystems in terms of anatomical relationships with other regions and in terms of behavioral functions. Isaacson adjures us to talk about limbic systems, not a limbic system (Isaacson, 1982).

THE HIPPOCAMPUS MODEL FOR SYNESTHESIA

What we can say about the triune brain in relation to our metaphor of synesthesia as a fundamental sensation characteristic of mammals is that the durable and stereotyped synesthetic response seems reminiscent of the "ancestral learning and ancestral memories" of the R-complex, which emerge through dysregulation of the paleomammalian limbic system. The emotional nature of the subjective conviction that the parallel sense is real and often "out there" derives from the limbic complex. All of this, of course, occurs without conscious effort on the synesthete's part.

We have singled out the hippocampus as the most likely structure to be involved with the production of synesthesia as well as the purveyor of its hypermnestic quality. One reason is that there are persons with hippocampal epileptogenic foci who have synesthetic experiences relatable to a seizure, but who are not synesthetic otherwise (Anderson, 1886; Gloor et al., 1982; Gowers, 1901; Horrax, 1923; Ionasescu, 1960; Jacome & Gumnit, 1979; Kennedy, 1911; Mulder & Daly, 1952; Penfield & Jasper, 1954; Penfield & Perot, 1963; Spiers et al., 1985; Weiser, 1983). This, of course, relates only to epileptic synesthesia. An important case of concurrent temporal lobe seizures with idiopathic synesthesia was just brought to my attention by Donald Rathbun, MD, in El Paso, TX. A woman with lifelong tactile-auditory-visual synesthesia also developed complex partial seizures, with a temporal focus, as an adolescent. Her seizures consist of staring, mouthing and facial flushing, but not synesthesia. Imaging demonstrates no anatomic lesion. She feels that Carbamezapine, given for her seizures, has made her synesthesia less vivid! What this case suggests is that although synesthesia depends on limbic mechanisms, her (and likely other people's) idiopathic synesthesia is not due to the epileptic spike itself. An analogous situation holds for the behavioral features seen in temporal lobe seizures (hypergraphia, hyperreligiosity, viscosity, humorlessness): we believe that the interictal behavioral features are an epiphenomenon of the spike.

The other reason is strongly anatomical. There very few places in the brain where it is possible to bring signals together from functionally different and geographically independent areas. There is a certain kind of togetherness in the thalamus; a certain kind of togetherness in the lateral frontal cortices; but the most important togetherness that virtually assembles every sensory modality as well as the internal milieu is in the anterior temporal lobe. The fact that the anterior temporal cortices utilize not the corpus callosum for their connections to the opposite hemisphere, but rather the anterior commissure, a commissure strongly associated with the limbic system, is further evidence of the close functional relationship of the temporal cortices to the limbic system. The brain is equipped with devices that permit the feeding of information both by stages and long relays into the medial aspect of the temporal lobe, converging on the entorhinal cortex (Brodmann area 28), which happens to be the primary gateway to the hippocampus lying immediately underneath. Furthermore, there is the marvelous opportunity for the hippocampal formation, via entorhinal cortex and the fornix, to respond back to virtually every element that is fed into it and to the hippocampus to start with. It is possible to bring information that was processed in geographically separate parts of the brain together as signals in a unique structure that knows about the internal milieu and about the fundamental goals of the organism as a biological entity. That structure can also respond back to the cortices that initiated the circuit and further act on autonomic structures that govern the internal milieu. One has, then, a fundamental yet ideal device that brings information together in the context of how the organism is what it wants to be. It is on this organ that I believe the expression of synesthesia depends.

The quintessential ability of the neocortex is to efficiently process information that has too many fine details to be easily handled by simpler and evolutionarily earlier brain systems. As derivative aspects of sensation separate in the cascade of sensory neural processing, there is the opportunity for these derivatives—color, directional movement, linearity, shape, texture, temperature—to recombine in limbic and paralimbic areas. Furthermore, it is here that the autonomic responses could join in to give the pleasurable sense that synesthetes experience in their parallel sensation.

As mammals evolved, overlap of function became less and less. So synesthetes may themselves hold clues to how the mammalian cortex evolved, how the intellectual brain of the neocortex dominated and overrode the emotional brain of the limbic system over eons, yet still infrequently yields to it, as when senses mingle in the absence of cortical processing. The synesthetic experience may be a result of a fundamentally mammalian process in which the cortex briefly ceases to function in the modern manner, permitting the senses to fuse, or, rather, we should say, perceive fusion that may be there all along but that never arises to consciousness. At its essence, synesthesia may be a remnant of how early mammals perceived their world. As Dr. Ommaya comments in the foreword, "Synesthesia is what we all do without knowing that we do it, whereas synesthetes do it and know that they do it."

Conclusion

We have looked at the neural basis underlying the detachment of derivatives of cognition, particularly color, shape, space, and emotion. These properties are the bulk of what synesthesia is about, although a similar analysis is applicable to the less common forms of synesthesia. What has changed in almost 200 years of examining synesthesia is both the conceptualization of synesthesia and our conceptualization and understanding of neural tissue.

The reader should now have a fuller understanding of the rich sensory experience known as synesthesia and understand why, in the face of little real utility, patients who possess it value the experience so much.

Having considered the historical, experiential, and anatomical aspects of synesthesia, we will now make a transition to more abstract considerations in the next three chapters. These are the relation of synesthesia to language, its relation to artistic appreciation, and its relationship to the concept of what is real.

6
Synesthesia and Language

The main task of this chapter is to explore the claim, stated explicitly and implicitly and in several guises, that synesthesia is ultimately related to language. That is, it is assumed or surmised that the connection between a stimulus and the parallel synesthetic sense is brought about by a linguistic-based cross-modal association (D'Andrade & Egan, 1974; Karwoski et al., 1942; L.E. Marks, 1974, 1975, 1978; Ortmann, 1933; Osgood, 1960; Rader & Tellegen, 1987; Ries, 1969; Riggs & Karwoski, 1934; Vernon, 1930). I believe that this claim is erroneous. There is an enormously strong bias toward calling on language as an explanation for many cognitive functions. It is difficult to shun its appeal. Langfeld (1926), for example, stated that "synesthesia is not due to an organic condition of the brain, such as a 'tangling of the fibers,' but rather is a normal and essential function for the subject, a cognitive process differing in no respect from any other process of *meaning*." Wheeler (1920) speaks of synesthesia as "an immediate and permanent conditioned reflex," whereas for L.E. Marks (1975) synesthesia is "a cross-modal manifestation of connotative meaning in a pure sensory form." This is pure conjecture.

It is easy for those of us who lack the gift of colored hearing or some other type of synesthesia to dismiss the synesthete's descriptions as a mere literary contrivance, the result of either a limited vocabulary or else a voluble one that fails to set conceptual limits. Enough examples have been given, I think, for the careful reader to conclude otherwise. In his autobiography, the musician Thomas Wood (1936) emphasized that his lifelong musical color association is something that transcends simple metaphor.

It brings a definite color to single notes, to notes in groups, to movements; it changes the color according to height or depth, scoring, key; over all this it lays a color that goes with the work as a whole, and at times a shape is added which is just as fortuitous as the colors themselves.

It is rare for synesthetes to attach any meaning to their synesthesiae. BB is one exception who also shows frank linguistic difficulties. His writing shows semantic-cognitive distortions and his errors in grammar and semantics make his writing appear at times like that of a partially recovered aphasic. The meaning that BB assigns to his colors is reminiscent of medieval religious symbolism:

A white color, of course, is clearity [sic] and truth. Blue is comfort with pleasure of completeness to any thoughts. Amber is a lingering beyound [sic] reality to emotion. Not a fault its self [sic] but a zone of balance. Green is caution, sensitivity, compassion, jealousey [sic], potentially tearing or conflecting [sic]. Red is also a flag of caution to which anger, strength, movement is at hand. To me both green and red require patients [sic] and effort.

In addition to the frank dyslexic and syntactic errors that BB demonstrates, other subjects have shown related analytical deficits such as acalculia, right-left confusion, and impairment of finger gnosis. Other spelling errors can be seen in the examples in Chapter 2. These impairments, together with the examples given in Chapter 4 of simple synesthesia in patients with left hemispheric brain lesions, are supportive of the notion that the neural real estate for synesthesia resides in the left hemisphere. This anatomical localization is not the same as saying that language is the basis for synesthesia. It is this latter point that needs clarification.

The Semantic Differential

Osgood et al. (1957) identified *meaning* as a representational mediation process and developed a particular kind of measurement operation, *the semantic differential*. They postulated a semantic space, Euclidean in nature, of unknown dimensionality. Each semantic scale, defined by a pair of polar adjectives, is assumed to represent a straight line function that passes through the origin of this space.

A subject "differentiates" the meaning of a concept when he judges it against a series of scales. For example:

FATHER

Good ___	: _X_	: ___	: ___	: ___	: ___	: ___	Bad
Fast ___	: ___	: ___	: ___	: _X_	: ___	: ___	Slow
Hard ___	: ___	: ___	: ___	: ___	: _x_	Soft

Each judgment represents a selection among a set of given alternatives and serves to localize the concept as a point in the semantic space.

Even with subjects who have considerable linguistic sophistication, almost half the total variance in meaningful judgments is accounted for by only three factors: evaluation, potency, and activity. These factors are stable. A pervasive *evaluative factor* in human judgment regularly appears first. Is it good or is it bad? Next, the potency factor is concerned with power and things associated with it—size, weight, toughness, and so forth. Third, the activity factor is concerned with quickness, excitement, warmth, agitation, and the like.

These three major factors of evaluation, potency, and activity are empirically rather than theoretically derived and reappear in a wide variety of judgmental situations. The relative weights of the factors are constant, evaluation accounting for double the amount of variance due to either potency or activity, and these two in turn being double the weight of any subsequent factors. A large portion of the total variance remains unaccounted for, however, and Osgood et al. (1957) suggested that there must be a large number of relatively specific semantic factors.

The semantic differential is a generalizable technique of measurement. There are no standard concepts and no standard scales, the concepts and scales used in a particular study depending upon the purposes of the research. Single words most often serve as a unitary semantic concept (e.g., *fraud*), but nonverbal concepts such as Rorschach pictures, representational or abstract paintings, sculpture, and even sonar signals have been used (Osgood et al., 1957).

It is precisely because the semantic differential taps the connotative aspects of meaning more immediately than the highly diversified denotative aspects that is should be readily applicable to aesthetic studies and concepts such as synesthesia.

The history of the semantic differential in relation to synesthesia is of some interest. The use of polar adjectives to define the terminae of semantic dimensions grew out of research on synesthesia by Karwoski and Odbert (1938). These researchers related synesthetic perception to thinking and language in general and believed that any difference from the general population was one of degree rather than kind. While synesthetes might picture fast, exciting music as bright, angular, red photisms, nonsynesthetic listeners would merely agree that *words* like "red hot," "bright," and "fiery," as verbal metaphors, adequately described the music. Osgood et al. (1957) said that "the relation of this phenomenon to ordinary metaphor is evident," a conclusion that is not, in fact, adequately justified. They did show that stimuli from several modalities— visual, auditory, emotional, and verbal—*may* have shared significates or meanings. Showing this, however, does little to clarify the underlying mechanism of synesthesia itself, nor is it justified to conclude that semantic mediation or shared linguistic meaning is the link in synesthesia. This point was argued in Chapter 3.

In explicating the logic behind the semantic differential, Osgood et al. (1957) cited Karwoski and colleagues (Karwoski, Gramlich, & Arnot, 1944; Karwoski & Odbert, 1938; Karwoski et al., 1942; Odbert, Karwoski, & Eckerson, 1942) and pointed to their diagram of "synesthetes" illustrating a rising and falling tone (Figure 6.1). They showed that "practiced synesthetes" (a term undefined) and *trained nonsynesthetes*

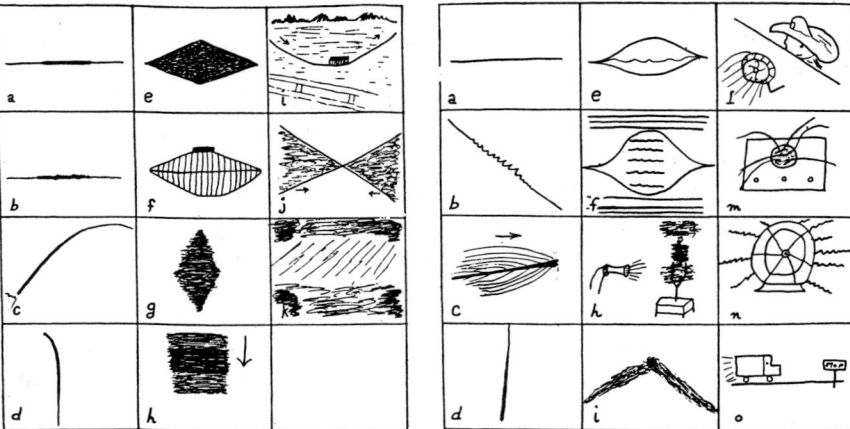

FIGURE 6.1. *Left:* Drawings of "photistic visualizers" responding to tones that simply get louder, then softer. *Right:* Drawings of unselected controls responding to the same stimuli. There is little qualitative difference between the two. Far from representing a synesthetic photism, these drawings merely represent the abstract concept of a crescendo-diminuendo. See text for further details. From *Journal of General Psychology, 26,* 199–222, 1942. Reprinted with permission of the Helen Dwight Reid Educational Foundation. Published by Heldref Publications, 4000 Albemarle St., N.W., Washington, DC 20016. Copyright © 1942.

would make similar graphic representations, and argued for cognitive similarity.

The first point is that their subjects are clearly not synesthetic but are using imagery at best. The second objection is that *they trained their controls* to make specific cross-modal associations. But the major point, which is clear from examination of the figure, is that what is being drawn is not the synesthetic sense of the sound but rather the underlying *concept* of the stimulus to which the subjects are exposed: namely, a rising and falling tone. *They are drawing the abstract concept, not the sound.* Osgood et al. (1957) stated "that these practiced synesthetes were not exercising a 'rare' capacity was shown in two subsequent experiments: In one, subjects who had never even thought of 'seeing things' when they heard music were played the same stimulus selections and told that they *had* to draw something to represent each stimulus—exactly the same types of productions were obtained" (p. 22). Figure 6.1 shows the drawings of "photistic visualizers" versus controls. One sees that there is little qualitative difference between the two. Many are either line or solid forms whose increased thickness corresponds to the increased intensity of the stimulus. The representations of the soft parts of the stimulus appear as the directly opposite characteristic used by the subjects to represent the loud central part. Karwoski et al. (1942) believed that these symbols seemed "conceptually adequate to represent the stimulus."

This is not synesthesia. Although "the same types of productions" were elicited, one needs to ask whether these subjects routinely *saw* such representations whenever they heard a rising and falling tone (a crescendo-diminuendo) or—to give a more likely occurrence—the Doppler effect of a passing siren. If so, one would rightly suspect that such subjects were synesthetic. Yet the information is lacking for the reader to make such a judgment. Did subjects who rendered these graphic representations for the experimenters render the same drawings when challenged at a later time with the same stimuli? There are no data to show whether these associations are stable over time.

Karwoski et al. (1942) thought that the ease with which the translations from the auditory to the visual may be reduced to verbal terms, and the fact that the translations nearly always occurred as related pairs of opposites, suggested a close relationship of these processes to verbal behaviors. This led them to differentiate the visual and mood poles of music and further suggest that the form aspect in colored hearing is "very closely related to common factors in our culture," such as "light or heavy music, thin strings and thick bass." In fact, they satisfied themselves that there was a "great repertoire of similies and metaphors for translating sound into sight" and that language was the key to this translation.

But what are these so-called synesthetic subjects actually responding to? I think the correct analysis is that they are giving a graphic representation of a concept—an abstract principle—rather than giving a graphic representation of the synesthesia they might experience (if they actually were synesthetic) when they heard such a sound. Karwoski et al.'s conclusion may have contributed to psychologists' view that synesthesia was not so rare. Karwoski claimed to relate synesthesia to thinking and language in general. Rather than being a freak phenomenon, colored music synesthesia was reported by Karwoski and Odbert (1938) as being "indulged in" by 13% of Dartmouth College students, "often as a means of enriching their enjoyment of music." An even larger number were reported to have such experiences occasionally. Their conclusions are unfounded, but it is easy to see how this fostered the notion that semantic meaning could be the link in synesthesia.

The high agreement of 100 nonsynesthetic subjects as to what the most appropriate visualizations of music might be yielded Karwoski and Odbert's conclusion that "the *capacity* to appreciate music in visual terms exists in a considerable proportion of the population." I think no one would argue with this, but appreciating music in terms of verbal metaphor is quite another thing from having an involuntary synesthetic photism.

Osgood and colleagues (1957) relied on Karwoski et al.'s synesthesia investigations in formulating the theoretical background for the semantic differential. I find it ironic and amusing that using the same instrument 30 years later should show that there is no correlation between the semantic meaning of a stimulus and a synesthetic response.

In 1979 Frank Wood and I (unpublished data) applied the semantic differential to subject VE and three controls. A sound-color matching task revealed that notes that she perceived as high generated predominantly pink responses while low notes were predominantly blue (see Figure 3.9). We used 10 colors (black, blue, brown, green, gray, orange, pink, purple, red, white, and yellow) as the concepts, and differentiated them across the 25 scales of pleasant-unpleasant, strong-weak, familiar-strange, good-bad, high-low, fast-slow, delicate-massive, fragrant-foul, animated-listless, large-small, clean-dirty, mellow-sharp, full-empty, nice-awful, sharp-dull, regular-irregular, active-passive, light-dark, sacred-profane, open-closed, angular-rounded, light-heavy, hard-soft, soaring-earth-bound, and voluminous-sparse.

Differentiating the 10 colors over 25 scales failed to show any similarity in the semantic space between pink and those notes that were perceived to be high, and between blue and those notes that were perceived to be low. In fact, blue was judged to be high, good, somewhat passive, and neither potent nor impotent. Pink was judged to be neither high nor low, neither good nor bad, neither active nor passive, and only slightly potent. We concluded that whatever caused VE to perceive high notes as pink and low notes as blue, it was not on the basis of any shared meaning.

The semantic differential did not seem to consistently explain matching of the three control subjects either. Control A seemed to have a clear relational effect in matching red, yellow, and pink to high notes. These were all perceived to be good, relatively potent and passive, while all being high. Control T showed no consistency in semantic meanings of colors that were associated with high and low notes, and control L was inconsistent. We did not pursue linguistic meanings further, having shown that there was no semantic parallelism.

Osgood (1960) studied cross-cultural generalities of visual-verbal tendencies (which he called "synesthetic") and explicitly stated that the bipolar dimensions for semantic evaluation derived from the bipolarity of dimensions obtained in the study of synesthesia. This is why, more than any other reason, falling back on cognitive linguistic mediation as an explanation for synesthesia is a circular argument. Osgood's own interpretation of his theory is that meaning consists of a process of mediation, whose connotative components correspond to the dimensions that obtain via semantic differentiation. The mediation processes themselves are treated as learned representations of responses that become attached to their signs through learning (reinforcement). More importantly, the representational components are complex rather than simple responses and are derived from several reaction systems.

Recalling our discussion of Aristotelian common senses, it is clear that we can perceive an object as light or heavy by the sound of its fall or can, for example, estimate the number of pins knocked over by the sound of a bowling ball as it crashes into them. Such cross-modal linguistic associations may be a cognitive shorthand that serves to highlight, conveniently, important sensory attributes that are held in common. However, these attributes are qualitatively different from the parallel sense of synesthesia and should not be confused with it.

Language and Cross-Modal Associations

The nature of language and cross-modal associations as it relates to synesthesia has been repeatedly confused and misunderstood. I take this opportunity to state it plainly: the development of speech itself depends on the ability to form stable intermodal associations readily.

The issue is one of priority, and the common error is to state that language arose de novo, and from it the ability to form cross-modal associations developed. This view, if correct, would support the hypothesis that the link between modalities in synesthesia is a linguistic intermodal association that depends on tertiary parietal association cortex.

The problem, however, is that this view is not correct. Geschwind (1965a, 1965b) argued this point carefully and in great detail, yet it continues to be misunderstood and misquoted. L.E. Marks, for example, argued from generalization when he pointed out that there are parallel psychophysical processes operating in different sense modalities (1978). It is, of course, true that there are common psychophysical processes accountable for analagous sensory dimensions (such as intensity, spatial and temporal features, and signal sensitivity). He then argued that psychophysical similarities among the senses "may in some instances demand the existence of analogies in the anatomical structures and physiological mechanisms that must mediate sensory perception in different modalities" (Marks, 1978, p. 143). He avoided the issue of what kind of perceptual information common anatomy and physiology (such as the multimodal cells discussed in Chapters 3 and 5) may convey, but rather supposed that linguistic-based nonlimbic-to-nonlimbic intermodal associations of the inferior parietal lobule of the left hemisphere are the basis for these similarities, and, by extension, for synesthesia. He *incorrectly* stated that "Geschwind has argued that cross-modal perception depends significantly on language, and in this function he has implicated the inferior parietal lobe of the dominant cerebral hemisphere . . ." (Marks, 1978, p. 162).

Geschwind (1965a) was explicit in discrediting the idea that "verbal mediation" is the means by which humans achieve cross-modal transfers.

As I have noted earlier, *it cannot be argued that the ability to form cross-modal associations depends on already having speech;* rather we must say that *the ability to acquire speech has as a prerequisite the ability to form cross-modal associations* (p. 275).

In other words, because man can form certain intermodal associations, he can develop speech, and "once he has developed speech, he can succeed in turn in forming other intermodal associations." It is these "other intermodal associations" that form the higher and most abstract cognitive functions in man, which seem to be the ones with which synesthesia is repeatedly confused.

When one looks at the phylogeny and ontogeny of cerebral development in man, it is not the expansion of the frontal lobes and the high brow that is most striking but, as Bailey and Bonin (1951) stressed, "the parietal and temporal lobe in the widest meaning of that term, and it is here that we should look for the substrate of certain functions which are supposed to be characteristic of man." The language cortex and heteromodal association areas of the parietal lobe are responsible for Geschwind's "other intermodal associations," associations occurring at that high level where we have already concluded that synesthesia cannot exist. The precise quote of Geschwind's position is given on page 72. With the evolutionary introduction of the angular gyrus region, intermodal associations become quite powerful and, in a sense, the parietal sense does free man to some extent from the limbic system.

There are other errors besides this most fundamental one that contribute to the incorrect attribution of synesthesia as part of language. Some have to do with sloppy terminology, as, for example, the analysis by Rader and Tellegen (1987) that explicitly defines synesthesia as imagery: "Although synesthesia, the occurrence of imagery in one sense modality in response to sensations in another, has long intrigued investigators . . ." (p. 981). Other glaring errors are the use of nonsynesthetes in constructing theories of synesthesia (L.E. Marks, 1974, 1975; Ries, 1969).

Synesthesia as a Disconnection

Consider a point of view that regards synesthesia as a disconnection from language modules of the brain. I am unable to do more than entertain some theoretical ideas regarding anatomical and physiological substrates for synesthesia and share them here. Although cases are too few and only a handful have been able to be studied in any depth, these ideas can help suggest the direction for future inquiry.

In formulating his ideas of disconnection, one of Geschwind's primary points is that language depends on stable intermodal associations, especially visual-auditory and tactile-auditory. These are, one readily sees, the most common modes of synesthesia. It is the nature of the cross-modal associations and where they might be represented in the nervous system that is of greatest interest.

I believe that the correct view is that synesthesia, as a product of the brain, antedates language. It follows that it is evolutionarily earlier and, as discussed in Chapter 3, less "abstract" and more concrete. Rather than synesthesia being merely a more intense form of metaphoric speech, one can look at cross-modal metaphor as an abstract, linguistic derivative of the stuff of synesthesia. A number of authors have discussed the idea that intersensory and intermodal associations are relatively inconspicuous and, with the development of conceptual thought and language, they tend to be suppressed (Boring, 1942; Hayek, 1952; Werner, 1948). Sophistication makes us overlook that which is obvious to naive experience. Children certainly accept synesthesia more readily as a product of genuine intrasensory attributes. Hayek believed that the development of transmodal metaphors in speech rested on more than just a turn of phrase and was a product of actual perceptual intersensory attributes.

It is interesting to see what happens when we invert this argument. The inverted point of view would hold that synesthesia results from a disconnection of language modules, by which the unelaborated cross-modal percept emerges. This point of view is similar conceptually with microgenetic theory.

The inferior parietal lobule (IPL) must be prominent in any conception of synesthesia as a disconnection. Since the IPL figures prominently in language, is athalamic, and receives afferents from association cortices, disconnection or inactivation of this region is consistent with our hypothesis of suppressed cortical activity during synesthesia. The maturity of this region may also be important. In keeping with its late evolutionary development, the IPL has a highly variable gyral structure. Flechsig (1901) and Yakovlev (1962; Yakovlev & Lecours, 1967) showed that it is late to myelinate, matures late cytoarchitectonically, and is one of the last cortical areas in which dendrites appear. G. Elliott Smith believed that the thin, distinctive cortical bands that he described above and below the parietal region were remnants of lower primates (1907). It is precisely this region of the IPL in which intermodal associations, cross-connections between primary nonlimbic sensory modalities, become powerful.

RELATION TO THE CONFABULATORY RESPONSE

Confabulation is filling in the gaps in the information available to the speech area, a recitation of imaginary experiences to compensate for perceptual loss or memory impairment. Split-brain patients and those who confabulate teach us that the ability of the speech area to describe is no guarantee that we get an *accurate description* of perceptions going on in another part of the brain. A patient cannot introspect about activities of a piece of brain that has no connections to the speech area. What he tells you, therefore, is of little value in elucidating the mechanism of a clinical feature and may be actively misleading. Confabulation is an attempt to explain what the patient cannot understand.

Part of the problem lies in perceiving the patient as an entity. Work with split-brain patients and disconnection syndromes shows that *the patient who speaks is not the same one who perceives. They are separate but usually unified.* If a patient's speech area is disconnected from a site of primary perception, why should the speech area be able to describe accurately what is going on?

This leads to consideration of the confabulatory response: Based on at least a partial disconnection of the IPL or other association cortex from the speech region, the patient is left to confabulate that something heard is really something seen. A disconnection of language modules implies a relative enhancement of temporal neocortex-limbic structures that would provide validity and assurance that the percept is real.

Weinstein (Weinstein, Cole, & Mitchel, 1963; Weinstein, Kahn, & Slote, 1955) and Geschwind (1965b) agree on several characteristics of confabulation: it does not occur in the absence of a deficit; it is less marked in the presence of aphasia; it is more likely in the presence of some general impairment of awareness such as dementia or encephalopathy; and it is more likely in the presence of disease of association cortex or association fibers (either commissural or intrahemispheric) than in cases of injury to primary sensory pathways up to and including the primary sensory cortex. The less dementia and clouding are prominent, the more confabulation depends on these lesions of association cortex or fibers.

Geschwind's explanation for confabulation is similar to that for release hallucinations. It assumes that the association areas never fail to send a message to the speech area and always send positive messages regarding circumstances. If the primary visual cortex is destroyed, the speech area still remains innervated by visual association cortex. In this case, the association cortex, receiving no stimulus from calcarine cortex, would send the "message" to the speech area that there is no visual "message"—that is, everything is black.

The destruction of association cortex or fibers is a totally unphysiological state—one in which *no message* is received by the speech area. In this abnormal state, the speech area may react to its own spontaneous firing or to random messages coming from subcortical pathways. A partial disconnection would mean that the neural signals are inadequate to convey all the information for the "true" stimulus to reach conscious perception. This may lead to errors less bizarre than in total isolation of the speech cortex. Thus, sound may be misspoken of as something seen.

Release of the anterior temporal cortex, which communicates to the opposite side via the anterior commissure, may mean that the connections to the medial temporal structures, particularly the hippocampus (which communicates with all sensory modalities) and the limbic structures, may be particularly enhanced. Frontal disinhibition may also be operative during this state, explaining the affective component of synesthesia and the certainty in the patients' minds that what they are perceiving is valid and true.

Thus, the cerebral blood flow data, scanty as they are, support the possibility that the supramodal cortex of the IPL region is not functionally active, but rather disconnected during synesthetic perception. The development of more advanced physiological techniques may further our knowledge of this issue without recourse to a verbal account from the patient. Specific attention to this question in future studies will be of great interest. Magnetic resonance imaging might, by virtue of its tissue sensitivity and spatial resolution, also disclose abnormalities, particularly if phosphorus spectroscopy can be employed. The presence of such pathology is implied by abnormal visual perimetry in MW and the neuropsychological deficits seen in various synesthetic subjects. Unfortunately, it is unlikely that any subjects will ever come to confirmatory postmortem cytoarchitectonic study.

Language and Consciousness

There is no unitary faculty of "recognition." Errors of recognition are thought to lie somewhere between defects of "perception" and those of "naming." However, we really show recognition when any appropriate response occurs. Recognition certainly occurs in synesthetic perception. Yet debating whether such recognition is conscious or unconscious, or presupposes language, is to me very much mistaken.

In taking the biological approach to human intelligence, one can say that the information content of both inherited and acquired knowledge can be extremely great. Without the background of inherited knowledge, which is almost all unconscious and which is incorporated in our genes, we would not, of course, be able to acquire any new knowledge. This disagrees strongly with empiricist philosophy that sees the mind as a tabula rasa until perception makes an entry. This idea is severely mistaken. It is probable that the huge amount of information that we can acquire in a lifetime through our senses is small compared with the amount in our inherited background of potential.

Various languages are man-made, cultural objects, although they are made possible by capabilities and needs that have become genetically entrenched. Every normal child acquires language through much active work, and a tremendous intellectual achievement goes with it. This effort has a strong feedback effect on the child's personality and his relations to other persons and his material environment. Thus we can say that the child is partly the product of his achievement.

Just as the child's mastery and consciousness of his material environment is extended by his newly acquired ability to speak, so also is his consciousness of himself. Becoming a fully sentient human being depends on a maturation process in which the acquisition of speech plays an enormous part. One learns not only to perceive, and to *interpret one's perceptions,* but also to be a person, and to be a self. To think that our perceptions are "given" is a mistake. Rather, they are "made" by us, the result of active work. As Popper pointed out, "it is a similar mistake to overlook the fact that the famous Cartesian argument 'I think, therefore I am' presupposes language and the ability to use the personal pronoun (to say nothing of the formulation of the highly sophisticated problem which this argument is supposed to settle)" (Popper & Eccles, 1977).

Is synesthesia culturally determined? Did it evolve with language? The development of cultural ideas in general is not in phase with the growth of the brain, but the brain achieved its great size millenia before the appearance of language. Surely, it developed far ahead of Popper's "World III," the world of abstract ideas that it was required to handle. One can only wonder about the evolutionary survival value of so large a brain in neolithic times.

Language and Electrical Stimulation of the Brain

The topographical extent of language cortex in an individual subject is likely to be wider than that indicated in the classic maps. Within this zone, language is discretely localized, with different sites variably committed to language as measured by naming (Ojemann & Whitaker, 1978; Whitaker, 1979). These researchers established that in a single individual language may occupy a very wide expanse of the left lateral cortex, even larger than identified by Penfield and Roberts (1959). Furthermore, there is a graded localization of the naming function (Whitaker & Ojemann, 1977).

These experiments show that the language function is not homogeneously distributed throughout the left hemisphere. Synesthesia is probably not either. Within the language area there are graded effects, so that at a uniform current level some sites always show naming errors, others only some of the time, and others not at all. The transition from an area of 100% naming errors to a site with none may occur over quite a short distance, sometimes within millimeters over the continuous surface of a gyrus. This pattern of localization seems analogous, over a much larger scale, to the columnar pattern of localization described for somatosensory and visual cortex. Five tasks that seem to be selectively disruptable in areas as close as 5 millimeters apart are naming, short-term verbal memory, reading grammatical words (close procedure), phoneme identification (stop consonants), and oral praxis (matching face gestures to a picture) (Whitaker, 1979).

A high degree of variability in localization between subjects is apparent. This functional variability may be a consequence of considerable variability in the detailed anatomy of the cortex. This is suggested by studies of striate cortex that were undertaken as part of the visual prosthesis project in which implanted electrode arrays produce phosphenes that the subject can see (Brindley & Lewin, 1968; Dobelle &

Mladejovksy, 1974). Contacts that are adjacent to each other may or may not produce phosphenes that are adjacent in the perceived visual field. Nonetheless, the phosphene map that is produced remains stable in each patient even though the phosphene maps differ between patients. This suggests that for striate cortex there is a high degree of variation in response to stimulation between patients but considerable reproducibility of responses in any given patient, a condition that is also quite true for synesthetic percepts. If such a degree of individual variation exists in the visual system, generally considered to be one the most "hard wired," then anatomical and functional variability certainly seems likely in other cortices. Studies of morphological asymmetries seem to point in the same direction. As Ojemann and Whitaker (1978) suggested, "the detailed functional anatomy of our brains may be as individualized as the detailed anatomy of our faces."

7

Synesthesia and Personality

At the very end of *The Mind of A Mnemonist,* Luria (1968) devoted a few pages to S's personality and asked the following:

Is it reasonable to think that the existence of an extraordinarily developed figurative memory, of synesthesia, has no effect on an individual's personality structure? Can a person who "sees" everything; who cannot understand a thing unless an impression of it "leaks" through all his sense organs; who must feel a telephone number on the tip of his tongue before he can remember it—can he possibly develop as others do? . . . Indeed one would be hard put to say which was more real for him: The world of imagination in which he lived or the world of reality in which he was but a temporary guest (pp. 150, 159).

One of the things that does seem surprising is that synesthetes appear to be such ordinary persons from all walks of life. As their histories suggest and the evidence supports, most are of normal or superior intelligence. They have superior memories and claim to be highly organized because of their synesthesiae. *Yet their cognitive skills are uneven.* Aside from the rare instances when the intensity of the parallel sense interferes with comprehension, there are lacunae in their intellect and quirks in their personalities. The most common complaints are poor mathematical aptitude despite a good memory for numbers; a poor sense of direction; and difficulty with certain types of abstractions, such as poetry or philosophy.

Almost all synesthetes have suffered ridicule or derision because of their parallel senses. As children they were accused of overactive imaginations, taunted by their classmates, even doubted by their own parents. Unlike the stresses of expectation that befall child prodigies, foreigners in a strange culture, or the sickly child, synesthetes shoulder those of the freak. This chapter looks into the influence of synesthesia on personality and what distinctive personality characteristics synesthetes might have. What is the effect of having a "sixth sense" on personality, memory, learning, organizational skills, and interpersonal relationships? The effect on childhood development, imagination, and creativity are of particular interest. Personality testing, visuospatial skills, and geographic knowledge and orientation are discussed. The number form, another oddity of synesthetes that involves visualizing numbers and other concepts in space, is also examined here.

One cannot assume that synesthetes represent a homogeneous population any more than other groups that are clinically defined, such as schizophrenics. The diagnostic criteria for schizophrenia and synesthesia each define a symptom complex by setting restrictions on who can and cannot be called a schizophrenic or synesthete, respectively. However, they do nothing more and certainly do not guarantee uniformity of brains or behavior.

Does this mean that searching for a unique synesthetic "personality type" will be fruitless? I think not. Because of the variety of synesthetic combinations, the best approach is a detailed description of individual cases in the manner of Luria's together with conventional psychometric instruments when possible. In this way, one gains insight into the personality of synesthetes and the influence of synesthesia on their thinking and organization of day-to-day life, their internal dialogue, and their level of creativity. Instruments such as the Minnesota Multiphasic Personality Inventory (MMPI) and Rorschach test can help answer whether synesthetes are unusually creative or even have a particular tendency toward purple prose. The Wechsler Memory Scale is one objective means to support their claims of hypermnesis; other measures are described in appropriate sections of the text.

Number Forms

Number forms occur with sufficient regularity among synesthetes that they might conceivably be regarded as a special instance of synesthesia. This curiosity was first noted by Sir Francis Galton (1822–1911), the British explorer, anthropologist, and eugenicist known for his pioneering studies in human intelligence. The association of colors and forms with concepts involving serial order was also noted by Suarez de Mendoza (1890), Holden (1891), Flournoy (1893), Calkins (1893), Bos (1929), Weller (1931), and Kloos (1931). Since this section deals with heritability of mental and personality traits, a few words on the birth of this subject are in order. Galton's nine books and some 200 papers deal with diverse subjects ranging from the use of fingerprints for personal identification to correlational calculus (a branch of applied statistics), in both of which Galton was a pioneer. Many of his works show a predilection for quantification and improving standards of measurement.

Galton coined the word "eugenics" to denote scientific endeavors that increase the proportion of persons with better than average genetic endowment through selective marriage and mating. In *Hereditary Genius* (1869), he used that word, "genius," to denote "an ability that was exceptionally high and at the same time inborn.'' His main argument was that mental and physical features were equally inherited, a proposition not accepted at the time. He eventually converted his skeptical cousin, Charles Darwin, to his point of view. Unmentioned in Darwin's *Origin of Species* (1859), Galton is quoted several times in Darwin's later *Descent of Man* (1871). Galton's *Inquiries Into Human Faculty and its Development* (1883 original; reprinted 1907) is a collection of some 40 articles of widely varying length that are based on his scientific papers between 1869 and 1883 and can be regarded as a summary of his ideas.

Since eugenics takes primary account of inborn differences between human beings, Galton's idea came under suspicion from those who believed that social and educational factors were largely responsible for differences in human performance. Accusations of class prejudice probably misrepresented his thoughts, since his aim was not the creation of an aristocratic elite but a population of superior men and women. His ideas, like those of his cousin Darwin, were limited by lack of an adequate theory of inheritance. The rediscovery of Mendel's work in 1900 came too late to affect Galton's contributions in any way.

Generically, Galton established that human ability was hereditary. One of the curiosities that he catalogued was the number form. Like synesthesia, it represents a parallel perception. A number form is the spatial organization of numbers, days of the week, months, and other concepts involving time and magnitude.

I was initially surprised when a number of synesthetes disclosed that they possessed a number form, and later began to inquire routinely of potential subjects. Ascertainment of number forms in synesthetes, therefore, may be incomplete. Table 7.1 shows the incidence of those who possess such forms without synesthesia, those with synesthesia without a number form, and those with both. Synesthesia and number forms share many characteristics. Number forms are always involuntary, memorable, discrete, and durable; they can be projected and emotional.

The most obvious similarity with synesthesia is the coloration of the form together with the capacity for projected visualization of numbers, days of the week, and so forth. Number forms do seem to have a hypermnestic quality and those that possess them claim that the forms help their "ordinary" figurative memory. The number forms are vivid and spoken of in the present tense. Those that possess this mental trait are consistently surprised to "discover" that others do not perceive this way,

TABLE 7.1. Subjects with synesthesia and number forms ($N=42$).

Subjects with synesthesia only	Subjects with both synesthesia and number forms	Subjects with number forms only	Number form projected?
33	4	5	6/9

a common response being, "Well how else could you visualize numbers?" or "But I assumed everyone saw numbers this way."

Figure 7.1 shows a rather simple number form from Galton. The numbers 1 to 20 are seen on a vertical line, then the numbers 30 to 100 appear on the horizontal step. At this point, the pattern repeats. Figure 7.2 shows a more erratic form in which the numbers from 1 to 20 receive more psychophysical space than those from 20 to 1,000. Figure 7.3 shows other types of number forms collected by Galton.

Galton (1907) spoke of variations in the various patterns:

> The pattern or "Form" in which the numerals are seen is by no means the same in different persons, but assumes the most grotesque variety of shapes, which run in all sorts of angles, bends, curves and zigzags . . . The drawings, however, fail in giving the idea of their apparent size to those who see them; they usually occupy a wider range than the mental eye can take in at a single glance, and compel it to wander. Sometimes they are nearly panoramic.
>
> These forms have for the most part certain characteristics in common. They are stated in all cases to have been in existence, so far as the earlier numbers in the Form are concerned, as long back as the memory extends; they come "into view quite independently" of the will, and their shape and position . . . are nearly invariable.

The only modern text in which number forms are discussed is Bowers and Bowers' *Arithmetical Excursions* (1961, pp. 244–247). They noted that "sometimes the numerals are not arranged on a form but are colored," a comment that suggests they might have confused synesthesia with number forms. Whether the two are distinct or whether the number form represents an instance of synesthesia is moot. Because of the similarities between them, I argue the latter.

Bowers and Bowers' initial diagnosis of this in one of their students followed the latter's comment that "I'm having difficulty because the digits keep going up to their places." They gave her a length of stiff wire and asked her to show them the figures' location.

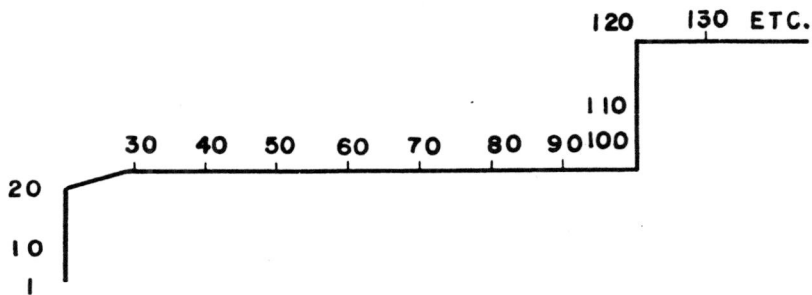

FIGURE 7.1. Number form. (From Galton, F. (1907). *Inquiries into human faculty and its development.* London: J.M. Dent & Sons.)

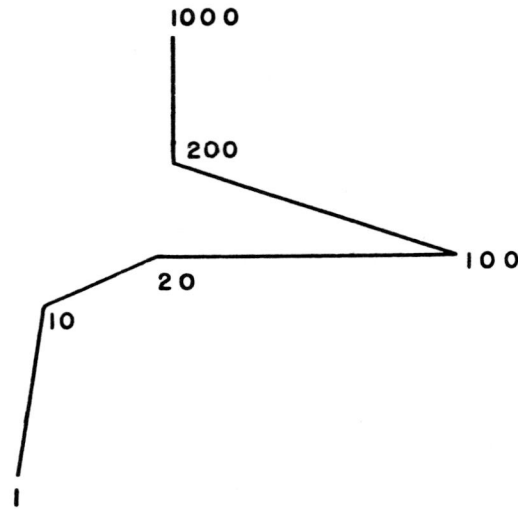

FIGURE 7.2. Note the greater psychophysical space given to the more frequently used numbers, compared to that for numbers between 200 and 1,000. (From Galton, F. (1907). *Inquiries into human faculty and its development*. London: J.M. Dent & Sons.)

Without displaying the least surprise, she took the wire and bent it here and there in three dimensions until it looked like a tortured thing. A number of times, she returned to previously made bends, correcting the angles precisely.

Their student then indicated where the numbers resided along the shape she had created. Her comment, "Is there anything odd about it? Everybody sees numbers like that, don't they?" was characteristic. They collected approximately 20 cases and estimated the incidence of number forms at 3% of the population.

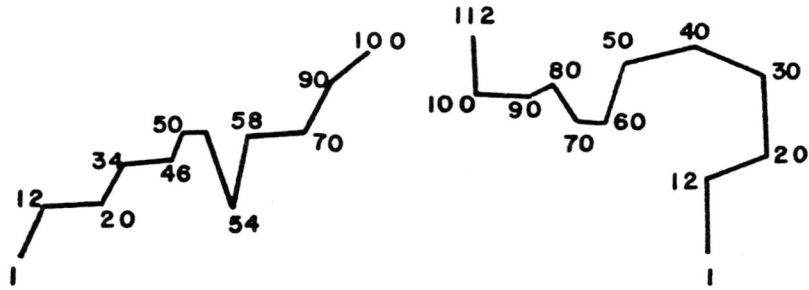

FIGURE 7.3. Two more examples of number forms collected by Galton. (From Galton, F. (1907). *Inquiries into human faculty and its development*. London: J.M. Dent & Sons.)

Neither Galton nor Bowers and Bowers speculated on the origin of number forms. They do not indicate high mathematical ability or deficiency, nor do they seem to be correlated with any specific intellectual talent or mental dullness. The current data do suggest a relative deficiency in arithmetical competency. Subjects DS and MW, however, are frankly acalculic and have some other features of Gerstman's syndrome. The forms help greatly in remembering numbers, in spelling, in organizing personal calendars, and in time management. None of the current subjects have been impaired by possession of a form; all find it beneficial.

Some people have forms for things other than numbers. Galton mentioned forms for the months and the alphabet: "It is a common peculiarity that the months do not occupy equal spaces, but those that are most important to the child extend more widely than the rest. There are many varieties as to the topmost month; it is by no means always January." Bowers and Bowers obtained an elliptical form for the days of the week with the weekend days being close together. They cite, but do not illustrate, examples dealing with ancestry and education.

The Canadian subject DB illustrates the unevenness of spacing for each contained segment of her number forms. Although one might expect at first that weekends or vacation months might occupy more psychophysical space, the examples from Galton and those of the current patients show no such orderliness. Figure 7.4 demonstrates this for the months, where the first 6 months have equal vertical spacing, and last 6 are horizontally unequal, and December is uniquely upended. The form has existed since DB can remember, and clearly before she recalls the regularity of school vacations or the arrival of warm weather in Canada. Figure 7.5 shows DB's form for the days of the week, which contains an internested time form for the hours. The detail of the time form is shown in Figure 7.6.

Number forms need not exist in isolation. DB, whose forms for decades and months are shown in Figure 7.4, also possesses a number and alphabet form, all of which are colorless. An examination of the complexity of these makes one wonder what use they could serve. Why not just rely on a calendar like the rest of us or counting on one's fingers if need be? The presence of DB's upside-down time form internested within the day of the week form is particularly complicated and would seem to require an undue amount of mental gymnastics to utilize. On inquiry, quite the opposite is true. "How else could I think? How would I know where anything is?" she asks incredulously. DB is highly organized, efficient, and detail oriented, much to the envy and admiration of her colleagues at the television station for which she works. "We could all take lessons from her," admits one co-worker who finds DB's forms amusing but concedes that she is highly organized and never relies on the bulletin-board-type production calendar that the rest of the television crew uses.

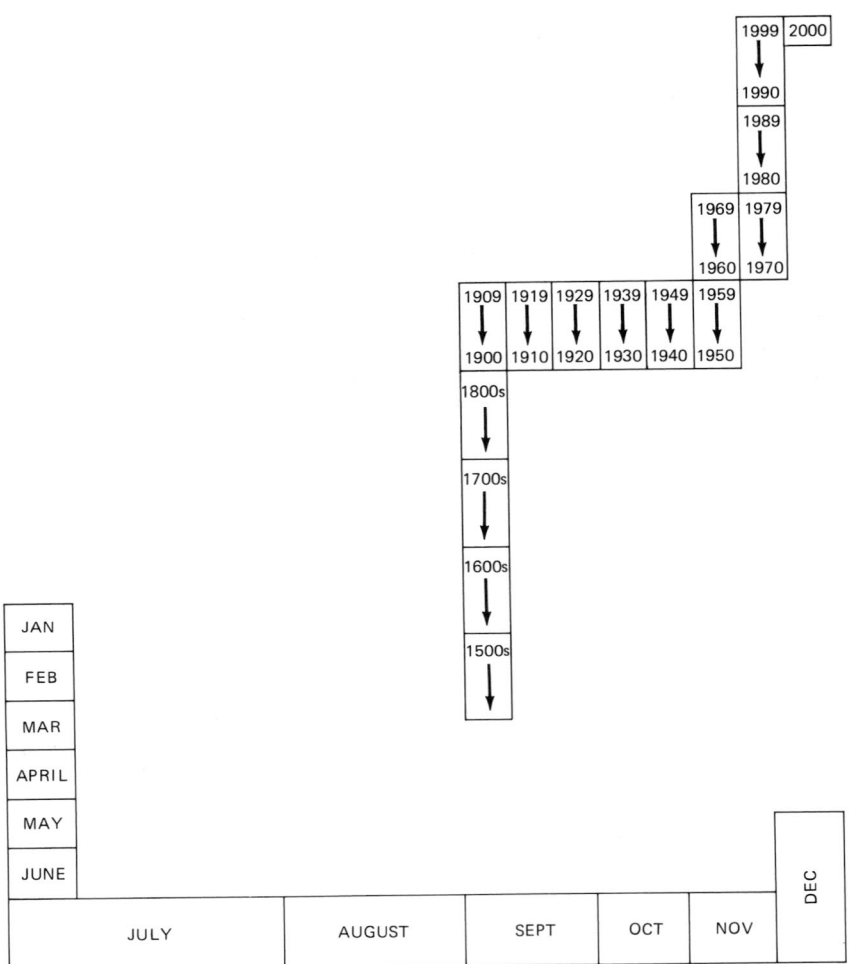

FIGURE 7.4. Decade and month forms of subject DB. *Top:* Decade forms. DB has no notion why the 1960 and 1970 decades are adjacent. The form stops at 2000. DB's birth year is 1960. Decades 1500 to 1800 take less psychophysical space. *Bottom:* Unevenness of month spacing. See text for further details.

The synesthete EW, whose chromasthesia extends over four generations, has number forms, as did a paternal uncle:

My father's brother, a history professor who died at 90, told me shortly before he died that he saw things in space as I did. He did not see in color. His younger brothers died before I thought to ask them, but maybe that shows further that it is hereditary. He said things arranged themselves in a pattern before him like on a chart.

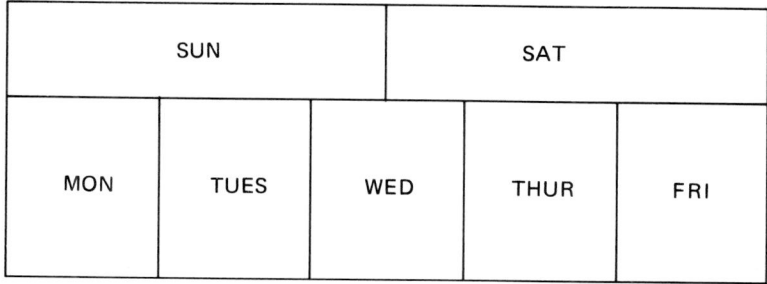

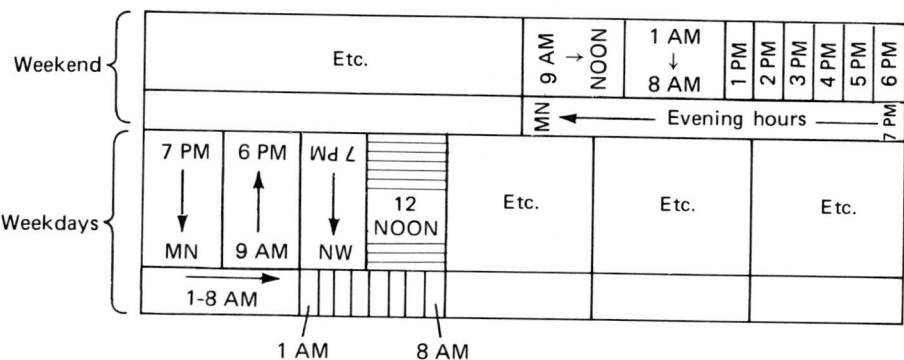

FIGURE 7.5. Days of the week and time of day, subject DB. *Top:* Days of the week. Weekdays are equally spaced, with Saturday and Sunday given disproportionate psychophysical space. *Bottom:* Time of day. Close inspection shows each day of the week to contain an upside-down time cell. Noon and 6 P.M. have more space than other hours, which are equal. Evening hours from 7 P.M. to midnight are on a fluid continuum without distinct separations. Relative orientation of time is different for the weekend and weekdays.

Figure 7.7 shows her pattern for the months, the days of the week, and numbers.

I don't know how anyone with synesthesia could be anything but artistic, in a way, because it has so much to do with color and symmetry and relationship to other appreciations. I find myself rearranging things in a more symmetrical form at home and, mentally, outside! My study of languages (I was a Latin and French major) has been aided by it, I think, because the "amo, amas, amat," etc. was so easy for me to *place* in space as I studied them. Can you understand my meaning here? I also think I can be annoying to others sometimes when I want things to be *just right,* as I see them. It makes me more exacting and "prissy," but I can't seem to help it! (9/19/85)

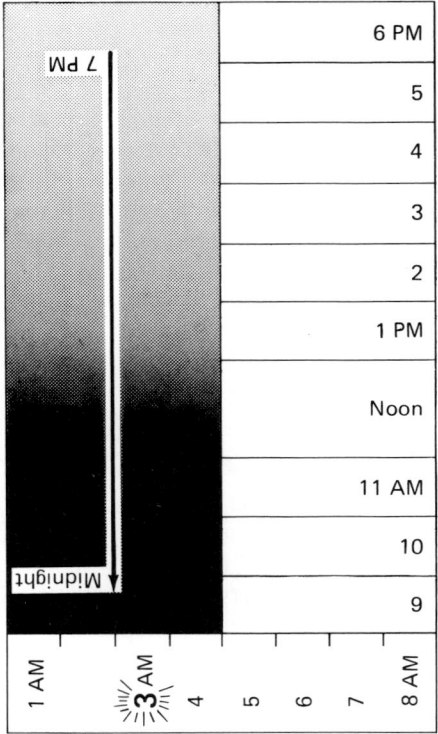

FIGURE 7.6. Detail of weekday time cell in DB's days of the week form. DB does a "mental inversion" when she sees the time cell in detail (cf. Figure 7.5, *bottom*).

DS, with colored hearing and hypermnesis, describes several ways of spatially perceiving items, from the simple to the complex. For her, *time* assumes the circular arrangement of a clock. "For example, 3:00 is always viewed as a physical place in its location on the traditional clock dial." The *days of the week* are linear, "perceived on a number line [*sic*]:

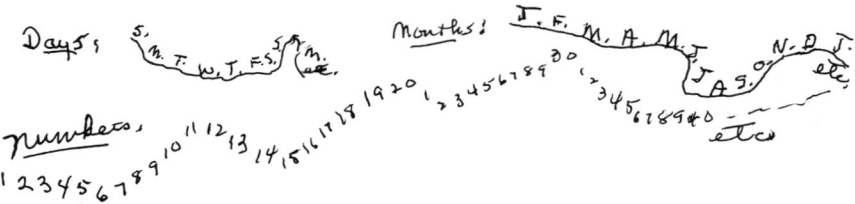

FIGURE 7.7. Day, month, and number forms for synesthete EW. Note tendency for downward slant in space for the days and months, and the undulation of the integers. Multiples of 10 do not occupy the apex of the sine wave shape.

Monday, Tuesday, Wednesday, Thursday, Friday, Saturday, Sunday.'' Figure 7.8 shows DS's months somewhat differently. "I always perceive myself somewhere on this month form.''

Although DS is a polymodal synesthete, some spatial aspects of her perception are worth noting here. One is the *visual perception of pain,* which can be a thin, metallic vertical line or a dense, low, dark fog-like sensation. (Parenthetically, the only other instance I am aware of in which pain has figured synesthetically has been in patients with closed-head trauma. In these patients, sound or light may produce violent pain unilaterally in an extremity, often associated with hemicranial pain. In my experience with eight such cases between 1983 and 1986, this audioalgesic or photoalgesic synesthesia has resolved over several months to a year.)

DS's visualizations are sometimes the making of *Schadenfreude:*

I also experience pain visually. Pain (and pleasure) sensations evoke visual/spatial perceptions which are also in color. In fact, I was recommended for psychological counseling in high school because I told the Assistant Principal that when I kissed my boyfriend I saw orange sherbet foam.

Both persons with synesthesia and those with number form disclose a need to visualize in order to ''think'' or ''comprehend.'' There is an awareness of the incongruity between their obvious intelligence and their apparent density in getting the gist of more abstract discourse or even the content of a lecture or business meeting. DS expresses this well:

I have discovered that I am a visual rather than an auditory learner. I MUST convert oral directions to the visual mode or I cannot function. When someone gives me a set of directions or informally tells me to do more than one thing, I cannot successfully complete the task unless I write it down or mentally visualize the words.

I see words when I talk, when others talk, and when I think. The words are similar to a [*digital*] clock display where each number flips down and is replaced by a new one. When someone asks me how to spell a word I must either write it or close my eyes and visualize it, letter by letter. (I am an excellent speller.) However, I have often left meetings without the vaguest idea of how to process what was said (9/17/84).

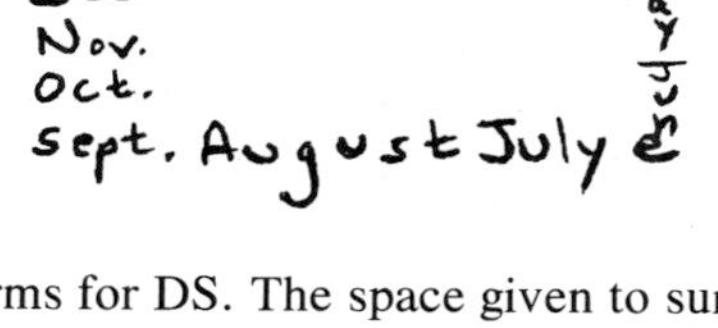

FIGURE 7.8. Month forms for DS. The space given to summer and fall months is not equal.

This visualization appears to give synesthetes excellent memories. For example, "I remember words in print very well, including their location on the page."

To summarize the features of number forms is to point out their similarities with synesthesia, for which reason I consider the form, even when it exists in isolation, to be an instance of synesthesia. Although the forms are not always externally projected (see Table 7.1), they are in all cases vivid. Patients talk about them matter-of-factly and in the present tense; they accept them as real and express surprise that everyone does not manipulate numbers and other concepts in space. The shapes and positions are durable and constant, although the point of view may change depending, for example, on the time of year or the subject's age (see MP below; DS's month box above). That is, although one perspective may change, the relationships between items of the form remain constant over the subject's lifetime.

Memorability is another feature of number forms and synesthesia. One recalls that Luria's mnemonicist remembered limitless amounts of material by recalling the synesthetic image that the item produced and particularly by "where he put the image." When he did make errors it was usually because the synesthetic image was "placed" somewhere where it was later difficult to see, where it was poorly illuminated or blended into the background. His defects of "memory" were really "defects of perception."

Sometimes I put a word in a dark place and have trouble seeing it as I go by. Take the word *box*, for example. I'd put it in a niche in the gate. Since it was dark there I couldn't see it. . . . The same thing happened with the word *egg*. I had put it up against a white wall and it blended in with the background. How could I possibly spot a white egg up against a white wall? (Luria, 1968, pp. 36–37.)

The hypermnesis leads to speculation about the neurology of other elevated functions. Do idiot savants, hyperlexics, and hypercalculics also visualize in space?

The need to visualize seems strong in synesthetes, particularly if they wish to remember.

DS: Reading is not sufficient if I want to remember information. I MUST write down what I want to retain. This is true also with taking directions. In my Tae Kwando [*sic*] class I must translate each "form" [*set of prearranged stances involving both arm and leg movements*] to a written code which I then VISUALLY memorize. I also verbally rehearse constantly when I need to remember, either vocally or sub-vocally depending on the situational appropriateness of talking to oneself. (This was also evident at our meeting.) (3/1/87.)

Synesthetic Forms

Following are four detailed examples from patients involving (1) uncolored spatial patterns for multiple concepts; (2) a simple color form for the days of the week; (3) hypermnestic colored numbers with spatial representation; and (4) an extraordinary case of "memory maps" that combines all these elements.

MULTIPLE VISUAL FORMS

Subject CS: Multiple Visual Forms, Projected, Without Color

The letter-color associations of JM (Chapter 2) showed that there is sometimes not so much color in those who have colored hearing. But the following subject has no color at all! There is not even much variation in light and dark. What her patterns lack in chroma they make up for in their profuseness. She is a 23-year-old American right-hander with 16 years of education, employed in an advertising agency. She has never used drugs. She "discovered" that others did not have spatial forms.

I have only been aware of my "patterns" as something special when I tried to explain to a friend how I see the days of the week (each with its own peculiar positioning and 3-dimensional shape), and he did not understand. My patterns have always been second nature to me, and that was my first attempt at vocalizing them (11/06/86).

Table 7.2 lists the kinds of patterns that she sees. These, she says, are some of her more common patterns, and she could probably enumerate more if she took the time to think further about it. Representative examples of these patterns are shown in Figures 7.9 through 7.11.

TABLE 7.2. Patterns seen by subject CS.

Patterns I See	
Numbers	Days of the week
Months of the year	History
Shoe sizes	Body measurements
Height	Weight
Salaries	Temperature
TV stations	Geographic maps
Body temperature	Multiplication tables
Time	The alphabet
Grades—a grading scale and pattern for GPAs[a]	
My life	
My ages All different patterns	
My school	

[a] Grade point averages.

Months of the Year

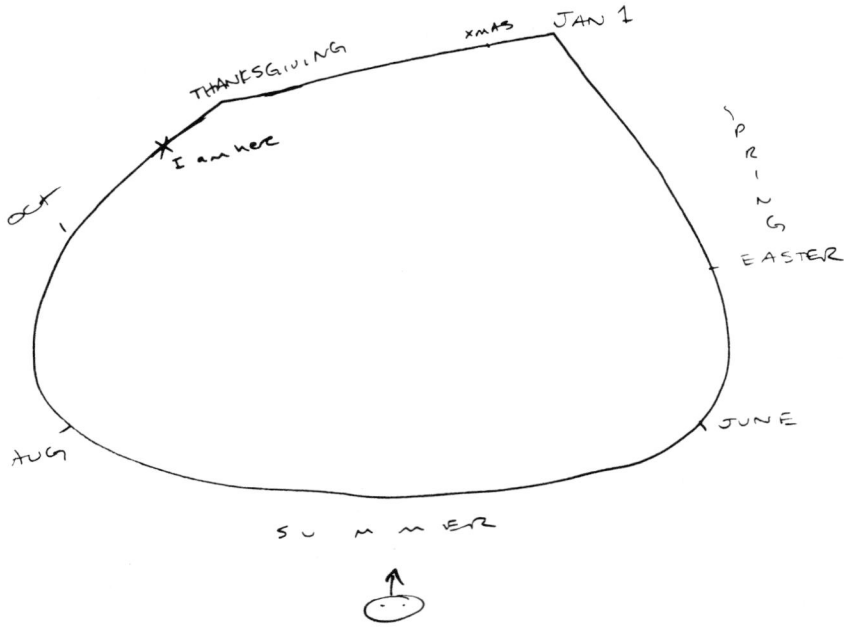

FIGURE 7.9. Months of the year patterns, subject CS. The "face" indicates one point of view, and changes with the season. "X" marks her position when she wrote to me in November. "My perspective changes as I move around within the pattern, i.e. looking up at Christmas or down to Summer or across to Fall."

Numbers

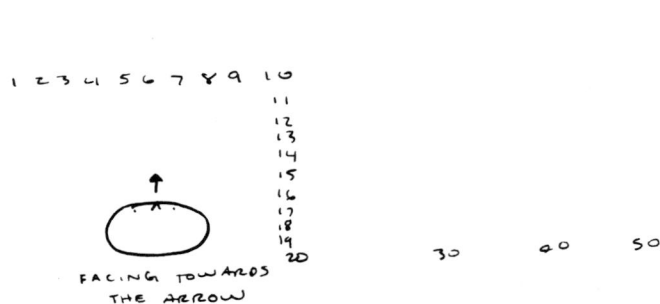

FIGURE 7.10. Number patterns for CS. Note the extracorporeal space behind her, which is usually noted by hearing or proprioception. "As a child, and even now of course, when I sang '100 Bottles of Beer on the Wall' my mind would travel physically down the pattern."

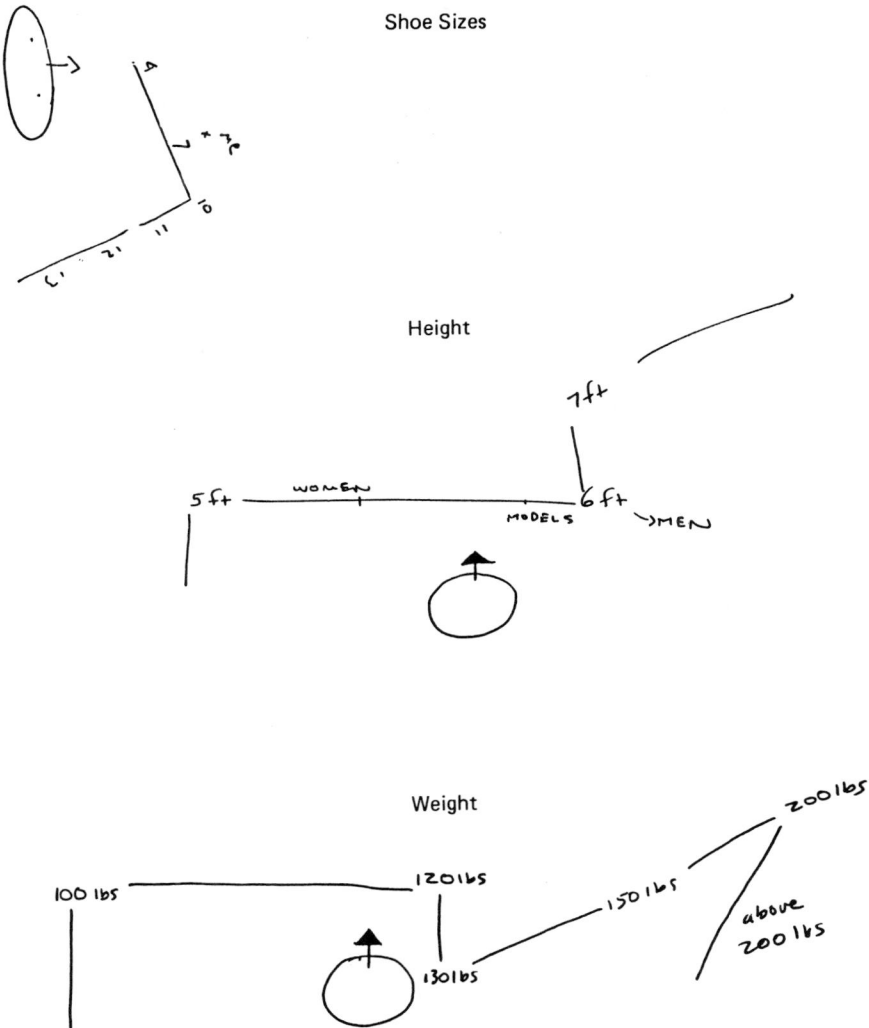

FIGURE 7.11. Shoe size (*top*), height (*middle*), and weight (*bottom*) patterns for CS. "Whenever I think of a shoe size larger than 10, I imagine the tip bent."

Characteristically, the forms have been present as early as she can remember and are invariable. They appear without any conscious volition on her part. Those that relate to her personal history grow from their terminal end, like a vine, as she ages. Her diagrams do not give a satisfactory sense of their expanse or three-dimensionality, but are like snapshots that afford only one point of view. The perspective changes as she moves about within the forms.

CS gives an excellent description of how the patterns are projected. Unlike afterimages, they do not move when the eyes or head change position. The form can be scanned. In explicating her pattern for shoe sizes (see Figure 7.11), she says "the arrow points in the direction I am *facing,* but not just the direction I am *looking.* For example, if I turn my head to the right the patterns don't move with me—they stay fixed around my body. They are fixed in space (around my body). Make sense?" Clarification discloses that it is not, for her, so much a shape that is projected as it is a space or spatial location to which she goes. "I'm not sure that I really see anything, but *I go to a place* where the number 1 or whatever is." With the days of the week, she has a sense of being inside something. The "wall" separating Friday and Saturday is very tall, for example, and on Friday morning she can "look up" at Friday night. Similarly, the alphabet is always on her right-hand side and goes back over her shoulder (Figure 7.12).

The simple line drawings in Figures 7.13 through 7.17, even though made by the subject, fail to convey the mental panorama or the depth they possess. "These patterns aren't accurate because in my mind they are 3-dimensional: either lying flat in a single plane or coming at me at an angle and crossing through other horizontal planes." What are some of the characteristics of these visual forms?

Location

I have always seen things in patterns—a sort of 3-dimensional map that stretches out in front of me at different levels and sometimes wraps around my head. They have always been there.

Durability and Change in Perspective

The Patterns are very defined, have always been in the same place (and are constantly getting longer) as I get older. History is a good example: I cannot think of a period in history (or my past) without simultaneously (but not necessarily consciously) thinking of where it is 3-dimensionally in my mind! For example, the Renaissance [Figure 7.15] is on a curve down to the left of my body. The idea, or thought, and the position are inseparable.

Chronology and Magnitude

Those periods that I know little or nothing about, but I know exist (something should be there on my time-line), are hazy. They are sort of gray, out-of-focus areas, but definitely not empty.

I have a different time-line for all chronological events—history, my life, the days of the week, etc. but I also "see" things like a geographic map, shoe sizes, and body measurements. These also have a linearness to them, with increasing and decreasing sizes and shapes, but why do I see my shoe size about a foot away from my right arm?

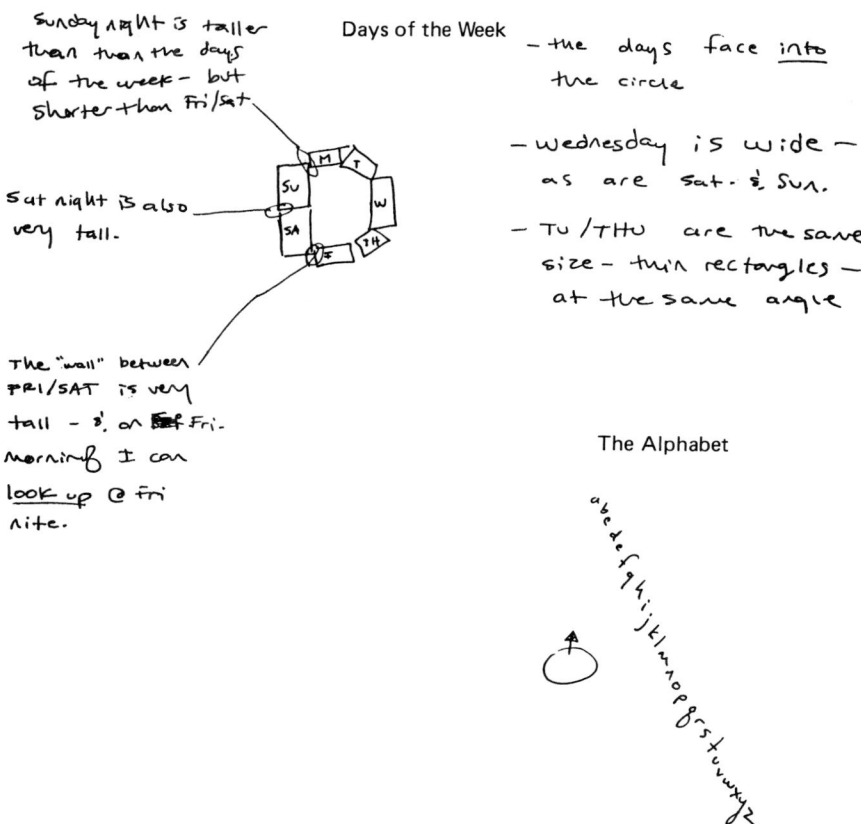

Days of the Week

Sunday night is taller than than the days of the week - but shorter than Fri/Sat.

Sat night is also very tall.

The "wall" between FRI/SAT is very tall - 3', on Fri. Morning I can look up @ fri nite.

- the days face into the circle

- wednesday is wide - as are Sat. & Sun.

- Tu /THU are the same size - thin rectangles - at the same angle

The Alphabet

FIGURE 7.12. Spatial relations of days of the week (*top*) and the alphabet (*bottom*) for CS. See text for further details.

Some schools of philosophy believe that thinking and perceiving are inseparable. For CS, her forms appear inseparable from thinking too. They have always been present. They are fixed in space independently of head or eye movement and occupy intersecting planes. There is no clue to why they are located where they are in her extracorporeal space (''but why do I see my shoe size about a foot away from my right arm?''). The growth of personal chronology versus social history is in opposite directions. The absence of color, which is so prominent in synesthesia, makes CS doubly valuable. Here was the first case without coloration, and her prolific spatial forms should not overshadow the proof that color is *independent of the synesthesia itself*. (The Canadian DB also has uncolored forms.)

CS provides her own best summary: ''My entire life, everything, has a place that goes all around my body.''

Salaries

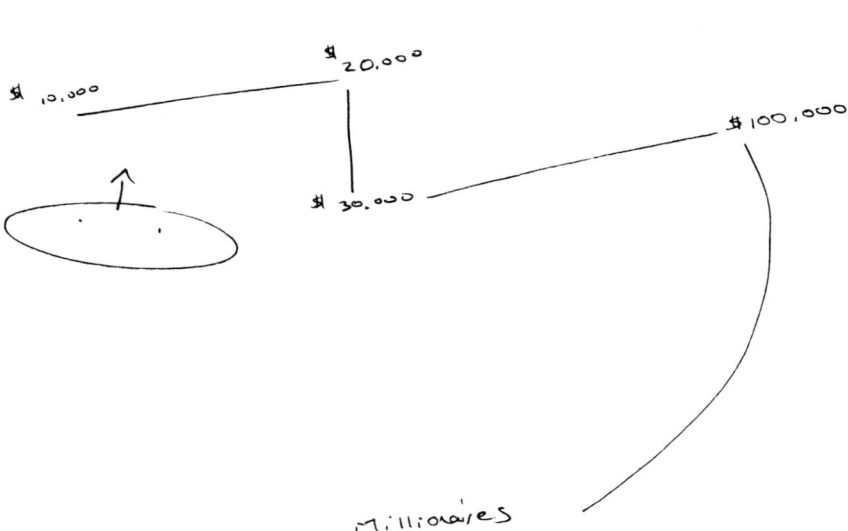

FIGURE 7.13. Salary patterns for CS. Compare with her integers (Figure 7.7), particularly in how large numbers are located behind her.

My Age

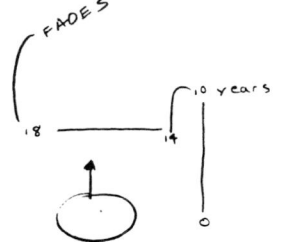

My pattern up until high school

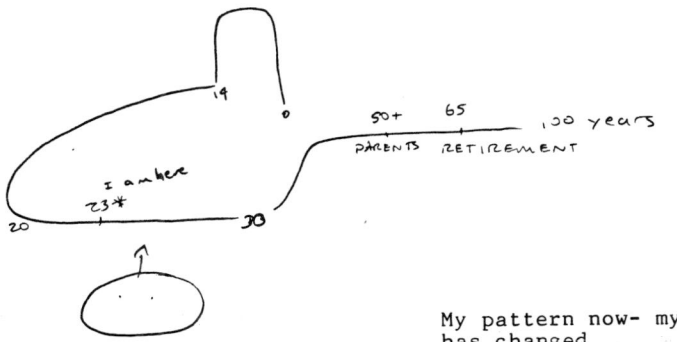

My pattern now- my perspective
has changed

FIGURE 7.14. Patterns of her own age for CS. *Top:* "My pattern up until high school." At this younger age, the pattern faded into the foreground. *Bottom:* "My pattern now—my perspective has changed." At age 23, the psychophysical space has enlarged posteriorly.

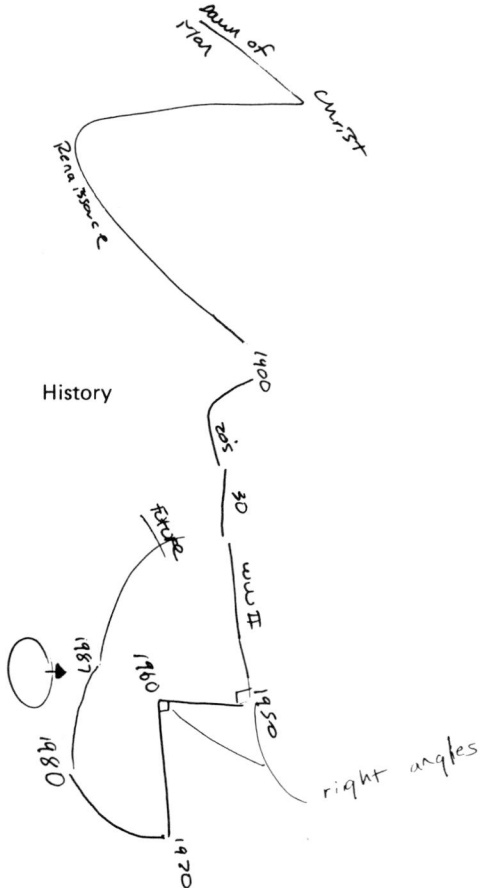

History

FIGURE 7.15. History pattern of CS. The growth and direction is opposite that of her personal chronology (Figure 7.14).

COLORATION OF SPATIAL FORMS

Compared to CS, other synesthetes may rely more on the color than the shape of their form as both an aid for memory and personal organization.

Subject AC: Colored Days of the Week

AC is a 30-year-old right-handed female physican who has a brother who is autistic. There is no family history of sinistrality or synesthesia. She has never used drugs.

AC has always seen the days of the week in an unchanging form. The days form a rectangle with cells of equal space. Monday is leftmost

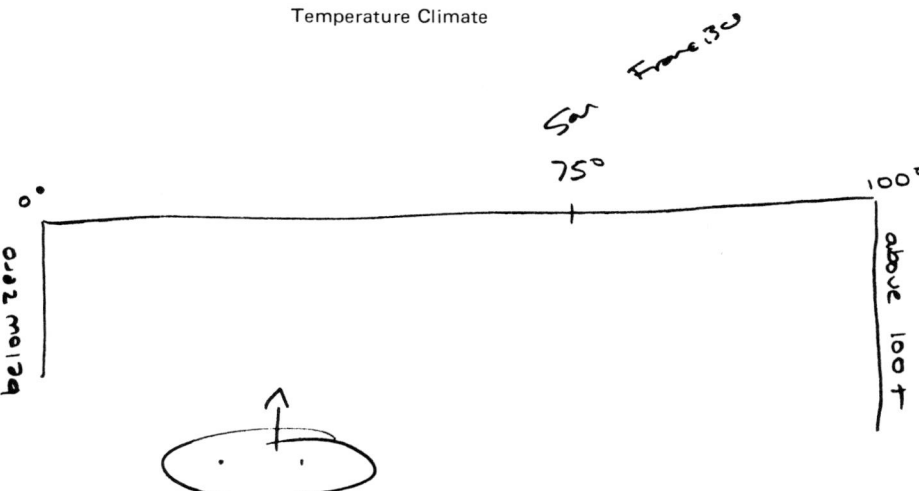

Temperature Climate

FIGURE 7.16. Climatic temperature pattern of CS. Note her use of acute angles with concepts involving magnitude.

(Figure 7.18). She has never mentioned her form to teachers or colleagues because "they would throw me out." Likewise, she feels that she would lose credibility with patients should they discover that she possessed such a form. She realizes such sentiments are irrational but "can't help it."

Her week form is useful for organizing her personal and professional schedule. It is primarily *through the colors* that she keeps track of "what I am doing and where I am supposed to be." She cannot offer any explanation for the origin of either the form or the colors. She boasts a good memory (Wechsler Memory Quotient = 125). Her MMPI (below) shows no elevation of the clinical scales.

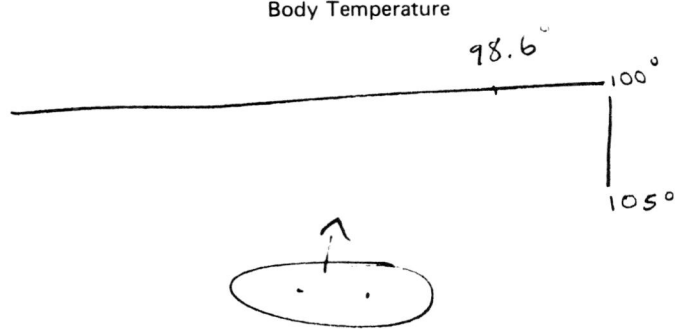

Body Temperature

FIGURE 7.17. Body temperature pattern of CS. "So if somebody says they have a temperature—my mind *goes* to the area above 100°—that corner."

MON	TUE	WED	THU	FRI	SAT	SUN
baby blue	lavender	bright green	maroon	blue	green	white

FIGURE 7.18. Colored days of the week help AC in organizing her personal schedule. The colors are more important than the shape.

Subject SdeM: Colored Visual Forms: Eidetic Memory; Navigational Incompetence; Olfaction No Longer Able to Stimulate Memory After Radiation for Pituitary Tumor

This 48-year-old right-handed female, born in Yorkshire, England, holds a doctoral degree in urban planning and organizational studies. She comes from a poor background and had a stern Victorian upbringing, but eventually became widely traveled and lived among many cultures. She has no history of psychiatric problems, hallucinations, or use of recreational drugs. Family history is negative for mental illness and synesthesia.

She has three sisters (two artists, one nurse) and she, herself, has two fraternal twin boys; there is no other family incidence of twinning. A younger sister is left-handed and all girls have math difficulties. ("It must be genetic, but it wasn't encouraged for girls to go to school.") SdeM is the first to go to a university.

SdeM's synesthesiae are an inextricable part of her life. Aspects are catalogued below.

Colored Numbers, Days of Week, and Months

SdeM was self-referred after seeing a television program on which I appeared called "I See Music."

Unfortunately, I only caught the tail end of the program, but what I did manage to see absolutely astonished me. I am 48 years of age and in spite of talking to everyone who would listen, I have never come across anyone who, like me, vividly sees numbers in colours and who uses the consistency of those colours as a memory aid.

These are *my* colours:

1 = gray black
2 = white
3 = green
4 = deepish blue
5 = pink
6 = yellow

7 = light rust/brown
8 = very pale blue
9 = earthy brown (04/06/86).

Age of Onset; Spontaneity; Psychophysical Locale

I've always had it. I've never not had it. It was very intense as a child and got in the way of doing arithmetic. I've contrived to repress it because when I started putting formulae together [*while studying physics*], all I saw were colours and it would get in the way of the conceptual basis of what the formulae were about.

When someone says "2," I see white. The number is incidental to the white. I know it's 2 because it's white.

I'm disquieted if I see an advertisement with a 2 in the "wrong" colour. I can't remember it.

My children had a book—Learn Your Numbers—but the colours of the numbers were all wrong. The world was wrong.

In school, if the teacher asked "what is 2 times 2?" I would blurt out "Blue." I couldn't disaggregate it. The teacher and classmates thought I was very silly. The colour would come to mind first and I would have to consciously think of the answer.

Integers larger than 10 combine effects. She explains:

Zero has no color, only a space. With 21 I see the black and the white. Beyond 100 it gets very confusing. It's helpful when I can see the individual colors. For example, if I'm knitting and the phone rings and I'm on stitch 95, I can remember brown and pink and pick back up when the conversation is over.

The labor involved in such thinking is striking. Why not simply remember "95" instead of remembering the translation to brown and pink? The difficulty in thinking is revealed when the colors are not there to help.

I have great difficulty with real numbers over a thousand. *I have to think hard because the colors aren't there to help me.* If someone says "Write down 4226" I have to think about it. It's difficult.

Shapes, with Some Color

When asked where the numbers and colors are seen, SdeM replies that they seem "internal," but there is a sense of looking at a screen down on another plane. "It's like an aura around the number, but the 2 is down on the screen. If I try to draw it, it goes away. It becomes very hard for me to see."

Figure 7.19 shows the spatial arrangement of the weekdays and the months. Numbers have the least spatial component. The days of the week are colored; only a few months are:

Monday—brownish   January—blackish
Tuesday—yellowish   April—mustard
Wednesday—orange   September—white

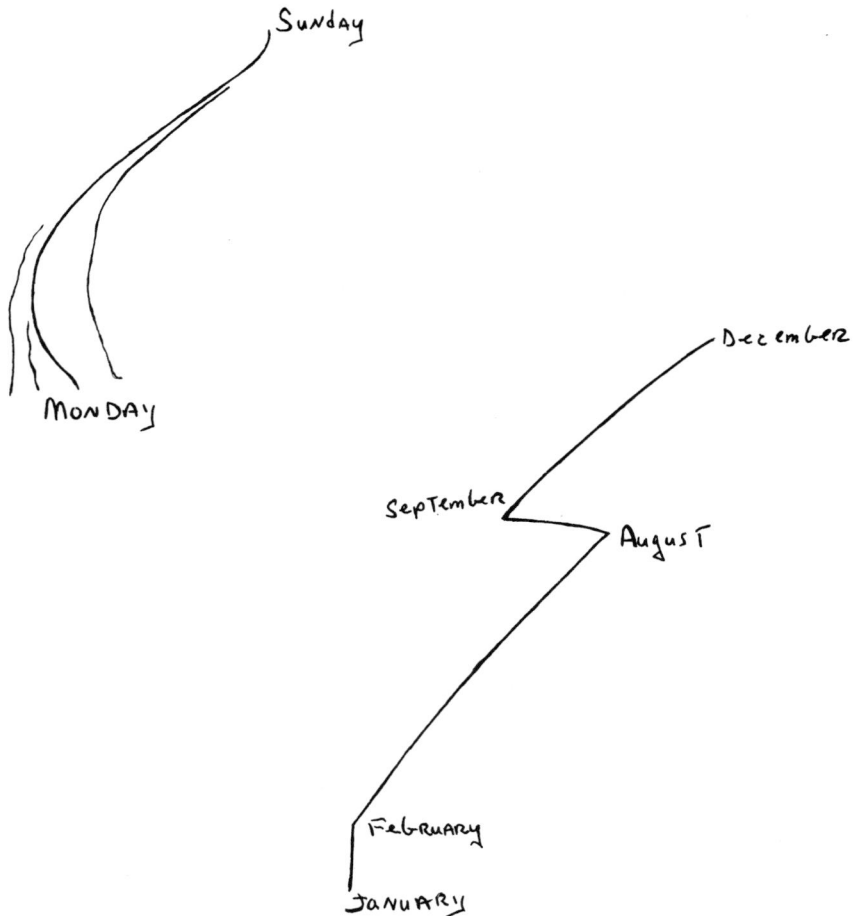

FIGURE 7.19. Weekday and month colors of SdeM. "I see the months spaced more than I see them in colours. The days of the week are curved and are fat at the beginning and get skinny as you approach Sunday [*note beginning with Monday*]. They start horizontal and become 'flat out' as they recede away. However, there is no parallax and Sunday is just as easy to see as Monday, which is closer. It isn't any harder to visualize because I'm looking down on it."

Thursday—ochre
Friday—grayish
Saturday—absolutely white
Sunday—gold

Music is perceived as "colours, moving like dots, like people in a crowd at a football game when the camera zooms in on them." This is vivid but not projected.

Failure of Volition

SdeM is able to manipulate or suppress her images very little if at all. They can often get in the way and, as they did in Luria's patient S, interfere with the semantic and meaningful attributes of everyday conversation.

I can do nothing to alter my immediate reactions. If I try to change the colour of the number—at least in my mind—it always slips back either to its own *colour* or to the *number* usually seen as the colour I tried to change it to. If someone gives me a particular number coloured in the "wrong" colour and then I close my eyes to see the number I feel I have to struggle to get the world right again.

I've had to impose other things on it for me to understand numbers for what they actually are instead of just these colours. I'm not good at math. I could conceptualize the physics, but I got the answers wrong. Numbers mixed with letters in physics formulae were very confusing.

Durability

The colors never change, their luminosity and intensity are constant, and all numbers are equally easy to visualize. Written and spoken numbers are perceived the same. She has no explanation for why there is no red among her colors.

Features of Her Memory: Eidetic Memory; Color Memory

SdeM's memory is vivid, durable, and appears to be equally good for auditory and visual modes. It is also highly detailed such that she can recall the doctor's complicated instructions by "seeing him speak," or visually recreate every schoolroom or house she has ever been in "right down to the cracks in the wall, or a piece of wallpaper coming off." Her conviction is firm: "I know it is totally, absolutely undistorted."

I have a very, very acute memory of environments, colours, people, clothes or whatever. I never have to take a swatch out to match colours. I can carry a colour in my head for years. For example, mother has had a favourite dress for years, and she was coming to visit [*from another country*]. I went out and bought her some beads that matched the dress exactly and I hadn't seen it for 7 years.

I can remember people's appearances very vividly and if I were an artist I would be able to paint almost everyone I know right down to the blemishes on their faces. Strangely, this facility has lessened since I lost my sense of smell (10/01/86).

She supplied an apt definition for eidetic memory, although she had never heard the term before. She describes this memory, which can be visual or auditory, as "that memory which does not require me to conceptually understand it but simply to recall it." She fulfills Haber and Haber's criteria (1964) for an eidetiker.

I remember places very, very well. We were in Europe this summer. When I close my eyes, I can actually see the hotel rooms, the furniture, the pictures, even though we were always in different places.

I always used to win those party games with trays and things. I can remember conversations if I want to, if it's important. As part of my research at [X] university, I have to interview people and I recall the words they say and even the inflection in their voices as long as I need to. I don't often take notes. At the Doctors, if he gives complicated instructions, I have no problem remembering because I have to. But I remember it because I remember hearing him saying it, I don't remember it conceptually. I can recall conversations down to the last jot, but they're always important conversations. . . . I hear them all over again, like a record.

If I'm studying and need to refer to something, I can go to that book and know exactly where to look for it. Yes, I can conjure it up in my mind, but I can't read it word for word. I can remember it in substance but not read it back. I can see the same, and how many lines the idea takes up, and where it is on the page. I can remember conversations word for word better than I can things I have read.

Olfactory Trigger for Memory; Loss of Memory after Pituitary Tumor

SdeM was treated with radiation and bromocriptine in 1977 for a pituitary tumor that had caused amenorrhea. She was still taking bromocriptine when examined. She has lost her sense of smell, but claimed that her sense of taste returned to normal. *The loss of smell has lessened the vividness of her memory.*

Her ability to "recreate," in minute detail, prior environments was particularly facilitated by olfaction. She also attributes the intense sense of conviction that her memories were "absolutely undistorted" to the olfactory facilitation. Upon encountering an odor, an image would flash in her mind.

The feeling was explosive. "Ah ha," I would say, "there's the bakery shop or the lake." It was a pleasant feeling, but I don't recall that there was any other physical sensation.

Now, anosmic, *these visualizations no longer force themselves on her,* although the memory does remain accessible. She has to think about it, much like we all do, and even then *the memory is different.*

It's not that the memory is diminished, but it has *affected* the way my memory works because I have to consciously imagine it. It doesn't come spontaneously like it used to before the operation.

One could rush to the conclusion that SdeM's memory impairment following loss of olfaction is not surprising because it is known that the entorhinal cortex and rhinencephalon participate in memory. For example, the olfactory cortex is markedly involved in senile dementia of the Alzheimer type, a disease whose hallmark is memory loss. Degeneration predominates in large cells, greater than 90 microns, and those of the association cortex (that is, those that make corticocortical connections). The primary isomodal cortex is little involved.

But SdeM does not have a cortical lesion. She has not had a temporal lobectomy or a hippocampal resection. She is likely anosmic from radiation and not the pituitary tumor itself. Her figurative memory remains normal and her current Memory Quotient is 135.

Her preoperative "memory explosion" illustrates a point often confused. Taste and smell are senses with low *gestalten.* With the possible exception of a vintner or perfumier, one never remembers a smell; rather it is a smell that leads to reminiscence. It is this spontaneous, explosive, emotional memory that was triggered by a smell that left SdeM when she became anosmic. For her, this memory was different from that which a smell might evoke in you and me. Synesthetes MW (geometric taste) and DS (polymodal) claim to remember actual scents.

Some memories are more vivid and carry more emotional baggage than others. The memory of what one did at work yesterday is likely to be bland. Recollection of a *faux pas* or a humiliating childhood experience can be accompanied by a physiological flush of vasodilitation or the emotion of embarrassment. SdeM's postoperative experience shows that there can be dissociation between the content of memory, the emotion of memory, and the conviction of a memory.

Absence of Screen Memory; Childhood Recollections

SdeM believes that she can recall things before she was able to speak and cites two reasons for her conclusion. The first is that the recollections are always from her point of view and that there are no screen memories. "I never ever see myself. I am looking at what I remember . . . seeing underneath the table in my home sitting room." Objects recalled from infancy are described as huge, while others are unexplainable or unrecognizable—lumps and shadows that she cannot identify. She apologizes, "I know it sounds odd, but I do, I really do."

An example antedating language convinces her that her memories are true memories and not something her family had described to her when she was older.

We lived in a house that was warmed by coal fires. The two downstairs rooms had fireplaces but we only burned one because it was cheaper, and we all huddled around the one. The other room was called the parlor. Because it was this gaping hole in which we occasionally had fires, we had a wooden screen with a cloth covering with pleats. I remember my grandmother sitting on one side of the fire and my father on the other and they had put coal on it and the fire was spitting sparks out into the room. Grandmother said "get the fireguard." Now the fireguard we had for the actual fire was iron with little grates. That was the one that prevented the fire from coming out. When Grandmother said "get the fireguard" I went into the parlor and dragged the cloth one into the room. Both my grandmother and my father laughed because I'd obviously brought what I understood to be the fireguard but it wasn't going to protect because it was cloth, not the metal one that was going to prevent the sparks. And I could remember my impotence at not being able to say "but you said fireguard" (although I didn't know the words at the time). My impotence at not being able to speak. I may have been able to say a few words, but I was aware that they were able to do something I couldn't to explain [*i.e., speech*]. I was walking, and was probably on the threshold of speaking but know I couldn't coherently put words together (10/03/86).

Visualization

Like DS and other synesthetes, SdeM thinks visually. Night and day her mind is full of images, bits of memories, words, and feelings. Although she often uses metaphors and analogies, "I don't know if the metaphors preceded the idea or follow it." She finds talking about her visualizations difficult because "you take what you are for granted. The only way I know about the [*coloring of my*] numbers is because it's come to the attention of others who don't function the way I do."

SdeM "materializes" ideas in a mental image "to better hold" them whenever she encounters difficulty in a concept. This is an automatic, unself-conscious act. As a not very able physics student at high school, the laws she had to learn would stay in her mind only when she could "see" images of perfect spheres on perfect planes, or density varying with pressure.

Physical Reaction to a Particular Color

To a particular shade of cobalt blue ("the colour of airport landing lights but without its luminousness") SdeM has an "unexplicable" visceral feeling of dropping too quickly in an elevator. She has experienced this feeling, even when thinking about the color, for as long as she can recall. What is one to make of her compulsion to look at the color, yet never to wear it or possess anything of that color?

What's strange is that occasionally I'll see people in the street with a scarf or a coat that [*cobalt*] colour and I have to follow them. I don't mean physically, but I have to look at it, look at them repeatedly. It's very attractive, and I have to do it. It's like bees going to a flower or something. I don't know. I feel it. It's not unpleasurable but it's not pleasurable. And I like the colour but I never buy it and I never wear it. I don't know why.

I saw a car when we were in Europe this summer that was that colour. And I had to keep looking at it for a while.

My family thinks it's very odd.

Sense of Direction

The hypothesis that synesthetes have geographic impairment is explored below. As an example, SdeM claims her sense of direction is "terrible."

On visiting my hotel for an interview she twice had to get instructions on how to find the elevators. Yet their location should have been obvious. She claims to be only slightly better at network maps than vector maps

. . . but I have to have a map of everyplace I go to. I have absolutely no sense of direction, even in cities I live in. Coming up out of the subway, I have to stop to figure out what side of the street I'm on. I'm always getting turned around. I've lived in [city] for 8 years now and I still get lost. No one in my family has this problem. They don't need maps.

MEMORY MAPS

MP uses the term "memory maps" for lack of a better term to describe how she sees the alphabet, numbers, months, and days of the week (Figures 7.20 through 7.22). Her drawings are a vague representation at best because they appear to her in a "flexible moving 3 dimension." Her drawings are therefore a *representation and not a reproduction of what she sees.*

In 1983 MP prepared a 25-page typewritten "explanation" of her "memory maps." Characteristic of these maps is the difficulty describing their panorama and three-dimensionality. It is also difficult to describe the color, although she rendered them with colored pencils, which she says are inaccurate because neither the subtleties nor transparent qualities are possible to render. Her colors are translucent rather than solid. Only after she discovered that others did not possess this did she start to inquire of others and verbalize her visions. They then became more concrete in her mind and easier to explicate, although they have always existed. Importantly, MP's diary, as far as it reflects her personality, gives no suggestion of a philosophical or cosmic orientation.

Her drawings for the alphabet and numbers are rendered on black backgrounds, which is close to her true vision. The x's in the figures denote points of view from which the form can be perused. "Looking back at my illustrations they look ridiculous, even to me. . . . I'm not used to seeing the map in one dimension or so finite with such limiting borders. The maps are larger than my visual range, like looking at the horizon." She likens her memory maps to a geographical map. One can get an overall view without any detail or zoom in to a specific section.

Her earliest recollection of the alphabet is age 4, when she recalls spelling M-I-L-K from a milk carton. She has a recollection that when her grandmother asked her how to spell TEA, she recalls that the letter "T" was in the dark part of the alphabet that she could not see. The alphabet was only just beginning to have form and still clouded in darkness. She learned to read before starting school and her alphabet pattern was firm by this time. The days of the week appeared shortly after the alphabet and her month form was in place at approximately age 7.

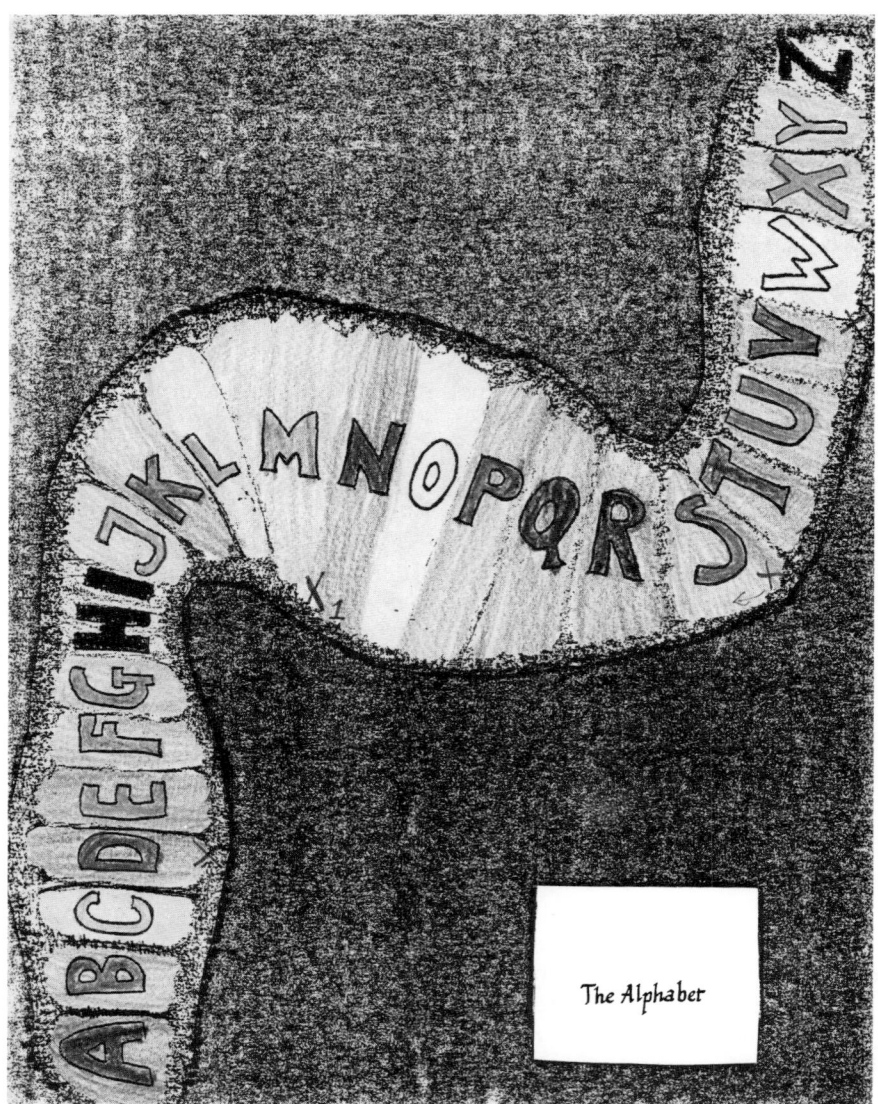

FIGURE 7.20. Subject MP, the alphabet. In this and subsequent drawings of MP the colors, of course, cannot be appreciated.

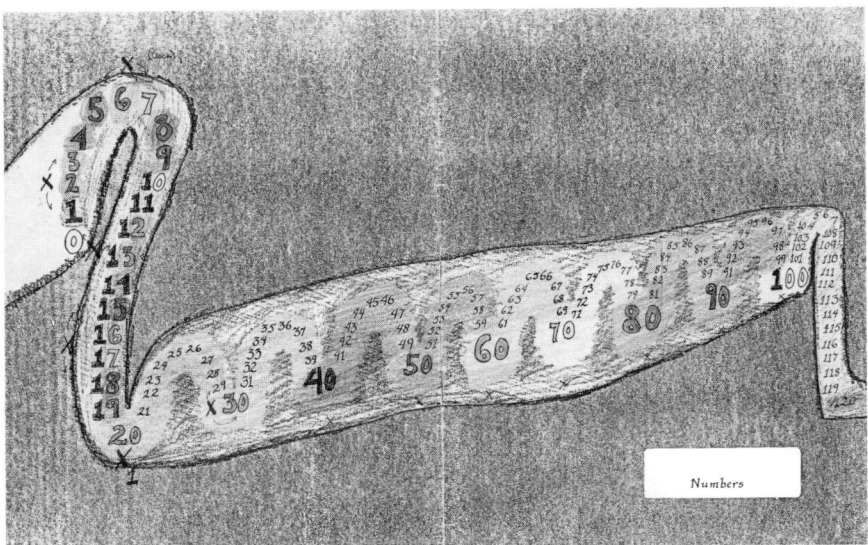

FIGURE 7.21. Number memory map of MP. 1 to 20 are seen singly, and 20 to 100 in groups of 10. After 100, the pattern repeats with a "1" in front of it. MP can view 100 numbers at a time (e.g., 50 to 150). Note the upside-down clock, a casualty of the number form on learning to tell time.

It is difficult for her to say exactly what the letters or numbers look like (i.e., typeset, handwritten, or Roman style). It as if she is more aware of the shape, spacing, and color than the graphology of the Latin alphabet or Arabic numerals. "It is like looking at your speedometer—you are so used to it that you don't really 'see' the numbers."

MP did not disclose her maps to anyone until in college. "I figured everyone did it this way! It was too much to fathom that it might be unique with me. Once I was asked when I would *need* to see the alphabet as a whole—my first response was, Doesn't everybody? It never occurred to me that it might be unnatural to visualize the whole alphabet (or numbers)."

The Alphabet

MP's alphabet forms a loop projecting out of the blackness, with A and Z anchored in the shadows and a spotlight on the letters J through S. This section includes several letters in her name (M, R, L, O, P, K). When learning a new word as a child she would pick out the letters as in a scrabble set and combine them. She is an excellent speller. The process then became automatic, except now in instances when she is requested to spell or define a word it appears letter by letter.

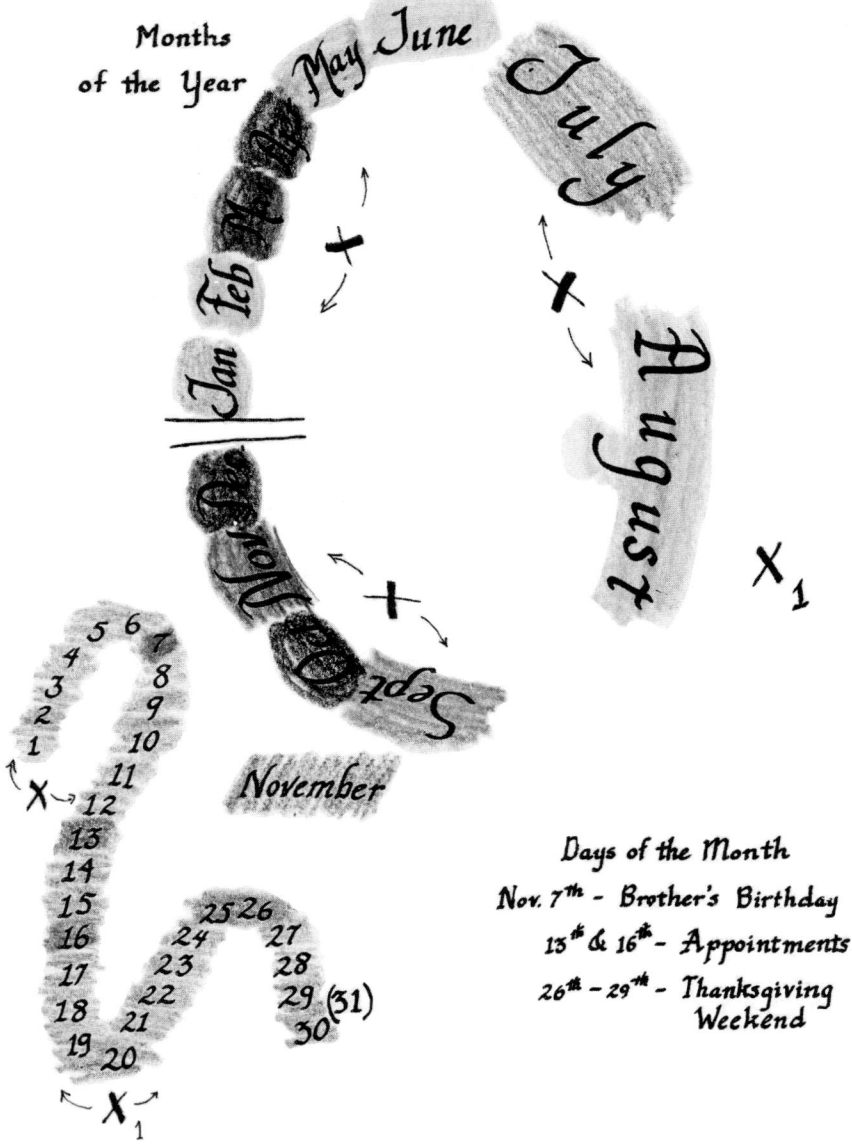

FIGURE 7.22. MP, months of the year. *Below:* The days of the month for November are shown. There is a blending of the usual integer color with an overall brown, the color for November. This helps to identify the numbers as belonging to that month.

Words and Names

In words the first letter influences the overall color of the word (Figure 7.23). Vowels, which have a paler color, shade the word: A and I darken it, E and O lighten it, and U is neutral. TIN is darker than TAN, TAN darker than TEN (although "10" is different), TEN darker than TUN. TUN (a large cask of wine) is in between TIN and TAN or TAN and TEN. If E is added to TUN to make TUNE, the word becomes much lighter. Next in importance are letters that are spatially big to her (B has *more color* than C, K than L) or have *more sound* (S more than R, G more than H). Hers is a good example of the fact that synesthetes and those with number forms visualize some numbers and letters as larger than others.

MP compares the process to threads in a tapestry:

The letter colors appear like fabric; pull the individual threads apart and you can see the various colors. Woven together, they become one, i.e. predominantly green ("T"), but influenced by the other "strands." For example, say you are looking at a rug. One or two strands out of 5 will be brown, the rest green. Look at the fibers running through the strands. Some are red (A—TAN), or perhaps yellow (E—TEN), or gray (U—TUN), or maybe black (I—TIN). Standing on it, you say that the carpet is green; sitting on it you might notice the brown, and examining it closely, you may see the red, yellow, etc.

The colors are helpful in remembering names, particularly if they have less common spellings. "Cathie" looks entirely different than "Kathy;" even "Brown" is different than "Browne" (Figure 7.24). Thinking about someone produces a different visualization than talking about them. She will visualize their physical features if imagining a conversation with them or recollecting them performing some task. But if speaking about them ("he believes such and such"), then MP *sees their name.* She will also see the name in color if searching for it on a list.

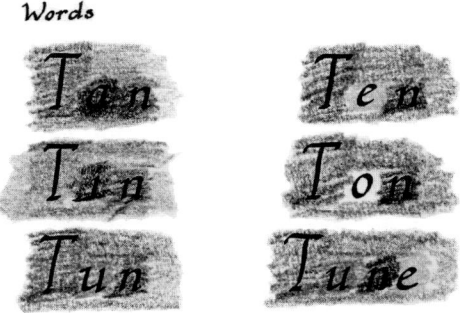

FIGURE 7.23. MP, influences of vowels on the coloration of a word. A = red, i = black, u = gray, e = yellow, o = white.

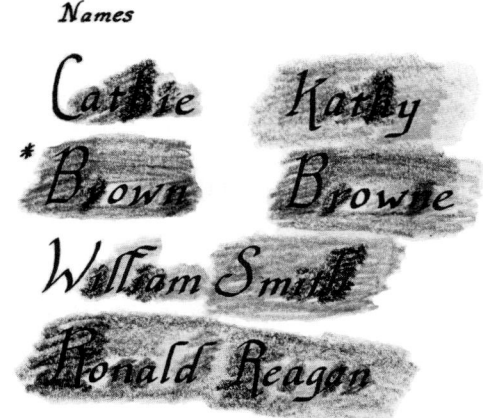

Names

* B is very changeable in color. In this case, it is brown, other times, it is blue, or black.

FIGURE 7.24. MP, coloration of names that are homonyms. For MP, the orthography influences the synesthesia. "Cathy" is blue overall, while "Kathy" is green.

The colors have no emotional meaning.

The colors are totally objective. I put no meaning into them. People frequently ask me to tell them what color their name is. If someone thinks "Ugh, what a terrible combination of colors; she must not like me," that is not at all true. I don't relate it with a person in that way at all. The colors have no meaning.

Colors will change if someone changes his name, by marriage or, more commonly for MP, who works in a film studio, if an actor changes a role. "It seems to be rather easy to jump back and forth between the character and the actor (both the name and the personality). Actually it helps establish the new personality or character in my mind."

Numbers

The visualized numbers (Figure 7.21) do not interfere with simple arithmetic, but they do interfere with more complex mathematics, such as algebra. "The numbers cannot be visualized for complex calculations. For one thing, they are not evenly or consistently spaced. There is some fluid or jelly-like movement to them." Six and numbers containing "6" represent the highest degree of magnitude for her, since "6" is physically the highest in her visual representation. When thinking of someone older than herself, she looks "up;" younger people are seen not "down" but "in back" of herself.

Numbers take on variation in coloration if they represent time. Decades (Figure 7.25) do not have the same color as integers (see 50 and 80 in Figure 7.21 *top*). Times before her birth year, 1954, are dark. The 1950s are black to gray, the 1960s yellow, the 1970s bright blue, the 1980s orange, and the 1990s dark blue. The decades of the centuries take on the color of the century. Thinking of each century as a whole, 1900s are black, 1800s yellow, 1700s blue, 1600s red, and 2000s pink. On close examination, the individual decade color then appears. This is an example of her map analogy of describing how she views the large picture and then is able to zoom in to view the details.

Months, Weeks, and Days

Figure 7.22 shows MP's months. Considering a particular month causes the view to shift to the configuration of the numbers 1 to 30, colored not with their integer color value, but with the overall color of the month. Birthdays and other dates are remembered first by the color of the month, then by the picture of the number.

The weekdays have the least pattern of any of MP's maps (Figure 7.26). They are simply a string of days. If MP is in a particular room regularly enough, the room will take on a aura depending on what day of the week it is.

Figure 7.27 illustrates the hours of the day and minutes of the hour. Again, she sees time as space. "Digitals drive me crazy." She looks

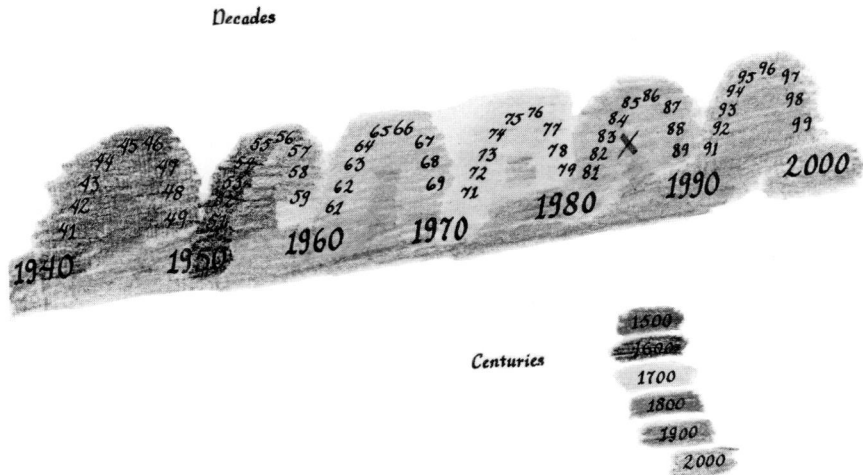

FIGURE 7.25. Integer colors (see Figure 7.21, *top*) are not the same as those for the digits representing decades, as in this figure. The "50" of 1950 is black, while the integer 50 is orange; the "80" of 1980 is peach, while the integer 80 is gray.

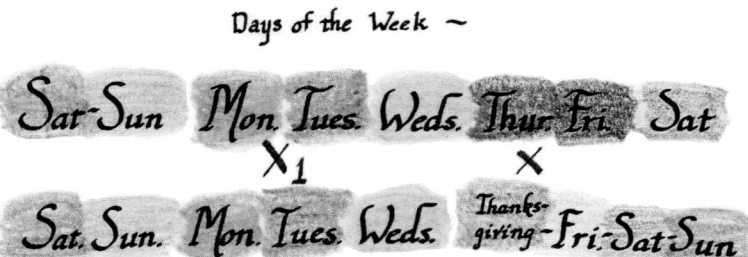

Days of the Week ~

Sat-Sun Mon. Tues. Weds. Thur. Fri. Sat
X₁

Sat. Sun. Mon. Tues. Weds. Thanks-giving—Fri-Sat-Sun

FIGURE 7.26. Weekdays memory map of MP. She can see ahead 2 weeks and backward 1 week. Appointment days are "marked" with a hump and a spotlight—"they are different in a way I cannot explain."

upward at time in a spiral, and when planning a day sees blocks of time as sections of the spiral. The density of coloration of the spiral changes should she have to do something at a particular time. "The difference is like that between a print and a solid—the more free my time is the more 'solid' color the time is. Sewing or vacation time is quite solid in color."

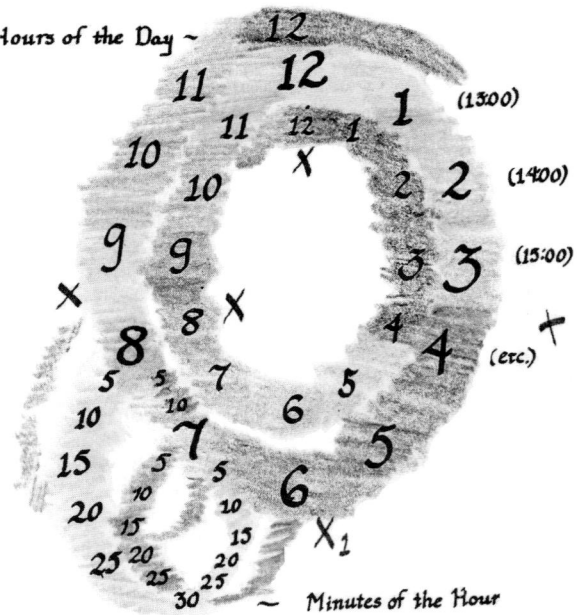

FIGURE 7.27. MP's hour and minute memory maps.

Obviously, MP is quite organized and her spatial and color scheme has practical benefits. Like any rigid scheme, however, it has its drawbacks. There are noticeable differences with a change of routine schedule and with the change of the seasons. Were she to change her schedule with a new job, for example, the appearance of the days of the week "would change radically. Even if things are going fairly routinely, there is a gradual change with the seasons . . . so over a 4 to 6 month period, there is a noticeable difference." Again, she has great difficulty verbalizing the difference and claims that it is "vague and hazy." She is certain, however, that the difference exists.

The Utility of MP's Memory Maps

MP's memory maps are important in her career as a librarian. Her specialty is cataloguing, and she finds her maps essential for remembering patrons' names, trivial facts, page and call numbers, and filing. When someone stands in front of the card catalogue reciting a portion of the alphabet, "it amazes me that people know the alphabet only auditorily."

One of the restrictions of such visualization is that, like Luria's patient, images tend to guide MP's thinking rather than thought guiding her figurative memory. When reading a book, she cannot describe the plot or characters without picturing the surroundings, usually by taking a room or a setting that she is familiar with and changing it to fit the description of the book.

A store in the book may be visualized as the living room (rearranged) of someone I knew at one time, especially one in which I had often visited. Of course, most frequently, it is *my own house*, either as I have it now or as I remember it when it was my grandmother's house.

Just like the actual card catalogue cases she uses in her job, her memory maps are becoming full and the material more cumbersome to manipulate. "The older I get the more I have to store—there just is not enough room for everything." Nor does she have a cross-reference system. "The maps are not connected in any way. I cannot see one from the other. They are completely separate, like different slides." DS makes a similar comment: "I visualize everything. There's always so much junk in my mind."

The emergence and retreat into the darkness is almost primeval. MP has often asked herself what is "behind" the maps, what is in the darkness. Although she does not have a philosophic or cosmic *Weltanschauung,* when considering the blackness that anchors the ends of her maps, her impression is that *what is behind the maps in the blackness is actually someone else's mind!* Her image of losing her mind or not being able to think would be to have all of her maps erased or vanish into the darkness.

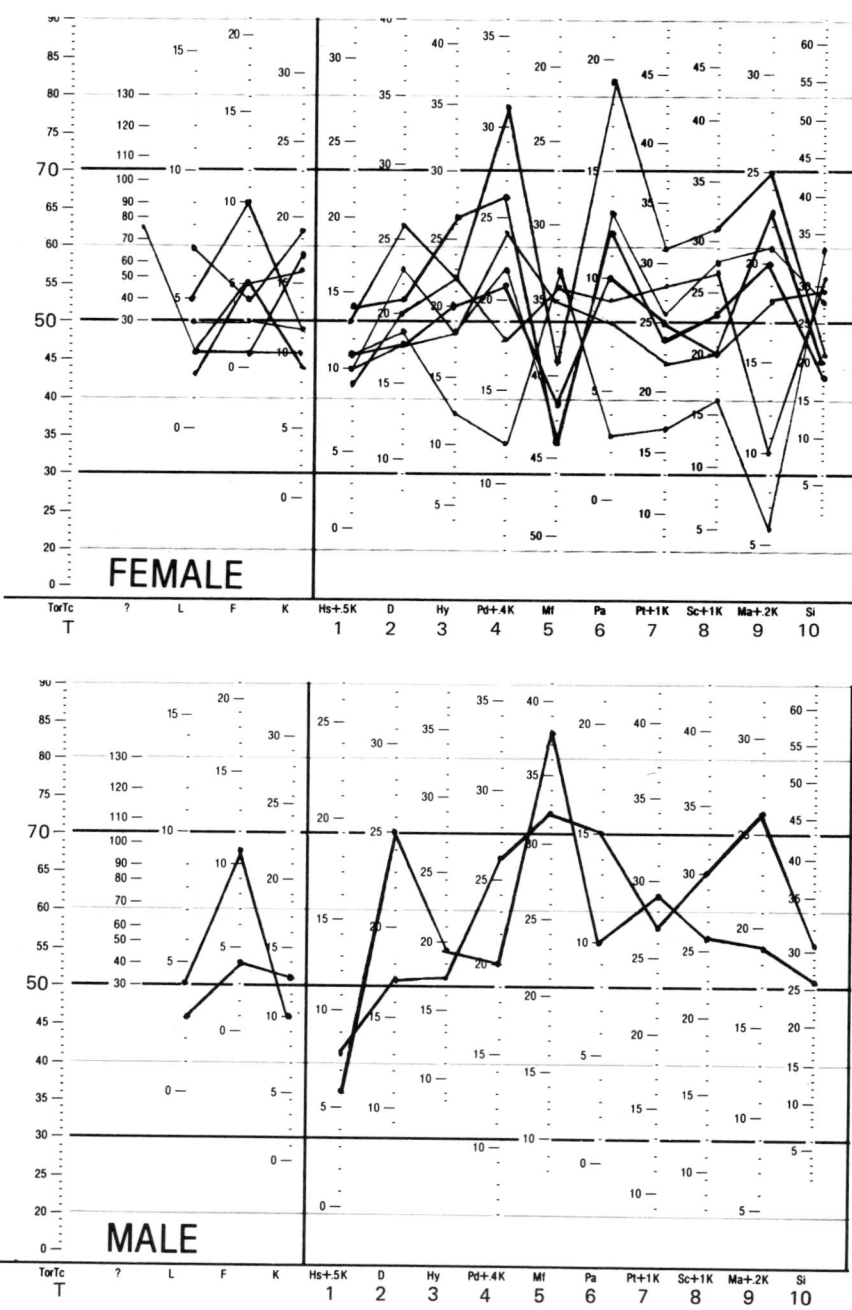

FIGURE 7.28. *T* score plots for the MMPI scores of two male (*bottom*) and six female (*top*) synesthetes.

Psychological Parameters of Synesthetes

PSYCHOLOGICAL TEST RESULTS

Eight synesthetes were given the MMPI. The results were unimpressive. None had significant elevations of the clinical scales. On clinical interview none were judged to have present or historical evidence of psychopathology. Eleven of the 42 subjects are artists or in artistic professions (medical illustration, television production, lighting design). Figure 7.28 shows plots of the MMPI T scores.

Results of the Weschler Memory Scale have been discussed in Chapter 4, which found that synesthetes report and in fact have good memories on psychometric instruments. It would be interesting to do a Stroop-type test on someone like SdeM who has colored numbers. Because of the normal MMPI results, Rorschach and other projective testing was not pursued in these subjects.

We can summarize here the favorable influence of synesthesia on organization, creativity, and memory. There is a tendency to prefer order, neatness, symmetry, and balance. Work cannot be done unless the desk is arranged just so, or everything is put away in the kitchen in its proper place. This fondness for order extends to other people's homes and offices as well, and this tendency persists even when their efforts are unwelcome. Synesthetes resort to mentally redecorating the environmental spaces in which they find themselves. The acalculia and other elements of Gerstman's syndrome in subjects were explicated in Chapter 4.

PERSONALITY OF LETTERS AND NUMBERS

Although MT's personality appears normal by both clinical examination and MMPI, it came as a unique surprise that letters, numbers, and punctuation marks not only have color, but gender and personality! Like the colors, these characteristics are durable over time. Comparison of her lists done in person and by correspondence show no variation over 5 months; neither did a list done for a friend when compared 10 years later.

Table 7.3 gives the colors, genders, and personalities of MT's letters, numbers, and punctuation marks. When asked to recite them, she names these characteristics without the slightest hesitation. Her descriptions are articulate and given with conviction. Referring to her color list, she says that it is as accurate as she can describe them, but is certain that the colors are at once very specific and yet quite difficult to define. It is interesting to note that the letters of her initials, M ("my favorite color for 'my' letter") and T, are both masculine.

With multiple-digit numbers and groups of letters forming words, there is a combination of effects. Numbers 11 to 19 retain the gender of the final digit, but there is a blending of the personality characteristics of the

TABLE 7.3. Color, gender, and personality lists of MT.

Alphabet	
A:	Bright-to-medium yellow; female; very feminine (always in dresses).
B:	Orangey-beigy, medium tonality; female; sturdy in character.
C:	Sky-blue or slightly deeper; male, a touch impetuous, but generally dependable.
D:	Deep charcoal, nearly black; male; dashing, a bit of a joker.
E:	Light lavendar; male; a soft-spoken type.
F:	Brownish-woody-colored, medium tonality; male; perpetually youthful, easy-going, casual dresser.
G:	Slightly lighter than medium purple; male; rugged good looks, and credible.
H:	Orange but toned down, (lighter than "B"); female; of a more formidable figure than "A", but just as feminine.
I:	White; with "dirty edges"; male; a bit of a worrier at times, although easy-going, sincere.
J:	Violet–red-violet (purple with reddish cast); male; appearing jocular, but with strength of character.
K:	Yellowy-beige (more to beige than to yellow); female; quiet, responsible.
L:	Beige/tan/khaki: a specific shade; male; handsome, easy-going, adult without a thickened figure.
M:	Blue-violet (my favorite color for "my" letter); male; secretive, powerful, handsome.
N:	Medium-to-deep green, but the lightest of the green characters (which include "T", "Z", and "2"); male; youthful, handsome, mediator-type.
O:	Clear; the color of (clean) water; female; quiet, warm, reliable, of balanced character.
P:	Orangey, browner than "B"; female; busy, fun, sisterly.
Q:	Cranberry; female; elegant, non-talkative, more earthy than the playing-card depiction of "Q" (as "Queen").
R:	Red; female; all-American woman, out-going, active.
S:	Pastel yellow (lighter and less yellow than "A"); female; independent but good at partnering; mature.
T:	Forest green; male; quite masculine, and quiet, gentle, mature, responsible, slim build, handsome, good in relationships.
U:	Soft pink; rosy but not "pinky-pink"; female; of rounded, not slim, figure; sweet, hard-working, quiet.
V:	Yellowy beige but subdued. (More beige than "A"; deeper than "S"; more beige than "L" or "K"); female; very feminine, unflauntingly sexy; sophisticated.
W:	Medium gray; "clean" gray; male; open-minded, seeming older than other characters; good-looking, friendly.
X:	Cheddar-cheese color but deeper; androgynous; easy-going and fun-loving; of balanced character; sometimes cheerful, sometimes worried.
Y:	Medium-to-deep gray; male, effeminate, attractive, responsible.
Z:	Deep forest green; male; dashing and very handsome because of it; mature but still playful; reliable.

Numbers	
1:	White; male; quiet character; youthful appearance but serious in character.
2:	Green with an almost bluish tinge; masculine; good-looking, somewhat outgoing, laughs easily, kind.
3:	Lighter lavender than "E"; masculine; teddy-bearish character, can seem gruff but isn't.

4:	Very yellow: deeper than "A"; female, feminine, playful (but not flirtatious); sisterly.
5:	Blue, deeper than sky blue but similar to "C"; male; a bit of a worrier but not without self-confidence; mature.
6:	Pink, soft pink like "U" but slightly deeper; masculine; youthful, quiet, smart.
7:	Dark grainy gray, with an almost beigey sense to it; male; playful and impressively handsome.
8:	Orangey-beige like "H", but more beige and somewhat lighter in tone; masculine; cheerful, modest, firm-figured.
9:	Dark, almost purplish, charcoal-gray; male; a bit of a "wise-guy" but nevertheless dependable; with a serious and powerful side.
0:	Zero is the same color as the letter "O", that is, transparent, like the color of water; female; more subdued than "O" as if the less dominant twin.
10:	(and powers of 10) Although like all other combinations of letters and numbers 10 retains the individual colors of its component numbers, it also has a redness that lies under the white of "1" and the transparency of "0". The powers of "10", "100", "1000", etc., are all female, and increasingly formidable (as "10" is formidable). They are all friendly, matriarchal, and independent.
11–19:	Retain the gender of the *final* digit, and a blend of the characters of the composite digits.

Punctuation Marks

?	Cranberry-purple; masculine; respectable, serious, mannerly.
,	Dark-gray; male; a bit irreverent.
. : and !	Blackish, charcoal gray; masculine
"	Beige; masculine
'	Black
+	Yellowish; female; subdued character
#	Beige; male, hard working

Groups of Similar Colors

A, S, V, 4, @, $, +	I, 1
B, H, P, 8	J, Q, ?
C, 5	K, X, #, +
D, (W), Y, 7	N, T, Z, 2
E, 3	O, 0
F, L, "	(R, 10)
G, M	U, 6

composite digits. Beginning with 20, however, the gender is determined by the first digit. Twenty is male, for example, while 40 is female. The 40s, 400s, 4000s, and so forth are all female. Similarly, *words* take on the gender of the initial letter, but not the color or any other attribute.

GEOGRAPHIC KNOWLEDGE AND PATHFINDING

Early on when I began collecting cases of synesthesia, several subjects commented that they had a profoundly poor sense of direction. I found this surprising since excellent memory seemed to be emerging as a characteristic of synesthesia. As I continued to collect cases I began to inquire into aptitude for geographical knowledge and pathfinding and decided to pursue the hypothesis that, like their apparent mathematical difficulty, synesthetes have a relative deficiency in geography and navigation.

Table 7.4 shows, in those subjects of whom it was asked, who has a self-reported good or poor geographic memory. Those who claimed a poor sense of direction went to unusual lengths to get around. Generally, subjects relied more on network than vector maps (Byrne, 1982), even in their hometowns. This was particularly surprising in those cities laid out on a grid system, such as New York or Washington, DC.

Below are two examples of the distress caused by poor sense of direction.

RB: I have no sense of direction, which causes me distress. I cannot visualize where one location is in relation to another, even though they are very familiar places to me.

   I can't tell you how relieved I felt when you told me this was comon [sic] with synesthesia. My husband says I'm the only person who tried to go through a turnstile in the wrong direction. If I'm driving and come to a dead end street I can't get back to a parallel street and get terribly lost. I worked in the same office building for 10 years and still had trouble finding friends' offices (5/6/87).

MN: I have no sense of direction. I cannot read a map. In driving to a new location (which has been murder for me this Summer looking for a new job and going to several interviews a week [in various new locations]) I must have very specific directions. Most of the time, I have to "practice" a day in advance before going someplace new. Then I must write it down, very specifically in my own words and descriptive phrases. Most people think I am an idiot because I cannot read a map. I don't feel I have any trouble comprehending abstract vs concrete books, speeches, poetry, philosophy and understanding their metaphorical or symbolic content, but I find it hard to verbalize it so that others can understand (7/7/85).

Theoretically, several issues are involved. The first is that a "good memory" does not apply to all aspects of memory. Episodic, semantic, visual, and geographic are just some of the different kinds of memory. In the face of boasting that they could easily recount conversations long since past, interview without benefit of note taking, and recall the location of reference material in the workplace even down to the specific page of a

TABLE 7.4. Sense of direction.

Good	Poor
13/42 (31%)	29/42 (69%)

book on which the desired information resides, the prospect that synesthetes suffer from poor spatial memory is provocative.

It would be paradoxical to have a spatial impairment when the synesthesiae are so often intertwined with number forms and other spatial concepts. Geographic knowledge is presumed to be an example of spatial aptitude that resides in the right parietal region. Since the linguistic and blood flow data suggest that synesthesia occurs in the language hemisphere, a right posterior lesion would appear at first to be incongruous in the scheme of understanding synesthesia. To the extent one agrees with Geschwind's thoughts on laterality and dominance, however, one could speculate that some event in embryonal neuronal migration in these predominantly female synesthetes would have an effect in the opposite right hemisphere. If so, the clinical manifestation could be one of selective spatial difficulty (Geschwind & Galaburda, 1985a, 1985b, 1985c).

This idea was explored in a number of subjects with the Fargo Map Test, a psychometric instrument developed by William Beatty of North Dakota State University (Beatty & Tröster, 1987). Two tests were administered, the Fargo Map Test and the New Map Learning test.

The Fargo Map test is a standardized means of assessing remote memory for spatial knowledge. The subject first reports all of the places (city and state for the United States) and city and country outside the United States) in which he has lived for at least 1 year throughout his lifetime and the age range during which he lived at each location. The subject then locates as accurately as possible target items such as cities, mountains, and rivers on a series of 18 outline maps. Each map contains 12 to 16 target items. The first map is of the continental United States and contains both items that require only gross localization of features (Atlantic Ocean, Canada) as well as items requiring finer discrimination (Chicago, New York City). The following 17 regional maps contain outlines of the 48 continental states in groups of two to six contiguous states. In addition to locating the various targets, subjects are asked to identify the individual states.

Normative experiments involving 1,800 undergraduate students disclosed that males more accurately located places on maps of the United States or its various regions than did females, and that they perform more accurately than females on measures of egocentric and allocentric spatial orientation, although performance on these tasks is only weakly predictive of accuracy on tests of geographic knowledge. Both males and females learned locations of unfamiliar places at similar rates, whether such learning occurred under intentional or incidental instructions.

The New Map Learning test consists of a study map of three contiguous fictitious states within which 15 hypothetical towns are located. The towns have concrete and highly imaginable names (Emerald, Rifle, Cotton) and only one exemplar of a particular semantic category appears as the name of a town on the map. The test map is an outline of the three fictitious states and 25 dots (15 towns and 10 distractors). Four trials are given for learning.

The results with three synesthetes and one subject with a number form only on the Fargo Map test and the New Map Learning Test are as follows. Female subjects AC and JM claimed to have a good sense of direction, and in fact were almost two standard deviations above the mean for North Dakota females of the same age and education in geographical knowledge and in learning new maps. DS, MT, and MW— who claimed "no sense of direction"—were also quite good at geography but somewhat impaired at learning new maps.

Family Cases (Pedigrees)

Familial examples were cited in Chapter 2 as evidence for the heritability of synesthesia. Its occurrence in the same or contiguous generations, without preference for sexual inheritance, argues strongly for an autosomal dominant mode of transmission. Several pedigrees serve as examples here.

PEDIGREE OF EW

Figure 7.29 shows the pedigree for EW, with synesthesia extending over three, and possibly four, generations (see p. 57).

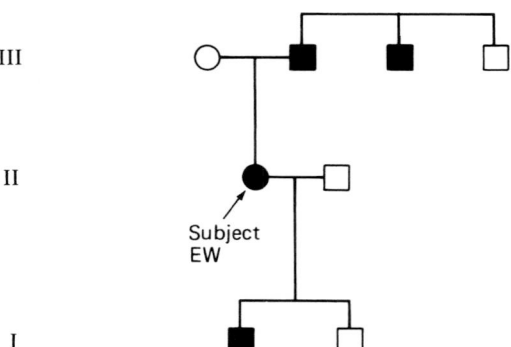

FIGURE 7.29. Pedigree of EW.

PEDIGREE OF MT

Colored numbers and letters are found in three generations of females in MT's family (Figure 7.30). The proband's mother has several hospitalizations for bipolar disorder with grandiose ideation. The mother was strongly synesthetic. MT was separated from her mother at 5 years and reunited at 21, shortly after which the mother died. This separation at such an early age would tend to discredit the notion that environmental exposure was causative of synesthesia.

MT recalls that she had synesthesia as far back as she can remember, "and I recall talking to my mother about it. My mother told me that she remembered my *saying* things to her that made me know I had it."

MT spoke with her maternal aunt in generation III and confirmed the presence of synesthesia in the aunt. Her maternal grandmother had right-left confusion. A maternal cousin in generation I (subject LF) has synesthesia. There is an unusual incidence of female offspring in MT's pedigree.

The cousin in generation I also has a letter-color synesthesia, but her colors merge so that the first letter influences the color of the entire word, unlike proband MT, for whom each letter retains its own color regardless of its context in a word.

MT's older brother has a sound-color synesthesia. He and his mother would "argue" about the colors of musical notes. Unlike her brother, MT is musically naive.

The maternal cousin in generation I suggests a particularly interesting point that the synesthetic trait might be inherited but not expressed. That is, her mother in generation II has no sign of synesthesia. The idiosyncracy of each synesthete's associations, the different kinds of synesthesia among MT and her siblings—and indeed the possibility of different

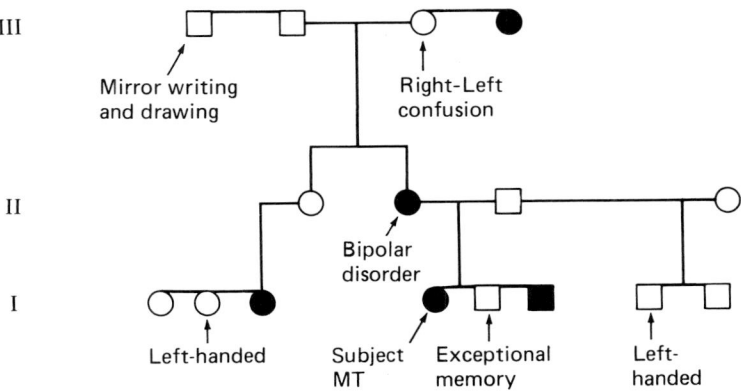

FIGURE 7.30. Pedigree of MT.

associations of modes within a single pedigree—plus the "skipping" of the trait in a generation, as evidenced by the seemingly solitary appearance of the trait in MT's cousin, can all be explained by penetrance. Penetrance is the relative ability of a gene to produce its specific effect in any degree in the organism of which it is part. A "skipped" generation is also found in the pedigree of FKD.

Siblings

Four female synesthetes have a synesthetic sister: LH, NM, SO, and SP.

LH, a 61-year-old left-handed white female with 16 years of education, has a typical story for synesthesia. She has an excellent memory, considers herself well read, but has poor arithmetical skills. She has other lacunae in her cognitive skills. "Philosophy is a closed book to me. I'm good in vocabulary, definitions, spelling and 'trivial pursuits' of all sorts including subjects not in my realm—the 'odd fact.' "

There are also lacunae in her synesthesia: letters and numbers that have no color. (Recall that the point was made with JM that the coloration is sometimes very pale, and that not all elements of a set are necessarily colored.) Her color list appears in Table 7.5.

I see some numbers and some letters in color, consistently the same colors, as did my now dead sister (only her colors differed from mine). I find this useful as a code for writing down PIN numbers, and getting a "feel" for telephone numbers and people's names.

Until my teens I thought this was quite normal for everyone, and it was only at the dinner table that my sister and I made the discovery that we two were "afflicted" and no one else was. Since then I have only met one other person with the trait and this was quite limited compared to mine. I am now near sixty but the colors shine as brightly as ever.

TABLE 7.5. Color list for LH.

a:	Cream	2:	Cream
e:	Green	3:	Yellow
f:	Light brown	4:	Blue
g:	Another brown	5:	Orange
h:	Reddish brown	6:	Red
j:	Brown again	7:	Gray
k:	Again brown, rather jaunty	8:	Green
m:	Red	9:	A hearty brown
n:	Orange		
p:	Green		
r:	Black		
s:	Yellow		
u:	Muddy brown		
z:	"Sharp" yellow		

CEREBRAL DOMINANCE

In favor of Geschwind's original ideas on cerebral dominance, we note (from Table 2.1) the incidence of left-handedness, familial left-handedness, dyslexia and other learning disabilities, migraine, and auto-immune illnesses in the subjects and their first-degree relatives (Geschwind & Galaburda, 1985a, 1985b, 1985c). An occasional instance of right-left confusion (alocria) will be unearthed in the synesthete's pedigree. MT, for example, shared from a letter from her maternal aunt that "your grandmother may have been ambidextrous; she always said the only way she could tell her left hand from her right was to look for her wedding ring." MLL considers herself right-handed, yet deals cards with her left hand; she also sews with her right hand but holds the material the "wrong way." "My mother complains that my kitchen is organized left handed." MLL's two daughters are left-handed; her paternal cousin is ambidextrous.

Clairvoyance and Other Unusual Experiences

It is difficult to know what to make of the following examples. Virtually none of them can be substantiated by any kind of objective measurement. Clairvoyant dreams, precognition, and a cosmic *Weltanschauung* occur in synesthestes more often than one would expect by chance. The experiences related below are quite distinct from the comments of oddballs, who relate experiences quite unlike those that are characteristic of true synesthetes. This leaves us with a group of patients who have additional unusual experiences that are best left to speak for themselves.

Seven of the current subjects have had such experiences. HC, TP, MG, and MLL have had clairvoyant experiences; JB has experienced psychokinetic phenomenon; VE has had clairvoyant and empathic healing experiences; and PP sometimes has the feeling of a presence accompany her synesthesia.

One is reminded that similar behavioral aspects are seen in ictal phenomena, particularly temporal lobe epilepsy. Such experiential manifestations of temporolimbic seizures may include memory flashbacks and illusions of familiarity or unfamiliarity, called *deja vu* or *deja vecu* (Gloor et al., 1982; Penfield & Jasper, 1954). These terms mean "already seen" or "already experienced" and convey the sense that what the patient is experiencing at the moment has been experienced or witnessed previously. This often leads patients to believe that they are clairvoyant or prescient ("I must have known it was going to happen, because it was all familiar to me") (Spiers et al., 1985). The opposite, *jamais vu* or *jamais vecu*, may also happen, leading patients to believe that events or people that are actually familiar are nonetheless alien. Like the subjects described here, such patients are reluctant to volunteer this kind of experience.

HC believes that she can read the moods of others.

I'm almost entirely intuitive rather than rely on logic and am particularly sensitive to mood vibrations from others. I can walk into a room and sense almost instantly what each person is feeling about himself or whether there is tension, hostility, "openness," pretense, etc. Perhaps this is not unusual. I don't know.

JB was quite frightened when things in her environment seemed to move.

At first, with movement of objects, I thought I was out of my mind, so I stopped talking about it. Lights would pop on. I would seem to affect electrical appliances. Plants would jump when I was near them. But I don't think about it as much as I used to. I was very skeptical. I used to think "this can not be happening to me." But it did. It did happen to me.

This sounds somewhat like metamorphopsia or macropsia. Our mechanism of perception is normally not reflexively directed onto itself, but directed toward the outside world. Thus we can forget about ourselves in normal perception. In order to become more clear about our subjective experience it is therefore useful to examine phenomena such as this in which something is out of the ordinary and appears to clash with the normal perceptual mechanism.

PP has the spontaneous appearance of blobs of color that "visit" her. One she calls "helping" and the other just "visiting." For example, a translucent but not transparent red blob covered the back of her writing hand while completing an examination of some difficulty; another time a blue light, warm as if the sun were directly shining on it, hovered about the left arm and shoulder as she wrote a letter on an emotional subject. The "visiting colors" are of three types: (1) a purple 3×4-inch oval that appears daily, (2) a smaller blue light that often appears when she puts her baby to bed, and (3) assorted other colors with magenta and silvery white sparks that seem to be all around.

I've thought of these as angels but who knows what they are. I've mentioned some of my experiences—no one so far knows what I'm talking about, but I love them. I'm grateful for it. For the record, I guess I'm "normal" otherwise, whatever that is.

Olivier Messiaen, discussed in the next chapter on art and synesthesia, is a devout Catholic. Yet he indulges in a magical thinking that Claude Samuel was able to touch on in *Conversations with Olivier Messiaen* (1976, pp. 20–21).

Claude Samuel:
    To understand your love of colours better, independently of psychic and psychological phenomena, should one recall the allure magic has for you?

Olivier Messiaen:

You're plumbing dangerous depths in me there! As a Catholic I should have no right to speak of magic but let's admit, it's not devoid of interest. I'm not speaking of black magic and of people who cast spells—that's just a joke, but there does exist a white magic, and that's a symbolical quest for the power of language, sounds or colours, for the influence of certain things we own or which surround us.

MLL has sent me numerous examples of her clairvoyant dreams. They are not frightening but are always ominous, portentious, and about bad news. Her mother also has clairvoyant dreams.

For further information, the interested reader may wish to consult Duplessis' *The Paranormal Perception of Color* (1975).

8
Synesthesia and Art

Colors are very important to me because I have a gift—it's not my fault, it's just how I am—whenever I hear music, or even if I read music, I see colors (Hume, 1979).

This aspect of composer Olivier Messiaen is discussed in nearly all of his major works. A trip to Utah came about when Messiaen accepted a commission from Alice Tully to write a work in honor of the United States. *Des Canyons aux Etoiles* ("From the Canyons to the Stars") (Messiaen, 1977) was inspired by Bryce Canyon, "the most beautiful thing in the United States. The piece I composed about Bryce Canyon is red and orange," says Messiaen, "the color of the cliffs."

Artists have always attempted to look at the universe as one side of a coin, while scientists are looking at the universe as the other side. But it is the same coin they are examining—the same principles of nature, in a sense. It is the purpose of this chapter to take the artist's view of synesthesia and see also how synesthesia influences the creation of art. We will change hats, discarding the scientist's thinking cap for the artist's beret. We will talk as a practicing artist, however, rather than posing as an art critic or historian. Indeed, art historians are not prepared to talk about art from a scientific point of view, or even one that is practical. Rather, they are trained to repeat what another art historian said aesthetically about something, or what they thought the artist was trying to convey emotionally, politically, or socially. There is a fear that discovering the mechanics of an artwork will spoil the mystery and magic. The art historian cannot talk about the technical or practical aspects of painting or sculpting. Curators and conservators in museums generally know much more about the technical aspects of the art they preserve than those who create it or the historians who critique it.

From the humanities, including ancient philosophy and mysticism, we will examine the propensity for geometry to appear in synesthetic percepts. Although highly mathematical, the fact is that both divine proportion and dynamic symmetry were developed not by engineers or mathemeticians but by artists to achieve aesthetically pleasing results. The artist's view of color, colored shadows, and the historical relationship between color and form is then examined. Just as we discussed derivative aspects of perception from the neurophysiologist's point of view, I point out here that "the arts" is also a burgeoning venture, with dozens of disciplines and specialties. In *The Two Cultures and The Scientific Revolution,* C.P. Snow (1959) viewed science and literature as culturally elite enemies separated by an incomprehensible gap.

For constantly I felt I was moving among two groups—comparable in intelligence, identical in race, not grossly different in social origin, earning about the same incomes, who had almost ceased to communicate at all, who in intellectual, moral and psychological climate had so little in common that . . . one might have crossed an ocean.

Society has since, I suppose, taken a view that one purpose of literature is not to oppose science but to humanize it. It is a cliché to reiterate, as Snow well knew, that scientific culture is a specialist culture. But perhaps it is not widely appreciated by the scientist that artistic culture is also multiplying, divergent, and in hot pursuit of loose ends. It has many paths of conceptualization each with its own *Weltgeist* and diverse means of investigation. Indeed, the artistic breakaway from synesthesia, as mentioned in Chapter 1, may be seen as a turning away from the romanticism of feeling that synesthesia represented toward a more "scientific" view of breaking it into its parts. The parallelism with the neurophysiological issues discussed in Chapter 5 should be clear. What we want is to better understand how the artist looks at the world. Both science and the humanities are about us.

One purpose of the humanities is to enlighten science. We have come finally to accept that science, despite all its pretenses to objectivity and truth, reflects individual, cultural, and philosophical prejudices. Artists and scientists may occupy different rooms, differently furnished, but it is indisputably in one house with a single roof that they live. Multiple historical examples show that scientist, poet, painter, scholar, and philosopher have lived side by side in the same head. Seamlessness, if only an illusion, never implied professions isolated by crocodile-filled moats. One often reflexly thinks of scientists and artists as alien breeds, reared apart, as if imagination were the domain of one and not the other, as if fact and instinct were exclusionary. Scientists trivialize artists, artists trivialize scientists. Both trivialize critics (and rightly so). Science is about how the heavens, the earth, and ourselves are constructed; literature about the meaning of the finished product.

Geometry, Color, and Form

Since ancient times, the universe was geometry and numbers, which represented heaven and earth, and the numbers and shapes all had assigned meaning. Rather than ask if the geometric and colored properties of synesthesia are not reflective of some inherent linguistic mechanism, we should rather ask: What is this inherent propensity for the human mind to find correctness or pleasure in these geometric proportions? The history of the ideal solids and divine proportion was not designed as an abstract philosophical construct and then forced down everybody's throat in the lyceum. It was developed because it appealed to the aesthetic sense. It appealed to the limbic brain's sense that this proportion and geometry was proper and correct. The same idea was applied many years later by Jung in his discussion of archetypal symbols. We have them, said Jung, because they appeal to a deeper level of our selves, to that part of our knowledge that does not reach consciousness, which is to say the majority of our selves, our essence. This is what we mean when we say that art speaks to the depth of our souls—it speaks to that greater formless part of ourselves of which we have no awareness.

Humans have a tendency to display an innate geometry. Although not as intense as the urge that children have to speak and acquire language, there also exists an inherent urge to draw. This visual urge is, I believe, universal. Children have a natural compulsion to scratch and scribble on the walls and elsewhere despite society telling them that they "shouldn't" act upon these impulses. This visual-manual geometry is discouraged by society, whereas linguistic murmurings are encouraged.

RELIGIOUS PHILOSOPHY

Historically, there is a relationship between color and form. This can be traced to Medieval times, and much of Medieval and early Renaissance concepts are based on knowledge of Greek and Egyptian mythology. Discussion of the relationship between shape and color can be found in the writings of the color theorist Johannes Itten (1888–1967) (1971a, 1971b, 1973).

In terms of components in artwork, color predominates over everything else. This is why in early training one is not allowed to use any color at all. The student works with charcoal in order to concentrate on line, thickness, thinness, texture, contour, light, dark, shadow, and shape in order to create form. Only when the ability to create space, shape, and form with black and white is mastered is one allowed to use color. Color is the overwhelming element—once you get involved with it you forget about shape, the line. The color becomes all important. In a practical sense, do we recognize common objects by their color or by their shape, size, or overall design?

Geometric symbolism is found in the Tarot, Egyptian mysticism, and Freemasonry, where the square, triangle, circle, and cross have esoteric meanings. These were later transformed into religious symbols during the Renaissance. Yellow was assigned the shape of a triangle because yellow was a sign of intelligence and the triangle stood for hierarchy as well as being a sign of danger. The circle was associated with blue because it was holistic, represented the heavens, and was godlike and spiritual. Earth was represented as a square because it comes from the Egyptian notion of solidity in the base of the pyramids. Earth and red were synonymous and so the square was red. Thus those three primary colors were based on three primary shapes: triangles, squares, and circles. Every other color and every other shape are derivatives of these three. Most of this formula stems from church theology, a shorthand way of identifying persons and their rank. Mary's robe is usually blue, sometimes purple, since red and blue combine: Heaven and earth is elevated to the place of royalty. There is much color symbology in religious paintings. Shape-note or fasola singing was popular in 17th- and 18th-century England and America. The four shapes of a triangle, circle, square, and diamond were related to the musical syllables *fa, so, la,* and *mi.*

Examination of master artists shows that they knew quite well the Greek and Roman principles of aesthetics and used them in constructing their paintings. It is no accident that they conform to the geometric ideals developed as part of ancient philosophy. When we examine, below, the geometric structure underlying the composition of a painting one may ask: Is not the template of divine proportion and Pythagorean stars artificial and forced? That is, is it not ridiculous rather than sublime to conceive of arithmetical relationships between lengths and widths, of interspaces between elements as equaling a segment or radius of a fundamental circle or pentacle? The answer is that it is no more forced than is the well-tempered musical scale, the latter being based on a proportion of even harmonies that is adjusted on either side to appeal to what our ear perceives as "harmonious." Geometric proportions are not forced upon the composition of a classical painting, a building, or a statue, but in effect the artistic eye agrees with this analysis of geometric proportion. Classical art shows a dedicated concern with manipulation of arithmetical relations between columns, capitals, interspaces, and relationships of lengths and widths that are perceived as beautiful and that are based on mathematics. The world of geometry is ordered exactly like the musician's lyre, and both speak in terms of basic numerical relations of the body. Music and the time arts, and geometry and the space arts led the Pythagoreans to conclude that order, rhythm, balance, and numerical simplicity were the foundation for personal and cosmic existence.

Divine Proportion and Dynamic Symmetry

ANCIENT PHILOSOPHY

Pythagoras, of the island of Samos, fled to Croton in southern Italy in 530 BC to set up a secret fraternity that was concerned with both cosmic and human issues. The Pythagoreans discovered the role of numbers in that enormous discipline we now call science. Number was the key to all reality. I am not referring to the divinatory number mysticism that confuses symbols with the thing symbolized, a numerology where manipulation of numbers bends back upon itself in a fantasy quite remote from the quantitative numbered world that we perceive and in which we live. Rather, I refer to the seemingly endless unity of proportion that so captivated the Pythagoreans and continues to influence us.

The two great discoveries of Pythagoras are the interdependence of the integers that add up to 10 and the musical properties of tuned strings. When one string is just twice as long as another, an octave, there was a unity in the blending of sound, and again when the lengths have a ratio of 3 to 2, and 4 to 3. With a four-stringed lyre the combinations 1 to 2, 3 to 2, and 4 to 3 were especially pleasing to the tone-loving ear. Simple numbers gave beauty; here was a direct relationship between arithmetical simplicity and what was perceived as beautiful and harmonious. The doctrine of harmony in nature followed from this, the dictum "all is number," meaning that all things can be ultimately reduced to numerical relationships. Pythagorean doctrine applied number relationships to music, acoustics, geometry, and astronomy. The dynamics of world structure depended on the interaction of contraries or pairs of opposites, and the soul was viewed as a self-moving number experiencing a form of metempsychosis, or successive reincarnations in different species, until its eventual purification through intellectual life. Finally, the Pythagoreans understood that all existing objects were fundamentally composed of form and not material substance. Thus they held that, at its deepest level, reality is mathematical in nature and that certain symbols have a mystical significance.

The sacredness of numbers was enormously accentuated by the discovery that the right triangle, familiar from Egyptian surveying, vibrated so with cosmic harmony that the square of the hypotenuse exactly equaled the sum of the squares of the other two sides. This relationship was not approximate or statistically probable but precisely an exact and eternal mathematical relationship.

Philosophers saw numbers as valuable guides not just to physical order but to aesthetic and ideal order. This led to mystical applications that neither the Pythagoreans nor the Platonists shunned. Indeed, Aristotle derived an ethical system from the theory of the golden mean and the Platonists saw man's moral fulfillment through the geometrical creation of the cosmos in the *Timaeus*. Number theory was perpetuated in the West through Plato's *Timaeus* and the Catholicism of St. Thomas Aquinas and his intellectual descendants. René Descartes invented analytical geometry, which showed that an orderly equation derived from the study of conic sections lays out on the plane as exquisite three- and four-petaled roses inherent in the bare abstractions of the equation. What more dramatic proof did one want of the Pythagoreans' belief that the realms of beauty, music, architecture and even the symmetry of human thought lie in the ordered relations of numbers themselves?

THE ARTIST'S USE OF COLOR AND FORM

Form and design, and light and color are rival tendencies in art. They hold the field by turns—the classic versus the romantic, the expressionistic and the impressionistic. After the turn of the century the theories of form and design once again became a chief preoccupation of artists in an age when measurement dominated science, when mechanism and machinery surrounded them on every side (the deco movement, streamlining), until it seemed almost every device manufactured, whether art or engineering, was an example of applied geometry. In a sense, artists became engineers and relations of shapes to one another was of great interest. Many think that this tendency found its extreme interpretation in the cubist movement, but it can be traced to all modern work from 1915 to 1930 (Richter, 1932).

This was also the time when dynamic symmetry appeared and rocked the world. This was largely the discovery of the Yale architect Jay Hambidge (Hambidge, 1920, 1924, 1926). The term refers to the symmetry and proportion of things that grow in nature, as opposed to the static symmetry of a snowflake, for example. It was a monumental discovery of its time, for it provided the lost key to much Classical Greek design and catapulted Hambidge to instant fame. Artists like George Bellows, Robert Gilles, William Sergeant Kendall, and Robert Henri came to study with him, learning how to proportion and arrange the elements on their own canvases according to his principles. Some sense of the popular excitement can be had by noting that Tiffany's designed a whole line of their jewelry, and the Chrysler Corporation designed several of their cars, using Hambidge's discovery of dynamic symmetry (*Saturday Evening Post,* January 19, 1924).

Hambidge checked his hypotheses in Greece during 1920–1921 by measuring and sketching the Parthenon, vases, and statues, and proving repeatedly that the proportions and ratios evident in the design of those things were identical to the ratios that govern all growth in nature (through the Fibonacci series and phyllotaxis, for example). There was a synchronicity in these principles—which are highly mathematical—being discovered simultaneously in North America by Hambidge and in Europe by the English scientist Sir D'Arcy Thompson. Others later applied these ideas of a constancy of proportion to specific applications, such as Denereoz (1931) to human form in *L'Harmonie des Nombres* and Richter (1932) to the visual arts in *Rhythmic Form and Art.* Richter illustrated and investigated the principles of dynamic symmetry in the visual arts. It was the goal of the dynamic symmetry movement to uncover a geometric scheme to help interpret the masterpieces. Knowledge of geometry alone cannot produce works of art, but the contention of dynamic symmetry was that a geometric scheme forms the basis of the composition of the great masters of classic art, and one could understand their work better by understanding this tool that they used. Richter noted that Piero della Francesca was a mathematician and that his paintings conformed to a geometric scheme. Fra Luca Pacioli was known to have derived his geometry from Piero and wrote a book called *De Devina Proportione*.

Thus, various authors deal contemporaneously with this fascinating subject and also give paramount importance to "divine proportion"—the artistic proportions that can be traced to natural formations and touch upon its profound significance from works of art. This dynamic symmetry of proportion underlies compositions of masterworks of art; it was used by Greek potters and by the architect of the Parthenon, and was also familiar to Egyptian craftsmen. From the beginning, this scheme had mystic significance. There are also philosophical and religious conceptions connected with the proportioning of space (Caskey, 1924; Ghika, 1927, 1930; Mössel, 1927; Zeising, 1854).

PROPORTION AND SPACE

Sculptors and painters are accustomed to conceive their compositions as part of an overall architectural design. Architects, sculptors, and painters work in close company and many have multiple talents. They were often employed to decorate walls and to adapt their compositions to tectonic spacing, and therefore the same rhythm that determined the work of the architect also penetrated the work of the painter and sculptor.

A Renaissance painting satisfies the eye by its unity, in which all details are coherently molded. The composition holds together and seems to be pervaded by some mysterious rhythm. Is this art done without rule and measurement, as the romantics would claim? The supposition that the Greeks achieved their works of beauty without a definite method is refuted by the titles of books on the theory of proportion written by Greek architects and artists. A comparison between arts clearly reveals underlying divisions of time and space. The Pythagoreans swore this to be so. What meter is to poetry, proportion is to painting and the plastic arts. Space in the plastic arts is analogous to time in music.

Architecture is the science of fine proportion, its only vehicle of expression from the laying out of the plan to the last detail of decorative molding. Proportion is the correspondence among the measures of the members of a work and of the whole to a certain part selected as a standard. From this results the principle of symmetry. Architecture, sculptures, and painting have space in common. The space of an artwork is divided into harmonious proportions just as the figures that it contains are built according to proportion.

All of this was known to the Greeks as far back as Euclid's *Elements*. Book V explains the theory of proportion and Book XII the five regular solids, earlier identified by the Pythagoreans. Euclid's textbook was the primary source of geometric reasoning at least until the invention of non-Euclidean geometry in the 19th century, and has remained in use practically unchanged for over 2,000 years. It is easy to see how arithmetic curiosities as illustrated below should have suggested intrinsic properties of numbers bordering on mysticism. A perfect digital invariant is an example of a narcissistic number, one that can be represented by a mathematical manipulation of its digits (e.g., $153 = 1^3 + 5^3 + 3^3$). A recurring digital invariant is illustrated by

$$55 : 5^3 + 5^3 \qquad = 250$$
$$250 : 2^3 + 5^3 + 0^3 = 133$$
$$133 : 1^3 + 3^3 + 3^3 = \ \ 55 \qquad \text{(Madachy, 1979)}.$$

An automorphic number is an integer whose square ends with the given integer: $25^2 = 625$ and $76^2 = 5776$. Strobogrammatic numbers read the same after having been rotated through $180°$: 69, 96, 1001.

Pythagoreans recognized that numbers had "shapes" or were "figurative." The triangular numbers 1, 3, 6, 10, 15, 21, and so on were visualized as points arranged in the shape of a triangle. Square numbers, such a 1, 4, 9, 16, and 25, are the squares of natural numbers that can be represented by a square array of dots. The sum of any two adjacent triangular numbers is always a square number. Oblong numbers are a similar example formed by doubling any triangular number (see Figure 8.1). Gnomons, which include all odd numbers and are represented by a right angle, were extremely useful to the Pythagoreans. They could build up squares by adding gnomons to smaller squares and deduced many interrelationships, such as $1^2 + 3 = 2^2$, $2^2 + 5 = 3^2$, $1 + 3 + 5 = 3^2$, $1 + 3 + 5 + 7 = 4^2$, or $1 + 3 + 5 + 7 + 9 = 5^2$. It may be that the Pythagorean theorem of $a^2 + b^2 = c^2$ was derived by contemplating the properties of gnomons and square numbers and observing that any odd square can be added to some even square to form a third square.

Of particular interest is the five-pointed Pythagorean star, in which every line and part of a line is interrelated in golden proportion. The golden or divine proportion deals with incommensurable lengths and cannot be accurately expressed by simple numbers. I will explain divine proportion by way of the Fibonacci numbers and the golden number.

In 1202, the mathematician Leonardo of Pisa, also called Fibonacci, published an influential treatise, *Liber abaci*. In it, he posed the question, "How many pairs of rabbits can be produced from a single pair in one year if it is assumed that every month each pair begets a new pair which from the second month becomes productive?" The results can easily be calculated as follows:

Month:	1	2	3	4	5	6	7	8	9	10	11	12
Number of Pairs:	1	1	2	3	5	8	13	21	34	55	89	144

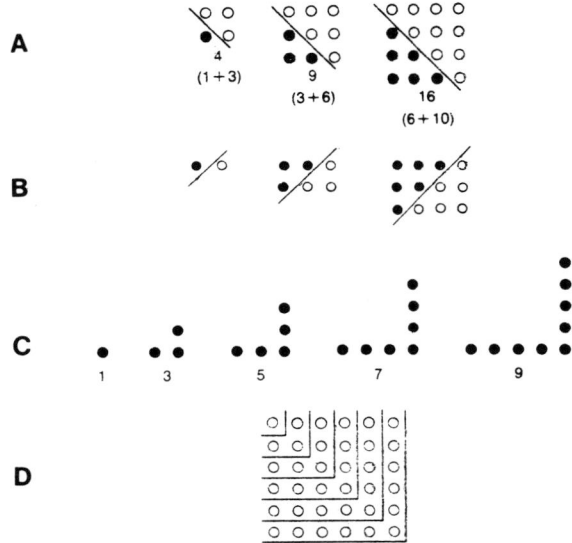

FIGURE 8.1. (A) Square numbers shown formed from consecutive triangular numbers. (B) Oblong numbers formed by doubling triangular numbers. (C) Odd numbers shown as gnomons. (D) Addition of gnomons to squares to form larger squares. From *The number of things: Pythagorus, geometry, and human strivings* by Evans G. Valens. Copyright © 1964 by Evans G. Valens. Reprinted by permission of the publisher, E. P. Dutton, a division of NAL Penguin Inc.

The second row represents the first 12 terms of the sequence known as Fibonacci numbers, in which each term (except the first two) can be found by adding the two terms immediately preceding it. In general, $x_n = x_{n-1} + x_{n-2}$, a relation that, incidentally, was not recognized until about 1600.

There is considerable literature on the Fibonacci numbers, and their properties seem inexhaustible. One of the many formulae for generating the Fibonacci numbers is Edouard Lucas':

$$x_n = \frac{1}{\sqrt{5}}\left\{\left(\frac{1 + \sqrt{5}}{2}\right)^n - \left(\frac{1 - \sqrt{5}}{2}\right)^n\right\}.$$

The ratio $(\sqrt{5} + 1) \div 2 = 1.618\ldots$, known as Φ, is the golden number. The reciprocal of Φ, the ratio $(\sqrt{5} - 1) \div 2$, is equal to $0.618\ldots$. Both of these ratios are related to the roots of $x^2 - x - 1 = 0$, an equation derived from Fra Luca Pacioli's *Devina Proportione* of the 15th century: $a/b = b/(a + b)$ when $a < b$ by setting $x = b/a$. In words, dividing a segment into two parts in mean and extreme proportion, so that the smaller part is to the larger part as the larger is to the entire segment, yields the divine proportion (also called the Golden Section), the concept of which we have

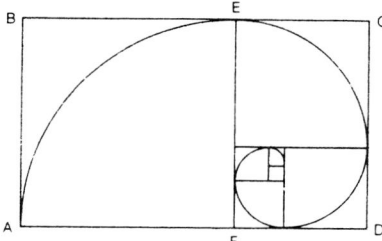

FIGURE 8.2. Golden rectangles and the logarithmic spiral.

spoken in both ancient and modern artistic and architectural design. A rectangle whose sides are in the approximate ratio of $3:5$ ($\Phi^{-1} = 0.618$ . . .) or $8:5$ ($\Phi = 1.618$ . . .) is believed to have the most aesthetically pleasing proportion.

Successive exponentiation of the golden number generates the following sequence:

$$\Phi = (\sqrt{5} + 1)/2 \qquad \Phi^4 = (3\sqrt{5} + 7)/2$$
$$\Phi^2 = (\sqrt{5} + 3)/2 \qquad \Phi^5 = (5\sqrt{5} + 11)/2$$
$$\Phi^3 = (2\sqrt{5} + 4)/2 \qquad \Phi^6 = (8\sqrt{5} + 18)/2$$

Note the successive coefficients of $\sqrt{5}$ are the Fibonacci sequence 1, 1, 2, 3, 5, 8, and so on. If a rectangle ABCD is constructed in divine proportion and the square ABEF removed, then the remaining rectangle ECDF is also in divine proportion. If the process is continued and circular arcs drawn, the curve generated is the logarithmic spiral so commonly found in nature (see Figure 8.2). The logarithmic spiral is the graph of $r = k^\theta$ in polar coordinates, where $k = \Phi^{2/\pi}$. Finally, we mentioned in passing above that the Fibonacci numbers are exemplified by the botanical process of phyllotaxis, where the arrangement of sunflower petals, whorls on a pinecone or pineapple, or branching of stems follows the series of fractions in Fibonacci sequence: 1/1, 1/2, 2/3, 3/5, 5/8, 8/13, and so on.

GEOMETRY AND ART

Several proportions are important to the artistic examples that follow. Figure 8.3(A) shows the divine proportion. When AB = BC + BD, the three lines are related in divine proportion.

The regular pentagon is intimately related to the divine proportion and can be inscribed in a circle. The diagonals of a regular pentagon cut one another in divine proportion and its sides are equal to the major section of the diagonals. Figure 8.3(B) describes a regular pentagon formed by dividing the circumference of a circle into five equal parts A, B, C, D, and E, and joining these points. If the five diagonals of the pentagon are

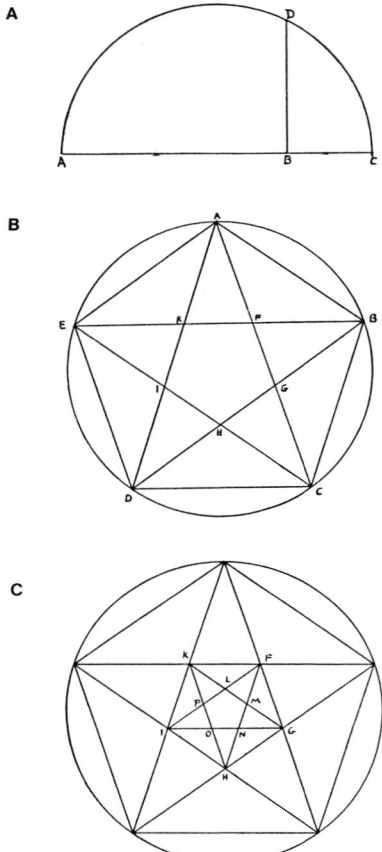

FIGURE 8.3. (A) The divine proportion. (B) Relationship of the regular pentagon to the divine proportion. (C) Concentric pentagons in proportional relations.

joined, a Pythagorean star is formed. One is at once struck by its beautiful proportions. Pythagoreans would doubtless feel that the whole figure is pervaded by divine proportion in a mysterious manner. For example, starting with the diagonal AC in Figure 8.3(B),

$$AC:AG \qquad AG:AF \qquad AF:FG$$

$$AC:FC \qquad FC:GC \qquad GC:FG$$

Furthermore, the sides of the pentagon are related in divine proportion to the diagonals because AG and FC are both equal to AB and all five diagonals and all five sides are similarly proportioned.

The intersection of the diagonals forms a second smaller regular

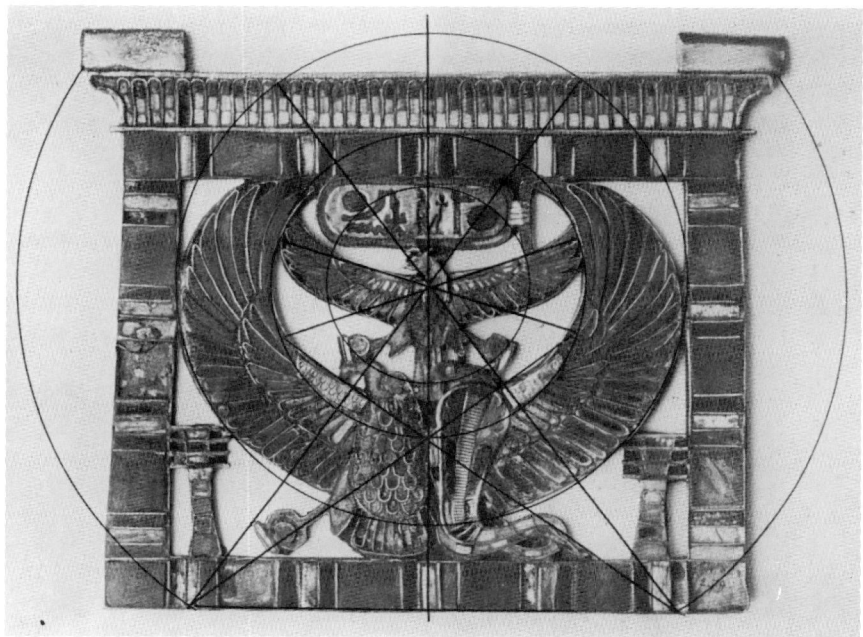

FIGURE 8.4. Pectoral of Khamuasit. The diameter of the smallest circle corresponds to the length of the cartouche. The next circle of the series fits into the outspread wings of the vulture. The third circle encloses the wings and corresponds to the total width of the design within the framework. The outer circle determines this framework. From *Rhythmic form and art: Investigation of the principles of composition in the works of the great masters* by I. Richter, 1932, London: John Lane The Bodley Head Ltd. Copyright 1932 by John Lane The Bodley Head Ltd. Reprinted by permission.

pentagon FGHIK near the center. Joining the diagonals of this inner pentagon [Figure 8.3(C)], a third pentagon LMNOP is formed that is in the same relation to the second as the second is to the first. In fact, a succession of concentric pentagons can thus be described containing an endless series of proportioned relations. Finally, this process can be reversed, where the sides of a pentagon can be produced until they meet to form a star. The points of the star are then joined to form a larger pentagon whose sides are again produced to form a larger star and so on indefinitely.

Mystical and magical properties were attributed to the pentagram. In the Judaic tradition it stood for Solomon's seal, and in Christian symbolism for Christ and the cross of salvation. It appeared as the stonemason's sign, was adopted by the Freemasons in the Middle Ages, and later occurred as a symbol of witchcraft. It formed an integral part of the magic circle that was drawn to protect the magician from evil spirits. In

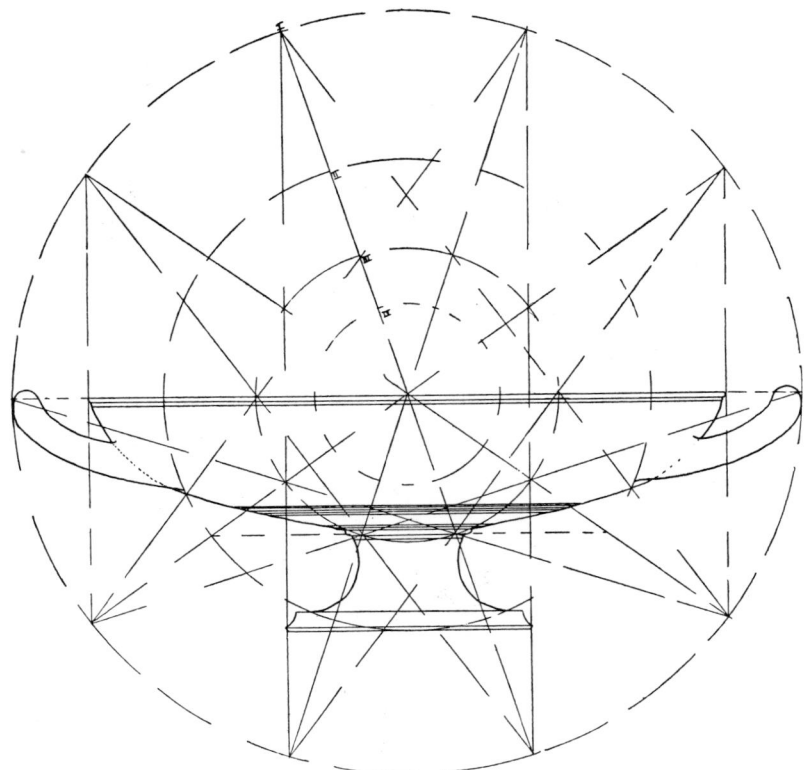

FIGURE 8.5. Kylix. From *Rhythmic form and art: Investigation of the principles of composition in the works of the great masters* by I. Richter, 1932, London: John Lane The Bodley Head Ltd. Copyright 1932 by John Lane The Bodley Head Ltd. Reprinted by permission. (See also Caskey, 1924, p. 176.)

Goethe's *Faust,* Mephistopheles is prevented from leaving Faust's study because of the pentagram engraved in the doorway (Part I, line 1394). Pentacles are one of the suits of the minor arcana of the Tarot.

In art one can overlay a rhythmic division of space on paintings. Compositions are usually based on the center of diameters of circles equal to the picture's width. Movement follows the direction of geometric lines. The size of figures and other important elements correspond to radii. The examples given below closely follow Richter's analysis (Richter, 1932).

The first example is the pectoral of prince Khamuasit, son of Ramses II of the XIX dynasty, who reigned in 1330 BC (Figure 8.4). The geometric diagram is based on a progresive series of four concentric circles related in divine proportion.

Greek vases have shown the principles of dynamic symmetry, as studied by its founder Jay Hambidge (Hambidge, 1920). Figure 8.5 shows a Kylix whose total width is the diameter of circle I. The other

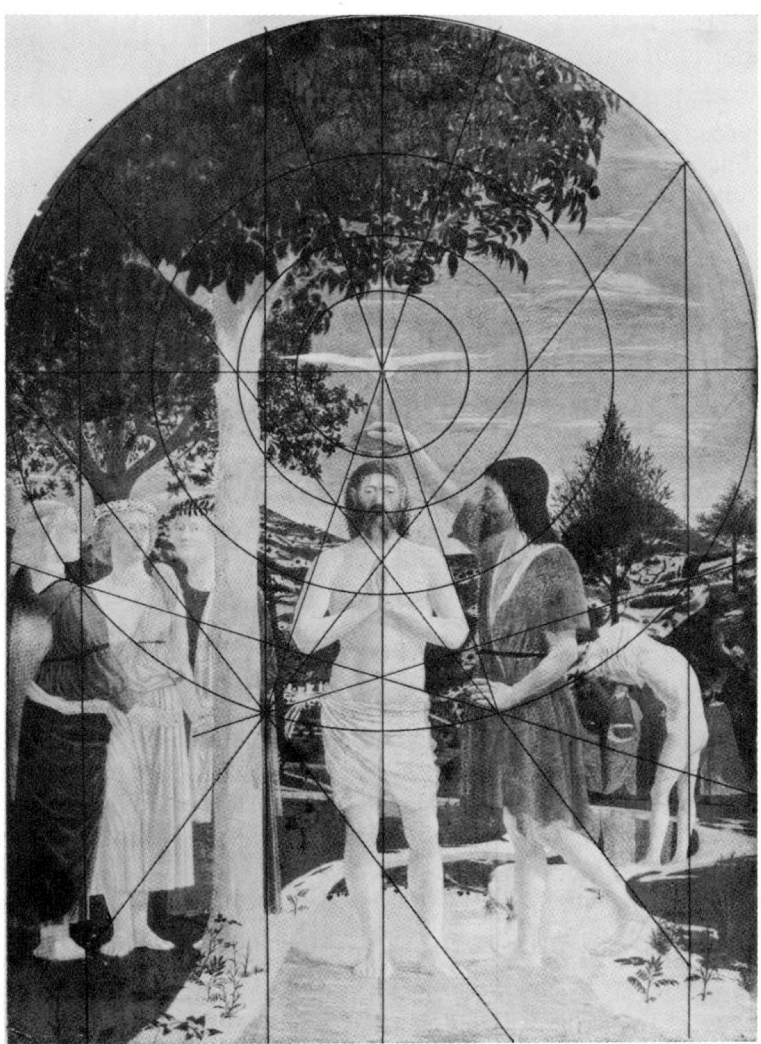

FIGURE 8.6. *The Baptism of Christ,* by Piero della Francesca. From *Rhythmic form and art: Investigation of the principles of composition in the works of the great masters* by I. Richter, 1932, London: John Lane The Bodley Head Ltd. Copyright 1932 by John Lane The Bodley Head Ltd. Reprinted by permission. Reproduced by courtesy of the trustees, the National Gallery, London.

measurements are taken from the radii and diameters of a series of four circles derived from circle I and related in divine proportion:

The height of the vase = radius of circle II
Total width = diameter of circle I
Diameter of bowl = radius of circle I + radius of circle II

Projection of each handle = radius of circle III
Diameter of foot = radius of circle II

An example from Italian art is the *Baptism of Christ* by Piero della Francesca (Figure 8.6). The geometry is based on a progressive series of four concentric circles related in divine proportion. The painting's width is the diameter of circle I, its height equals diameter I + radii II and IV. Note that the dove is in the center of the concentric circles. Also,

Height of Christ and Saint John = radius III + diameter II
Height of Saint John is divided into divine proportion by his belt
Height of two of the angels on the left = diameter II

Piero della Francesca was a mathematician as well as painter and experimented in problems of perspective and proportion. "He dreamed of an art which might proceed, like science, by pure calculation to discover the qualities which command beauty" (Richter, 1932, p. 102). He wrote two treatises to provide a mathematical foundation for future artists. One of these was on perspective (*Petrus pictor orgensis, d'prospectiva pingendi,* Codex in the Royal Library at Parma), the other on the five regular solids (*Libellus quinque corporibus regularibus,* which resides, amusingly, in the Vatican library).

This mathematical fine proportioning of painting extended out of Medieval and early Renaissance art. A final example is *Saint Jerome in his Chamber* by Dürer from 1514 (Figure 8.7). The geometric design is based on a series of six concentric circles related in divine proportion. The picture's width is the diameter of circle II; its height equals the radius I plus radius II. Unlike the Italians, Dürer was more interested in mastering representation, on rendering things as they are in nature rather than on their relation to each other. This is well illustrated by the study of Saint Jerome, which is filled with objects of daily use and appears very much to have been drawn from nature.

The chamber is perfectly constructed. All lines receding at right angles to the picture plane converge toward one vanishing point. The ceiling beams, window mullions, window seat, and step along the wall all point that way. Although the table is placed at right angles, it shares the same vanishing point, which itself is concurrent with an important point on the section of the circumference of circle II, namely, the point of a regular pentagon inscribed within it. This scheme of perspective, then, is related to the geometric diagram, and the motion of the perspectively converging lines toward that particular point is concurrent with five lines of the geometric diagram, all parts of a regular pentagon that also correspond to five focal elements of the composition. Further measurements of interest include:

Circumference of the hanging gourd = circumference of the innermost circle.
Saint Jerome's hat hanging behind him is formed by two circles: the

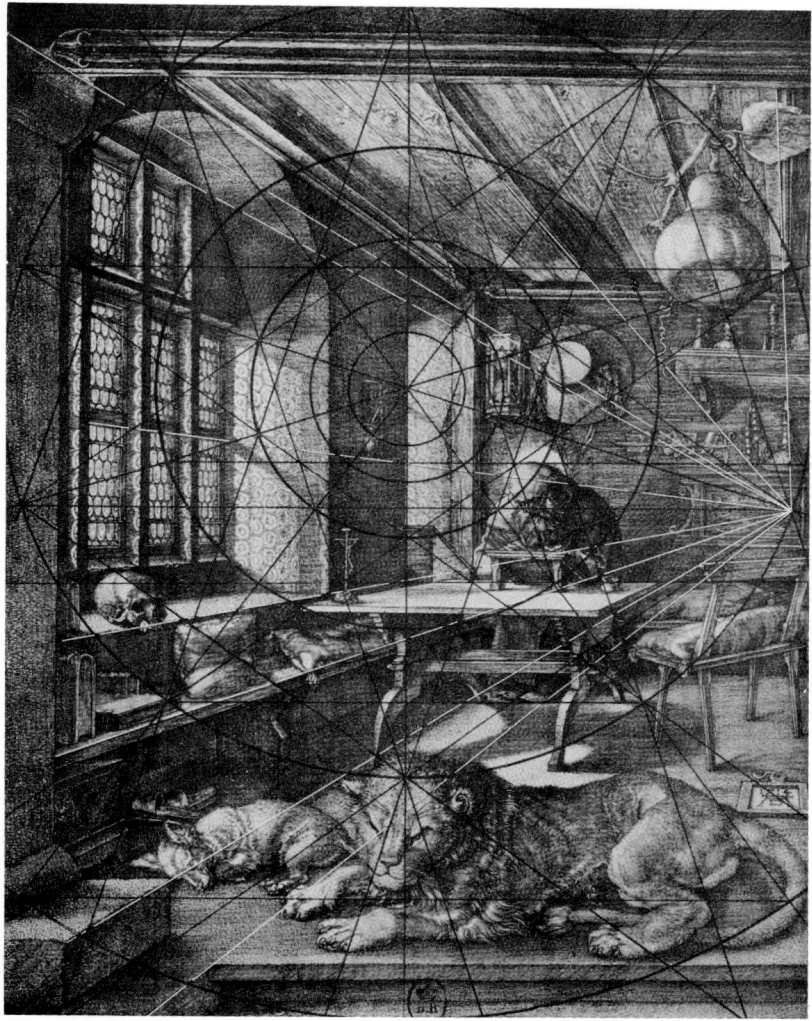

FIGURE 8.7. *St. Jerome in His Chamber,* by Albrect Dürer. From *Rhythmic form and art: Investigation of the principles of composition in the works of the great masters* by I. Richter, 1932, London: John Lane The Bodley Head Ltd. Copyright 1932 by John Lane The Bodley Head Ltd. Reprinted by permission.

diameter of the larger one around the brim = diameter of a pentagon inscribed in the innermost circle, while the diameter of the smaller circle forming the crown = radius of that same pentagon.
Length of table top = radius III + radius V

Geometry means "the measuring of the earth." Plato's *Timaeus* gives a mythical account of creation by geometry. The Pythagorean pentacle that gives the golden proportion is connected with the fifth Platonic solid, which stood for heaven and the all-permeating ether. To see things together, to recognize relationships, was the aim of Plato the philosopher, and he created a perfectly ordered cosmos from the chaos of the phenomenal world. The Greek search for cosmic harmony was in conformity with the striving of artists and craftsmen after fixed relations, clear proportions, and concentration toward a powerful unity of effect.

Thus viewed, artistic creation seems to become a matter of infinite importance. The explanation of psychology, that a reaction to harmonious arrangements of form may be a matter of "mere sensation," seems inadequate. The deep emotions seem, to those who experience them, to have a peculiar quality of reality remote from the superficial sensations of daily life.

Color

The retina has a remarkable ability to alter its own sensitivity. These internal adjustments permit most mammals to see effectively in sunlight or starlight, a 10-billion-fold range in light intensity. The rod cells of the retina function at light levels 1,000 times weaker than those required for cone response. Below so many lux, when only the rod system of the eye is operative, color does not exist (Land, 1977). This condition can be easily achieved by wearing neutral-density dark adaptation goggles that reduce the incident light by a factor of 30,000. After wearing them for half an hour in an environment illuminated to 20 foot-candles average, the effective illumination is 1/1,500th foot-candle. Objects in this environment are not only devoid of color but also distorted by the range of lightnesses from white to black that replaces the normal color sensation. We will see in Chapter 9 that in this colorless world the nature of the image is not determined by the flux of radiant energy reaching the eye. For now, however, we will the examine the artist's view of color, and ask: Why does color figure so prominently in synesthesia?

From the artist's point of view, all color theorists stress, but M. Jacobs (1924) particularly emphasized, that neither color nor the combination of colors alone is art: *there must be some form to be delineated.* Color is both a graphic and a plastic art, and must express some form to satisfy our aesthetic sense. The emotion of color is elusive. Many have found that the same color does not induce the same emotion in all people.

Some argue that all artistic perception is relative, and things are measured, seen, or felt by the relationship of one thing to another. Color is no exception to this law. One note of music in itself has no beauty, but by the sequence of tones we can create harmony or discord. So in color, more than one tone or hue must be visible at the same time so that we can appreciate the relative sequence. This is what makes color a graphic art.

What Jacobs did was devise a way to use the then-new Young-Helmholtz theory of color, a theory based on the spectrum. Newton's prevailing theory was based on the mixture of pigments. Jacobs wrote about the effect of light on color and also technically exploited the use of colored shadows in painting, textile design, theater lighting, the color separation process of color printing, and other areas of design.

Monet appears to have been the first to discover colored shadows, in the sense of trying to write a formulaic approach to them. In this sense, he was like a scientist in approaching the derivative aspects of color relationships. The principle of colored shadows is simply this: all shadows of any object, no matter what color, will be a different color than the lighted side. Not only will it be darker in black and white value, but the shadow will have a color toward the complement of the lighted side. Again, there is the appreciation of one sense by its relationship to others. The more light that is cast on an object, or the more brilliant the color, the nearer the shadow will be to its complementary color.

All color in nature is dependent on its surroundings. A sky that looks blue is composed of predominantly green and violet light. But if we look to this seemingly blue sky through yellow-green foliage, the color of the sky will appear to be purple with white. The same sky will look green seen through scarlet autumn foliage. This is known as simultaneous contrast. Colored shadows are an important example of consensual illusions. We will examine the neurophysiology of colored shadows in Chapter 9 when we discuss illusions and what is "real." A telling anecdote about the synesthetic painter David Hockney is that in the spring of 1983 Hockney's workshop was reproducing some photocollages for simultaneous exhibition. He summoned his photo technician to complain that a particular print was inaccurate. "The color's gone wrong here," he said. "Can't you make it darker?" The technician explained that the original prints had been incorrectly developed and that he was just trying to compensate "to make it look more like the true color." "I don't ever want to hear you say that to me again," scolded Hockney. "There is no such thing as 'true color.' Duplicate the prints as they are in my original drawing. I've used their misprintings in building up the collage" (Hockney, 1984).

We saw in Chapter 5 that physiological and anatomical findings in the primate visual system, as well as clinical evidence in humans, indicate that different components of visual information processing are segregated into largely independent parallel pathways. Different subdivisions of the visual system can be correlated with, or at least predicted by, interactions of color, shape, depth, and movement in human perception. Cytochrome oxidase staining of area 18 (V2) shows alternating thin dark stripes, pale stripes, and thick dark stripes, each with distinctive physiological properties. The thin dark stripes have high color opponency and are not orientation selective; the thick dark stripes are selective for binocular disparity and orientation, suggesting they are concerned with stereopsis (depth vision); and the pale stripes are orientation selective with more than half of them end stopped. Furthermore, each of the three subdivisions receives a different input from area 17: the thin stripes from the blobs, the pale stripes from the interblobs, and the thick stripes from layer 4B (Livingstone, 1987, 1988).

These neurophysiological differences between major subdivions of the visual system predict that brightness contrast and color contrast contours should convey different types of information, and indeed artists have known this in their own terms. Vision is a multipartite process involving one system for shape perception, another for color perception, and a third for movement, location, and spatial organization. They all differ in their contrast sensitivity, temporal resolution, and acuity. The color system has a three- to fourfold lower acuity than the form system does, for example. Therefore color can "bleed" off of shape boundaries, as often happens in watercolors, without interfering with the assignment of colors to objects in the image. This is, of course, the same thing that happens in hallucinations when colors melt off object boundaries, as we will discuss in Chapter 9. Color can take on a life of its own, as we have seen over and over again in the phenomenon of synesthesia.

Color influences form, contour, and perspective, and vice versa. Edge detection, boundaries, contrast, and depth are all modified by color. We take many aspects of color perception for granted. Color illusions are quite easy to produce and should disquiet us about what truly is "real." If any colored light is thrown onto the same colored pigment and no other light is visible, all colors that are in harmonious sequence will appear white if no other colors are within vision for comparison. This kind of demonstration must be actually seen to appreciate its drama. It is possible, for example, to paint stage scenery so that by illuminating it with different colored lights the scene takes on an entirely different effect— "really" an entirely different scene. An autumn scene painted in scarlet, red, orange, yellow, and their complementaries (blue, blue-violet, and violet) can be made to change into a winter snow scene if illuminated with red light. This is because the first three colors are in harmony to the red light and appear white, while the complementaries appear as different shades of gray. Therefore, the autumn trees lose their foliage of yellow, orange, and red, and the tree trunks become bare. This phenomenon is based on using complementary colors.

Artists have tricks of the trade for achieving the *illusion* of shape and texture. All art, after all, is an illusion of space and dimension. The retinal image produced by a painting of a tree is different from that produced by the tree itself. Consider the techniques of the Impressionists, who worked around the time of the Young-Helmholtz theory. When you look at the Impressionists, particularly the pointilists, you have a good example of how artists break up light, of how they use all the colors *surrounding* what we would ordinarily think of as a single color to create the illusion of that single color.

Borders, contours, and lines do more than just indicate the outline of objects: they can also determine how we perceive their three-dimensional shape, position, and movement. In this, the artist and scientist concur. Both the artist and scientist are aware, as the public or casual viewer is not, that although a contour formed by two vivid colors may be quite noticeable, it is remarkably ineffective in generating a sense of position, depth, or movement. A much stronger effect is achieved with two different shades of the same hue or even two shades of gray. A common example is that converging lines in a flat plane give a strong illusion of depth; stippling can give the impression of a three-dimensional object to a flat outline; and the apparent shape of a torso can be altered by lines in a garment that draw the eye along one direction. While colored and colorless contours have low and high ability, respectively, to generate a sense of three-dimensional shape, position, or movement, the identical contour can be more or less effective in generating these properties depending on what colors form the border. Margaret Livingstone has given demonstrations of this relationship (1987, 1988).

Few academic books on the artist's view of color have been written since Michael Jacob's in the 1920s (Jacobs, 1924) or Johannes Itten, who originally made his impact in the 1940s (Itten, 1971a, 1971b, 1973). The dearth of technical books may be a reaction from the 1950s, in which the prevailing mood was that emotional expression was the primary language of art, and that the technique of painting would be revealed to the artist as long as he could express himself emotionally.

Even Itten gives the impression that color should be a native instinct in the artist, who therefore needs no instruction. If for some reason he should lack the skill for color sense, then there is a way to learn it. This is the premise behind even writing such a book. Both Jacobs and Itten provided an explanation for how and why color functioned the way it did. Both are very strong in saying that in the end, from the artist's point of view, one has to rely on an emotional response for the color to be correct. You can have a paint-by-numbers concept that will produce all the colors in the world, but in the end will not produce an artistic work, therefore the need for individual interpretation, sensitivity, and perception. This system is just a tool.

One can ask why artistic interest in synesthesia declined in parallel with the scientific interest. That is, as the psychologists turned to more "objective" areas of inquiry, why did the artists and symbolist poets stop being interested in synesthesia?

A separation of arts and sciences in a truly clear-cut way then happened. Part of it had to do with the fact that science was trying to look at "real" facts; things had to be factually established. The artists, carrying over from the fauvist movement into the abstract expressionist movement, were not looking for facts, but were looking for sensuality and personal sensitivity. The artist's personal vision of the world was far more "real" than some scientist pointing out that "this is real wood or real marble." One was not concerned with what the properties of wood or stone were but with what sensations wood gave him when he touched it.

It was about this time that artists seemed unable to talk about their work. The climate against verbalization got worse and worse as we move from the 1930s toward the 1940s and 1950s. An artist just could not talk about his work. It was his experience and if the viewer could not see it, it was the viewer's problem, not the artist's. The artist had a vision and one had to be able, somehow, to see this inward vision. It was all internalized. The symbols and glyphs became very personal, and unless one knew what the artists' symbols were all about he could not understand their art.

This is quite unlike the kind of symbolism one finds in medieval art, where everybody knew exactly what the colors meant, what the shapes meant, and what the religious significance was. But from the 1920s until the 1950s (and it is starting to recur again in painting) each individual developed his own set of symbols that represented his own vocabulary, his signature. Look at the works of Paul Klee, Jackson Pollack or, much later, Mark Rothko—their symbolism is all highly personalized. It is like trying to read a writer's manuscript made up of scribbling. Although it may have meaning to the writer who scribbles the same way every day, it is opaque to someone who does not understand the scribbling. There is no way for an outsider to understand this process. This was probably the beginning of a schism between the sciences and the arts. Science was saying, "What does this mean, how does it relate to the history before, or the whole vocabulary of symbolist painting?" The artist replied, "I don't know. It doesn't matter. It's my symbolism."

Synesthesia seems first to have interested the artist, then the philosopher, and then the psychologist, but no one was very successful in making much real sense out of it, and all camps ceased to be interested. Of course, even today when one talks about synesthesia it is doubtful whether many people really understand what is meant. They immediately try to associate it with "If I'm hearing this piece of music I can imagine a beautiful landscape." It is not likely that people were much different in the 1920s and 1930s. However, the important point is that back then the explanations were all psychological, based on "associations," "meanings," and "feelings." That was simply the conceptual level of psychology at the time.

What happened in the field of music or art was that a fascination with synesthesia was considered too romantic. Thomas Cole, Constable, Turner, Beethoven, Schumann, and Mahler were all very romantic artists. The movement away from them was the impressionist movement—which was actually quite scientific! The Monet paintings of the Cathedral at Notre Dame at different times of day are an example of the impressionists' interest in illumination, color, and light. They were quite scientifically oriented.

Perhaps they got away from the romanticism of feeling that synesthesia represented and turned to a more scientific view: let's look at light, let's look at color, let's look at shape. That was the Impressionist movement. It began in the early 1870s and ended in the early 1930s with the American Impressionists. There was then a gradual shift from that to more abstract paintings. Artistic taste and ideology changed and the artist said, "To hell with this scientific analysis. Let's just paint." I think this is a very interesting parallel.

Art and Synesthesia

PERSONAL VISIONS ARISING FROM THE SYNESTHETIC SENSE

We see what our culture tells us to see. This gives rise to the many shared illusions, such as color constancy. Other illusions are more culturally determined. Different cultures can literally perceive the world in different ways. The 1898 Cambridge anthropological expedition to Torres Straits found that the natives were not fooled by optical illusions that uniformly deceived Europeans. To some degree, then, we see only what the culture tells us we can see and know.

Our lives and behaviors are much more profoundly affected by the beliefs we hold unconsciously than by those we hold consciously, and processes of interpretation are also influenced by these beliefs. An example is the well-known experiment in which rapidly exposed playing cards with reversed suit colors are perceived as the subject normally expects them to be.

Imagery offers us a direct clue to the nature of the creative process. It is no concidence that our culture equates creativity with imagination. The ability to imagine, to conjure up images or visions different from our ordinary reality, has always been recognized as the hallmark of the innovative mind.

All of us have visions to some degree or another. Those whom we call "creative" will make their private vision public while those at opposite end of the spectrum, unfortunately, will deny the originality of their thoughts and conform to what the masses dictate is "supposed to be." By their own words, synesthetes tell us how strong was the pressure to deny their sensations as children. Those whose egos were stronger trusted what their senses told them.

Critics traditionally suppose that the images of Arthur Rimbaud (1854–1891), one of our major symbolist poets, sprang from the *sortilege* of a submerged and surreal life. Rimbaud may well have been synesthetic and simply declarative in what he saw. Referring to his *"Sonnet des Voyelles,"* Rimbaud claims to have *invented* colored vowels.

I invented the colors of the vowels. A black, E white, I red, O blue, U green. I determined the shape and movement of each consonant, and with instinctive rhythms, I flatter myself to have invented a poetic verb form that is accessible one day to all the other human senses and I am serving as the translator.

Les Voyelles (1871)

A, Black hairy corset of gaudy flies
That bumble around cruel stinks,
Gulf of darkness

E, Canyons of vapors and intense spears of proud glaciers
White kings
Flutter of flower clusters

I, Deep reds. Coughed up blood
Laughter of lips, beautiful of anger, of petulant ecstasy

U, Cycles, Divine vibrations of seas growing green
Piece of the pasture sown with animals
Piece of the wrinkles that alchemy stands on studious brows

O, Supreme clarion full of strange silences
Silences crossed by worlds and angels
O, omega. That violent ray of his eyes.

Examples from three of the current subjects show how their synesthesia influences their personal creativity.

MLL (Colored Hearing)

MLL's synesthesia probably contributes to her sensitivity for artistic endeavors. It helps her see connections among seemingly disparate things, aiding her creativity in other areas. She has, in her adult years, been a pot mender at the Smithsonian, sign language docent at the National Air and Space Museum, and a docent for a county historical society. She has studied archeology and rock petrography. Aware of something extra when she hears music, MLL is sensitive to those with perceptual handicaps. Realizing that there was nothing for the blind to buy at the Smithsonian shop, she became the inventor, producer, and seller of souvenir postcards for the blind that are sold at the Smithsonian and at the Statue of Liberty, among other places. Because she wanted to give better tours, she learned sign language and was the first sign language volunteer at the Air and Space Museum 3 months after taking her first class. She also helped develop a sound tour with satellite bleeps and a greeting from astronaut Mike Collins. MLL's clairvoyance is discussed in Chapter 7.

MMo (Polymodal)

MMo is a polymodal synesthete for whom sounds or specific words stimulate visual shape, color, and, very often, flavors. The influence of his synesthesia is perhaps an amplification of that of MLL. While both are creative persons, his creativity is his livelihood. MMo designs toys and eventually became the creative director for the company that made Cabbage Patch Kids, a role that involves visual and personality development for new doll characters.

My particular experience in cross modalities tends to naturally stretch itself into an educational motif, with an inkling that such early nurturings might well destroy the tenacious concept of intellectual division or discrete disciplination.

MMo may represent a transition between synesthesia and imagery. His associations are not projected, although he fulfills the other four criteria for the diagnosis of synesthesia. It may be that his job as a creative designer of toys naturally encourages him to "stretch the limits" of what society has taught are logical and permissible associations. Creativity by definition takes items out of context and the flash of inspiration finds relationships between seemingly disparate items. Examples of his polymodality are given in Chapter 2. Its integration into his creative work is complex, and it is sometimes difficult to know where synesthesia stops and figurative thinking begins.

I would say that ideas for toys never come through a concerted effort and they never come to me in any one way. Sometimes they seem to come out of thin air or they may come *from a pun on a word* like 'fingermajig,' a little colored satellite-shaped ball with pushable buttons coming out of it—a toy which helps develop finger coordination (8/2/85).

MMo defends incongruous if not loose associations. "It's crazy, but there's a logic. I believe that somewhere within the human psyche there are equivalent associations between shape, form, color, sound, movement, that it's possible to look at a square and feel mashed potatoes. I enjoy this kind of lunacy and I've cherished and perpetuated these crazy associations."

MMo may provide a good example of the transition between synesthesia and nonsynesthetic imagery that can be found in creativity, because some of his associations are clearly not synesthetic. An analysis of Steve = poached eggs reveals multiple associations rather than the sound or orthography of "Steve" equaling some *sensory quality* possessed by poached eggs. MMo's father had a partner in his restaurant business named Steve, who was always unshaven. The roughness of Steve's beard became associated to the poached eggs that MMo ate there, which were always on toast that was burnt. The roughness of the toast was associated with Steve's beard. This circuitous route of multiple associations is clearly not synesthesia. While MMo may serve as an example of a transitional state, he is also a reminder that synesthesia and abstract thinking are not mutually exclusive.

The toughest thing we have to do is think like a kid thinks, to regress. Or maybe it's not regressing. Maybe it's really getting to another order of perception and response. People don't grow up, they just grow old.

JB (SIMPLE SYNESTHESIA)

JB has had simple, projected synesthesia all her life. She had 15 years of formal education, came from a talented family, and had studied ballet. Like Luria's patient cited in Chapter 4, she was searching for what to do with her life. Nothing seemed to fit or to be real to her. There was a sense

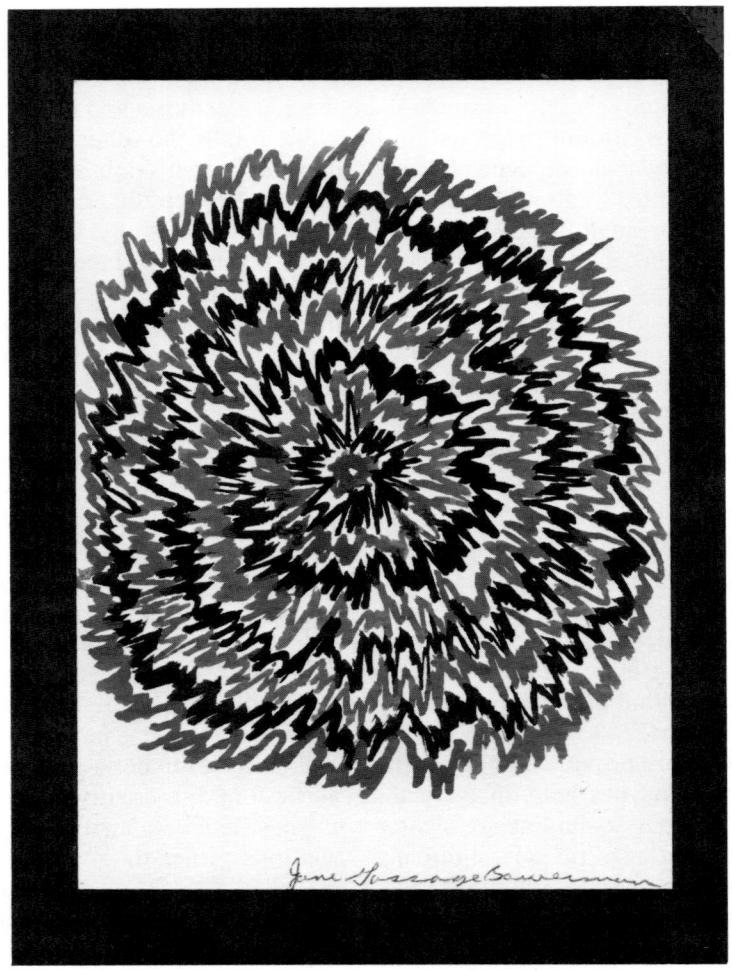

FIGURE 8.8. Painting by JB of one of her simple synesthesiae. (Courtesy of Visionary Images, 1516 Grant Avenue #212, Novato, CA 94947.)

of portentiousness that at any time something wonderful or important would happen to her. It was only after the occurrence of unusual experiences as an adult—what some refer to as psychic abilities—that she became an artist late in life. Here, then, is the influence of synesthesia on the development of artistic expression and talent. Figure 4.14 showed a Christmas card produced from a painting of one of her spontaneous projected synesthesiae. Its similarity to organic simple synesthesia, hallucinogenic visions, and migrainous photopsias was pointed out in Chapter 4. Figure 8.8 is another example showing a characteristic central pulsation and radial symmetry.

This is the only kind of painting JB does. She is completely self-taught and commercially successful.

I think I had this from childhood but I thought everyone had it. I never thought about it. One day waiting for the bus I saw little yellow balls jumping all around and I thought "I remember seeing that as a little girl," but I never mentioned this to anyone.

There is a consistent thing I see on my left side of 4 to 5 blue squares and it flashes once in a while. This is outside, no question, beyond my eyes. Most of things are outside. The flashes are always outside because I never know when they are going to happen.

OLIVIER MESSIAEN

While I have not personally examined the French composer Olivier Messiaen (1908–   ), he illustrates well the relationship among synesthesia, art, and number. In his case one could say that synesthesia does not merely influence his art, but drives it. In his invention of a unique rhythmic structure, the modes of limited transposition, Messiaen relies on highly mathematical relationships that have a personal mystic significance.

We will examine in close detail first the structure of Messiaen's music, how the structure is itself colored, and then how he manipulates the structure to achieve the desired coloration. There is a considerable precision behind Messiaen's method: nothing is arbitrary or capricious. "I try to convey colors through the music; certain combinations of tones and certain sonorities are bound to certain color combinations, and I employ them to this end" (Samuel, 1976, p. 125).

It may seem odd for a composer to explain the sources of his language by speaking first about color, but color is extremely important to Messiaen. As a child he would paint cellophane with colors and hang the pieces in the window, fascinated by the patches of colored light. His aesthetic for color is strong and carries over to his taste in painting, preferring "one painter to all others," Robert Delaunay, who established "in a very subtle and forceful manner the rapports between complementary colors, especially by the principle of simultaneous contrasts" (Samuel, 1976, p. 21).

Composers have been writing pictorial music for centuries, but no composer has, over such a long period of time or in such exhaustive detail, filled his music with passages specifically arising out of his study of nature's colors and birds as has Messiaen. Messiaen was influenced not only by nature and birdsong but, particularly as a child, stained glass. Visiting monuments, museums, and churches, Messiaen acknowledged that the stained glass "certainly exercised an influence on my career. I have remained dazzled forever at the marvelous colors of this medieval stained glass" (Samuel, 1976, p. 14).

In the acknowledgments of his textbook, *Technique de mon Language*

Musicale (Messiaen, 1956), Messiaen thanks those who influenced him, including "all that evokes stained-glass window and rainbow." In *Colours de la Citie Celeste,* material is allowed to interact so that one idea can be modified by the characteristics of another to produce the "stained-glass window" effect which is important to the concept of the piece. While the form of this piece arises from Messiaen's synesthesia, the idea has no immediate importance to the listener. Nonetheless, it permits the musical interaction and transformation to take place as a result of that synesthetic perception and is, in fact, rather similar to the same time characteristics of the postwar serial composition methods. This private device has influenced other composers; the time characteristics of *Colours de la Citie Celeste* are similar to the musical serialism of Messiaen's students Pierre Boulez, Karlheintz Stockhausen, and other postwar serialists.

When he was 6 years old, Messiaen taught himself to play the piano and began to compose. He felt that the greatest influence he received was from his mother, "an influence all the more extraordinary in that it preceded my birth." He refers to the prematernal poetry *l'Ame Bourgeon* by his mother, the poetess Cécile Sauvage, in which she addresses the child she is carrying. She writes to her child with premonition of future greatness. "Carry within me the love of mysterious and marvelous things." His father, Pierre Messiaen, had a reputation for his translations of the classics and Shakespeare. "Indeed, such a climate enormously developed the imagination of a child and guides it toward intangible expressions which find their true end in music, the most intangible of all arts."

Messiaen discovered at a very young age that he was able to hear a score. At the age of 6 he was looking through Gluck's *Orphee* "when I realized I was 'hearing' it. I could actually 'hear' the score—and I had only been doing music for a few months" (Samuel, 1976). Thus, Messiaen was a musical prodigy with an obviously well-developed aural sense. It was perhaps his early education that did not have the usual logical confines that permitted him to develop the paradox of his creative ideas, the "charming impossibilities," as he later called them in *Technique.*

Messiaen is a composer, performer, and educator. Five decades ago he invented his original "modes of limited transposition." He was a brilliant organist for more than 47 years, professor of music at the Paris conservatory, and has had considerable influence on 20th-century music. His works are so stylistically original that they are often immediately recognizable. It is impossible to understand his music without understanding the intense influence of Roman Catholic theology, Messiaen's devotion to nature, and his firm belief in his own creative powers.

Much of Messiaen's music is highly conerned with mathematical, particularly rhythmic, organization. Messiaen uses permutations and interversion to create rhythmic tension. Permutation is the exchange of order or the manipulation of a group of chromatic rhythms. A chromatic rhythm is a series of note values that move progressively to the next larger or smaller value, using the primary note value. This is what he does in *La Merle Noir,* a highly mathematical 12-tone composition patterned after the melodic contour of a blackbird. The irrational measures, Greek rhythms, and inexact augmentation convey more naturally the reproduction of birdsong in its precise but irregular rhythms. His use of permutation in *La Merle Noir* vividly illustrates the process of superimposition, of layers of rhythms. The variety of rhythmic patterns of ancient Greece, and the neumes of plainchant "will instill in us already a marked predilection for the rhythms of *prime numbers, 5, 7, 11, 13, etc.*" He also replaces the notion of a measure or beat by the feeling of a short value, such as the 16th note and its free multiplications, which leads to ametrical music.

Messiaen's music consistently uses a polymodal form based on our present "chromatic" system, a tempered system of 12 sounds. His invention of "modes of limited transposition" provides a wide variety of harmonic color and forms the basis of melody as well. The harmonic logic behind his modes is consistent and it is "mathematically impossible to find other modes that follow the structural laws inherent in these" (Messiaen, 1956, p. 58). The modes draw their special coloration from the fact that the harmonic modes are limited to a certain number of transpositions. Through this, Messiaen suceeds in "putting wheels of color in opposition, and to intervening rainbows, finding complimentary colors in music."

In Chapter 1 of *Technique de mon language musicale* Messiaen (1956) explained some of the mathematics behind his rhythmic and harmonic structures in a section titled "The Charm of Impossibilities and The Relation of The Different Subject Matters."

It is a glistening music we seek, giving to the aural sense voluptuously refined pleasures. At the same time, this music should be able to express some noble sentiments. This charm, at once voluptous and contemplative, resides particularly in certain mathematical impossibilities of the modal and rhythmic domains. Modes which cannot be transposed beyond a certain number of transpositions, because one always falls again into the same notes; rhythms which cannot be used in retrograde, because in such a case one finds the same order of values again—these are two striking impossibilities. . . . Immediately one notices the analogy of these two impossibilities and how they complement one another, the rhythms realizing in the horizontal direction (retrogradation) what the modes realize in the vertical direction (transposition).

In the nonretrogradable rhythms of the modes of limited transposition are found a highly detailed and self-contained mathematics. These modes cannot be transposed because they are—without polytonality—in the modal atmosphere of several keys at once and contain in themselves small transpositions (like Pythagorean stars that contain smaller stars within themselves); these rhythms cannot be retrograded because they contain in themselves small retrogradations. The modes are divisible into symmetrical groups; the rhythms also, with this difference: the symmetry of the rhythmic groups is a retrograde symmetry. Finally, the last note of each group of these modes is always *common* with the first of the following group; and the groups of these rhythms frame a central value *common* to each group. "The analogy is now complete. . . . The impossibility to transpose the modes makes their strange charm. They are at once in the atmosphere of several tonalities, without polytonality. Their series is closed. It is mathematically impossible to find others of them, at least in our tempered system of 12 semitones."

Speaking of the listener, Messiaen says "to be charmed will be only desire. That is precisely what will happen; in spite of himself [*trying to inspect the nontranspositions and the nonretrogradations*] he will submit to a strange charm of impossibilities; a certain effect on tonal ubiquity in the nontransposition, a certain unity of movement where beginning and end are confused (because they are identical) in the nonretrogradation, all things which will lead him progresively to that sort of *theological rainbow* which the musical language, of which we seek edification in theory, attempts to be" (Messiaen, 1956, chapter 5).

My secret desire of enchanted gorgeousness and harmony has pushed me toward those swords of fire, those sudden stars, those flows of blue-orange lavas, those planets of turquoise, those violet shades, those garnets of long-haired arborescence, those wheelings of sounds and colors in a jumble of rainbows of which I have spoken with love and the preface of my *Quatuor pour la Fin du Temps*; such a gushing out of chords should necessarily be filtered; it is the sacred instinct of the natural and true harmony which, alone, can so charge itself (Messiaen, 1956, p. 52).

Messiaen is absolutely convinced that his association of color and sound is a valid experience for him. Mode 2 of the limited transposition, for example, is a certain shade of violet, blue, and violet-purple, and mode 3, orange with red and green pigments and spots of gold, and also a milky white with iridescent reflections like an opal. As a consequence of these associations, one can speak of "color chords," and a melody that has harmonies associated with it can be said to be "colored" by these harmonies rather than "harmonized" in the classical sense.

Movement 7 of his symphony *Des Canyons aux Etoiles* is titled "Bryce Canyon And The Orange Red Rocks." That is, the music is the color of the cliffs. The music is much more than pictorial, however. As a Steller's jay flies over the canyon Messiaen noted that

His belly, wings and long tail are blue; the blue of his flight and the red of the rocks takes on the splendor of Gothic stained-glass windows. The music of this composition attempts to reproduce all these colors.

For the Steller's jay, chords with "contracted resonance" (red and orange). . . . Chords with "transposed inversions" (yellow, mauve, red, white and black) render the colors of the rocks. . . . Next, polymodality superimposing the three 4-mode (orange-colored with red strips) to the six 2-mode (brown, reddish, orange-colored, purple) bring to a fortissimo conclusion the sapphire blue and the orange red rocks (Messiaen, 1977).

When one understands that this is not metaphoric speech, not artistic license but what he is actually seeing, that this is his synesthetic perception refined by his intellect and his artistic craft, then one can only wonder what is going on in his mind.

Messiaen himself talks of harmonies in this way in connection with *Chronochromie*. In *Sept Haikai, Colours de le Citie Celeste,* and *Des Canyons aux Etoiles,* he names colors in the score in connection with particular chords. *Chronochromie* comes from two Greek words: *khronos* (time) and *khroma* (color). It means color of time. The integral parts of *Chronochromie,* its "strophes," are based on symmetrical permutations which are juxtaposed, superimposed, and further colored in three ways: subdividing note values, altering timbre, and using colored chords.

One note-value will be linked to a red sonority flecked with blue—another will be linked to a milky white sonorous complex embellished with orange and hemmed with gold—another will use green, orange and violet in parallel bands—another will be pale gray with green and violet reflections—another will be frankly violet or frankly red. Juxtaposed or superimposed, all will be made prominent by colorations, color serving to reveal the cut in Time. The durations and permutations of durations made perceptible by sonorous colorations is truly a "color of time," a *Chronochromie* (Samuel, 1976, p. 91).

Messiaen does not use the modes melodically, but as colors. They are not harmonies in the classical sense of the word, nor are they even recognized chords. "They sound like colors." They are colors, and their power springs "primarily from the impossibility of transpositions and also the color linked with this impossibility. The two phenomena are simultaneous."

In composing *Colours de la Citie Celeste* Messiaen was influenced by quotations from the Book of Revelations, which he describes as "extraordinary, extravagant, surrealistic and terrifying;" for example, "And to the star was given the key of the bottomless pit." The title, the colors of the celestial city, are the colors of celestial Jerusalem, that is to say, Paradise. Paradise is represented in Revelations as a shimmering of colors "and here again we come across the stained glass which fired my enthusiasm in my youth." It is worth examining in some detail Messiaen's color perception here.

To a medieval glassmaker a glass window was a religious lesson, a "holy history and a catechism." When the window is viewed at a distance the figures are too small to distinguish but one is dazzled by colors. For example, a window dominated by blues and reds (even with a few patches of yellow and green) produces in the eye a sensation of an enormous violet. It happens that Saint John, in his book of Revelation, described his celestial visions in the same way: So, when he spoke of divinity he didn't name it but said: "And there was a rainbow round about the throne", the idea of majesty being associated with the idea of dazzling color. When he spoke of the holy city, he said "And her light was like unto a stone most precious, even like a jasper stone, clear as crystal." Here note the jasper is mottled with various colors: as for jasper crystal it's an extremely rare stone which should not only support all the colors of the rainbow but also be translucent. Finally, Saint John says "and the foundations of the wall of the city were garnished with all manner of precious stones: Jasper, Sapphire, calcedony, emerald, sardonyx, sardine, chrysolite, beryl, topaz, chrysoprase, jacinth, and amethyst." (I'd ask you to note that the colors these stones give us all the colors of the rainbow.) (Samuel, 1976.)

Messiaen wanted to express in his work the colors mentioned in Revelations. "I think I've never been so deep into the sound color relationship. Certain sound combinations really correspond to certain color combinations, and I've noted the names of these colors on the score in order to impress this vision on the conductor who will, in his turn, transmit this vision to the players he directs: the brass should, dare I say it, play 'red,' the woodwinds should 'play blue' etc."

In *Conversations With Olivier Messiaen* (Samuel, 1976), Messiaen likens his colored composing to painting and, in fact, mentions his painter friend Blanc-Gatti who suffered from what he calls "synopsia." He fixes the "very brief and fugitive" glimpses of color on to the canvas. These colors turn, mix, and intermingle exactly like sounds. "When I hear music, and equally when I read it, I see inwardly, in the mind's eye, colors which move with the music and I sense these colors in an extremely vivid manner, and I sometimes even precisely indicate these correspondences in my scores. . . . I see them inwardly: This is not imagination, nor is it a psychic phenomenon. It is an inward reality." Messiaen paints with these colors "juxtaposing them and putting them in relief against each other, as a painter underlines one color with its complimentary."

To talk of an exact correspondence between a key and a color is not possible because colors are complex and linked to equally complex chords and sounds. Therefore, Messiaen invented the modes of limited transpositions to better represent this relationship. The two main modes are linked in very precise colorings for him, as described above. Messiaen thinks that "one should of course be able to prove this relationship scientifically, but I am incapable of it." He still feels that it "rests on scientific fact modified by the personality of whoever is subject to the phenomenon, to which may be added something of imagination and of literary influence difficult to express." I do not disagree with his analysis.

We mentioned earlier the religious symbolism of color, and it is not surprising that Messiaen should find a very "natural" mystic symbolism in color. Violet, his favorite color, is a complex color "because it blends blue, an extremely cold color, with red, an extremely warm color. But violet is capable of many nuances." There is, for example, a violet in which red dominates that is called purple, and at the other end of the scale there is a violet containing more blue than red called hyacinthe blue. These two violets have a great importance: in the symbolism and stained glass of the Middle Ages, according to Messiaen, the one represented the Love of Truth and the other the Truth of Love. "This reversal of terms is certainly not just a play on words but corresponds without doubt very closely to these nuances of violet."

Medieval masters of stained glass passed secrets from father to son for the same reasons as master architects and master masons. There could be some influence of magic or primitive initiations but as Messiaen says, "this doesn't gainsay that the symbolism was of great beauty and has produced extraordinary results."

Many think that Messiaen's mysticism is expressed in his use of unusual instruments with prolonged resonance, such as gongs, tam tams, the Ondes Martenot (an electronic instrument with a metallic timbre), the percussive gamelon, bells with their harmonic halos, the resultants of false fundamentals and complex overtones "which bring us close to some of the enormous and strange noises in nature like waterfalls and mountain torrents." Such sounds capture the unreality and mystery that so fascinate Messiaen. Mystery and magic meet at every turn in his process as a creator when he throws color, harmony, rhythm, and timbre in the caldron. What seems and sounds so complex is actually a few ideas crystallized around his synesthesia and its intellectual refinement, which constitute the very essence of both his human and his musical personality.

CREATIVITY AND SYNESTHESIA

It is not possible to do more than just touch on other synesthetic composers and artists. More important is what synesthesia can say about creativity. Although not a product of the imagination, synesthesia does give testimony to a product of the brain and an appreciation for where poetic imagination may arise in our minds. Synesthesia is far from being an "intellectual" act, although it can certainly be the stuff from which creative dreams are made. An appreciation of the synesthete's world, particularly those who make their synesthetic visions public, can help explain the eureka sensation of insight or the exhilaration of being seized by the creative muse. For a handful of artists, synesthesia is the creative fuel for creative transformation. Artists have always claimed a more direct perception of the world, a directness that is characterized, for one, by the synesthetic percept. Madness has also been linked to creativity, and the ability to see visions with the power to heal. Although they are not our private visions, the visions of the poet can also heal.

Subject JB says that her art is that of a visionary, that she is "of that group of specially gifted artists who do not construct their images but visualize them as completed wholes from the very first." Her works are, thus, products of inspiration, and they exhibit an unexpectedness and coherence that is unique. This is an example of closure in creativity, the ability to combine parts into a whole or to identify parts in a whole and to shift from one whole to another. Other features of the creative process include simultaneous rather than sequential thinking, removing the constraints of the intellect upon the imagination, and a suspension of evaluation. The invention of the modes of limited transposition and nonretrogradable rhythms by Messiaen shows an example of bi-sociation, the linkage of two conceptual frameworks that had hitherto appeared to have nothing in common. What we see in the contribution of synesthesia to creativity is similar to the universality of all archetypal sources, such as myth. The beauty of myth and symbol lies in their synthetic power. They can combine in one presentation disparate elements that would be self-contradictory if put into a declarative sentence. For synesthetic artists, and for most of their audience, I believe, there is an apperception of a connectedness and universal identity, an immediate apprehension without cognition or rational thought for touching a special truth that only metaphor can offer us. A good metaphor implies an intuitive perception of the similarity in the dissimilar. The metaphor seems to transport us closer to a world of absolute understanding that is more real than reality. The point is that we perceive something true, universal, mystic, correct in this art that is a result of the synesthetic vision.

Vasilly Kandinsky (1866–1944) was a synesthete who eliminated objective representation in his paintings after 1911. At 45 years of age, he had already been a professional artist for 15 years, had previously trained in law, for which he had been offered a professorship, and was fluent in several languages. Kandinsky was among the first to step off the path of representation that Western art had followed for 500 years, and his model for this new "symbolic" art form was music. Kandinsky explored harmonic relationships between sound and color and used musical terms to describe his paintings, calling them "compositions" and "improvisations."

Kandinsky studied piano for a time in Moscow, where he was captivated by the promise of artistic fusion in Symbolist transcendence. His one-act opera, *Der Gelbe Klang* ("The Yellow Sound," 1912), specifies a complex mixture of color, light, dance, and sound. The actual music was composed by Kandinsky's friend Thomas De Hartmann, who along with Kandinsky, Klee, and Schonberg, was connected with the avant garde *Blaue Reiter* group in Vienna.

Although what we think of as typical Kandinsky works were not produced until mid-life, they embodied ideas he held from his earliest years. With quantum theory and relativity published in 1900 and 1905, modern science was painting its own picture of the world, one that was as different from its classical predecessor as were Kandinsky's paintings from those of the renaissance artists. Kandinsky absorbed the teachings of Theosophy and Eastern thought, and the ideas he encountered in scientific and spiritual writings confirmed a spiritual view of the world that he had held since his student days. In essence, Kandinsky's conviction was that art, if it was to portray reality, should not concentrate on objects but on the direct and intuitive process that he exercised in abstract painting, and in which he believed the spiritual could be found (Kandinsky, 1910). His adjuration was:

lend your ears to music, open your eyes to painting, and . . . stop thinking! Just ask yourself whether the work has enabled you to "walk about" into a hitherto unknown world. If the answer is yes, what more do you want?

For the Russian composer Alexander Scriabin (1871–1915), the interest between color and sound grew not only out of his own synesthesia but also from his professional association with Nikolai Rimsky-Korsakov, who also saw sounds and musical keys in various hues. Their tone colors, of course, did not match. While Rimsky-Koraskov appears not to have specifically composed any colored music, Scriabin composed *Prometheus, The Poem of Fire* (1911) for large orchestra and piano, with organ, choir, and *clavier a lumieres*. The *clavier a lumieres* was a then-nonexistent instrument, a mute keyboard that could control the play of colored light in the form of beams, clouds, and so forth, flooding the concert hall and culminating in a white light so strong as to be "painful to the eyes." In the score, its part is written in conventional musical notation (Figure 8.9), Scriabin providing the code between notes and colors. Keys also had specific colors: F minor was blue, "the color of reason," D major a sunny golden, and F major "the blood red of hell." The first performance with lighting effects was March 20, 1915, in New York, just 5 weeks before the composer's death. Technical difficulties were insurmountable. As a compromise, which Scriabin rejected, the colors were merely projected on a screen above the orchestra. Interesting technical reviews are given in *Scientific American* (Plummer, 1915; Sullivan, 1914).

A more ambitious and all-embracing *Mysterium* was never completed. The work was planned to open with a "liturgical enactment" in which music, poetry, dance, colored light, and scent were to unite, inducing the worshipers to a "supreme, final ecstasy." Finally, one should mention Scriabin's invention of the "mystic chord," a chord consisting of a series of five fourths (note again the numerology): C, $F^{\#}$, B^{b}, E′ A′, D″, which forms the harmonic basis of *Prometheus* and other of his works.

The mysticism inherent in this colored music is, of course, not unique to it, for the idea of a harmony of sound and color is actually typical of the final phase of post-Wagnerian romanticism. Schonberg, who was not

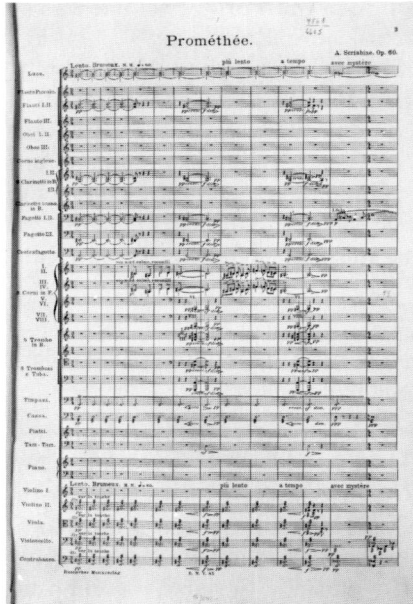 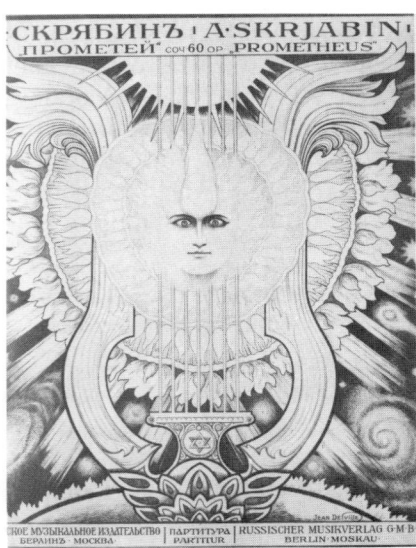

FIGURE 8.9. *Left:* Title page of Scriabin's *Prometheus*. Notation for the light instrument is on the top stave, marked "luce." *Right:* Cover of the score, to which Scriabin attached enormous importance, shows a huge, flaming sun with an androgynous male-female face enclosed in a world lyre and surrounded by magical and cosmic symbols—stars, comets, and spiraling clouds. It was designed by the composer's friend Jean Delville, artist, poet, and theosophist. The cover is orange, the color of fire. The illustration reflects Scriabin's increasing interest in mysticism. In Scriabin's symbolism, the androgynous eyes "express the will surrounded by primeval chaos from which the world-will calls everything to life." The first material life dissolves into spirit and in an orgiastic dance is united with God.

synesthetic, experimented with colored music in *Die Glückliche Hand,* a short opera written at nearly the same time as *Prometheus.* Schonberg wished to eliminate any distinction between waking reality and dream reality. The score calls for shifting colors to accompany the music and mirror the emotions of the characters.

One supposes that an aesthetic based on synesthesia can be only marginally meaningful to a general audience. Literally cut off from the artist's personal vision, we can appreciate such works sympathetically but without full understanding of their inspiration. This hardly means, however, that the artworks themselves are unable to move us, for they certainly do, and music, perhaps more than any of the arts, can easily transport us to that transitory and mystical change in self-awareness that is known as ecstasy. Ecstasy is simply any passion by which the thoughts are absorbed and in which the mind is for a time lost. In *Varieties of Religious Experience* (1901), William James spoke of its four qualities of ineffability, passivity, noetic quality, and transience. We should note that these are also qualities of synesthesia itself.

These examples hardly exhaust the topic of colored music, and the interested reader should consult musical and other sources (Critchley, 1977; Klein, 1926; Wood, 1936). The origin of color music comes from a theory, prevalent in the renaissance and systematically set forth by the Jesuit music theorist and mathemetician Athanasius Kircher (1602–1680), that each musical sound has a necessary and objective correspondence to a certain color. From the 18th to the 20th century experiments were made by adapting various keyboard instruments to devices that would, by pressing a key, project colored light in addition to producing a musical sound. Some of the works cited above stem from true synesthetic experience, such as those by Scriabin and Arthur Bliss (*Color Symphony*, 1922).

The topic of color music has received scholarly treatment in Scholes' *Dictionary of Music* (1900). In here, and in some other musical sources, an undertone of scepticism implies that synesthesia is purely subjective and the result of psychologic associations. It for precisely this reason that neurologists are concerned.

There is, finally, a complete category of colored music that is deliberately contrived. Although not without intrinsic interest, the notion that color and music can be translated into each rests, as mentioned above, on a fallacy, and it is important to distinguish color music that is deliberately contrived from that which is the result of synesthetic experience. Moreover, mixed media is not a modern invention. Odorama, smellavision, *son-et-lumiere* and laser light shows all have their historical place. The mixed media of *son-et-lumiere,* sometimes with odors, was popular in late 19th-century Paris. Mrs. Astor, at her Beechwood mansion in Newport, poured perfume into the glass cups of her crystal chandeliers to stimulate her guests as they danced in the ballroom. One doubts that there is much, if any, influence of synesthesia on these polysensory artworks. These are deliberate inventions.

Just as there are deliberately contrived sound-color compositions, so too have painters been *inspired* by music. *Music—Pink and Blue II* (1919), by Georgia O'Keeffe, is such an example. O'Keeffe created a series of pictures inspired by music. Yet they are inspired rather than synesthetic, and the distinction needs to be emphasized. It is interesting to note, however, that O'Keeffe was influenced by Kandinsky's *On The Spiritual in Art*. Without knowing the directness of synesthesia herself, perhaps she experienced in a more circuitous way the emotional experience that is the essence of art. Her discovery that colors could convey psychological and emotional states of mind and her convictions about the expressive power of abstract art are clearly stated in a letter from 1930.

I know I cannot paint a flower. I cannot paint the sun on the desert on a bright Summer morning but maybe in terms of paint color I convey to you my experience of the flower or the experience that makes the flower of significance to me at that particular time (O'Keeffe, 1987).

Here may be an example of the directness of perception characteristic of both synesthesia and the artistic experience. Both are ineffable, and both truly indescribable by language. Both may be examples of fundamental intermodal associations that are directly understandable.

A discussion of sound symbolism and synesthetic metaphor in poetry is beyond the scope of this chapter, although the subject is of interest in relation to synesthesia. Such works are often of a mystic nature. A discussion of it is given by L.E. Marks, a sensory psychologist (1978, chapters 7 and 8). The idea of synesthesia can be found in the invention of Zoltan Kodaly (1882–1967), the Hungarian composer and educator. Kodaly invented a method of teaching music to deaf students by the use of hand signs, each hand position representing a note value. Popularly, this auditory-manual yoking was given the nod in the film *Close Encounters of The Third Kind,* in which an alien spaceship visits Earth. The alien message to Earth is a melody played in conjunction with colored lights that emanate from the ship. The earthlings respond by parroting the melody and colors even though they have no idea what they are "saying." At last, a wise scientist uses Kodaly's formula for sound and hand motions, and deciphers the message as a gesture of greeting and handshake.

Critchley suggests that the doctrine of the unity of the senses took root in an obscure work by Von Hornbostel, which first appeared in *Melos, Zeitschrift für Musik,* Berlin (Von Hornbostel, 1926). He described a sensuous state called a supersensuous sense perception, the essential component of which unites all the senses "among themselves, unites them with the entire (even with the nonsensuous) experience in ourselves, and with all the external world that there is to be experienced!" How similar the objective scientist sounds to a symbolist poet.

David Hockney (DH)

The last example will be a visual artist who has been personally examined, the English painter David Hockney (1937–   ) (see subject DH in Table 2.1). Hockney is a painter, printmaker, photographer, and stage designer whose works are characterized by economy of technique, preoccupation with light, and a frank realism. There is for Hockney a synesthetic association between sound, color, and shape. It is not, of course, evident in the paintings that made him famous, since these are "silent" works. Costume and stage set for the Ballet de Marseille and the Glyndebourne and Metropolitan Operas revealed a new element in Hockney's artistry that was critically acclaimed. This acclaim is due, in my opinion, to Hockney's synesthesia, since he quite explicitly conceived his designs *to the music*. Certain comments by the artist made me suspect that he was synesthetic, and this suspicion was confirmed by later examination. Unless otherwise noted, all quotations are from examinations of September 11–12, 1981.

I find that visual equivalents for music reveal themselves. In Ravel, certain passages seem to me all blue and green, and certain shapes begin to suggest themselves almost naturally. It's the music that attracts me to doing the set designs rather than the plot. (*Architectural Digest,* September 1980, pp. 192–197).

Unable to read music, he plays it over and over. "I'll listen to the specific music constantly while I'm working," says Hockney. "You want to soak it in." Instead, he paints to the music itself, his arm guided by the kinetic sense of the music itself. In painting Ravel's *L'Enfant et les Sortileges* for the Metropolitan Opera in 1981 the "musical description of the tree in the garden has actual weight, like a tree has. I drew the form of the tree to the music" (*New York,* February 23, 1981, pp. 36–37). "I painted the sets to *Rossignol* the same way—to the music."

Hockney is not like MW or Luria's S, synesthetes who are so overwhelmed by the sensory experience that they find it hard to articulate. He has spoken in some detail about his feeling for color and space as they relate to stage works set to music. He is, I believe, an example of the process that Olivier Messiaen alluded to, namely the innate talent of synesthesia itself modified by personal intellect and creativity. One finds in Hockney an extremely intelligent man who is a master of his craft, has a firm sense of its history and classical foundations, and is above all else articulate enough to convey to the rest of us some sense of the process that occurs that permits him to translate his private synesthetic vision into a public artwork that moves us.

His Synesthesia

Dear Dr. Cytowic:
    I know it seems a long time to take to answer your interesting letter, but I have carried it about with me for a few months sometimes thinking of replying and then putting it off, then thinking I've put it off for a good reason. Would it tell me anything—or do I really want to know, etc.
    I must admit my first reaction to it was that you were trying to describe academically something I'd always thought and explained away as "poetic." I'd never heard of synesthesia.
    Anyway here I am replying to your note. Curiosity has got the better of me and so perhaps we could arrange a meeting (8/10/81).

Hockney's synesthesia involves an association of music, shape, color, and space. In my interviews it was not clear that he has projected photisms, although he does fulfill the other criteria for synesthesia. There is, furthermore, a kinesthetic sense that is active when he actually paints to the music itself. There was not much music as a child and Hockney has no musical talent. "It wasn't until I was forced to do something about it in 1974 with *The Rake's Progress*." He was very apprehensive about having to conceive a visual piece to accompany the opera, finding it difficult to "get" the actual music even after multiple hearings. By relinquishing the intellect and not trying to analyze the music he was listening to, he discovered that he experienced something else. "But then it was largely *involuntary* and I do 'get it,' something clicks and all of a sudden you hear and feel more of the music." Public reaction alerted Hockney that there was something unusual in his creations, some extra element.

The kinesthetic sense is present while actually painting to the music. In the Ravel, the tree music (of *L'Enfant et les Sortilege*) dictated the volume and weight of the tree that he painted. By this, Hockney means an expanse, a volume and visual area that corresponds to the physical shape of the music. He would actually paint with a long 3-foot brush, articulating at the arm, while he listened, the music dictating his arm motions—the lines, curves, blots, and dots as well as the color and overall dimensions. "In all operas I've done, the music gives me the set—the color and the shape. In [*Stravinsky's*] *Oedipus Rex* there was not much color but lines and sharp things which suggested cross hatchings." Note the reference to geometry.

A pilot study was performed September 11–12, 1981, at Hockney's home in Los Angeles. It confirmed the existence of absolute and relative effects in a sound-color matching task similar to that described in Chapter 3. This was a forced-choice task using 120 trials for each stimulus. In the study with Hockney, however, actual Munsell color chips were used instead of verbal labels. In addition to the effect of pitch (single tones) on the effect of color matching we were able to examine melody by using major and minor arpeggios and triad chords. Chords are more like tones than they are like arpeggios; arpeggios are just ascending tones strung together. Tones that were perceived as high tended to evoke warm colors, while the minor arpeggios showed a very restricted response and evoked blues and purples. For Hockney, the thing that most predicts a restricted response is melody. Thus, our pilot studies seemed to merely confirm what the artist himself acknowledged, that the music itself, the melody, provides the shape, color, and movement.

Color and Space

David Hockney is an example of a very specific type of creativity, that is, one that involves the translation of forms of one modality into forms of another modality *in a creative act*. Because he is gifted and skilled at this and verbal, we have an opportunity to observe this translation of the creative process much more readily than in other persons who are synesthetic. The pilot studies from 1981 discovered some trends in the way Hockney does this translation. To be sure, they are elementary trends regarding melody as well as some dynamic trends, but certainly it is not a random form. Even if it were possible to learn a complete translation algorithm it does not mean that just anybody can do it. People like Hockney and Messiaen are some of the few people who can do it, and the interest here is in trying to learn something about how they do it. From what we have discovered about the general principles of synesthesia, it is probably not possible or fruitful to ask questions such as, "What part of a picture emerges from which parts of the score?"

Once Hockney's attention became focused on these issues as a result of painting stage sets to music, he became preoccupied with color and space in a new way. The addition of metaphor derived from the geometric science of fractals gives his preoccupation an air of mysticism.

What Hockney wants is a space in which one can walk around corners as distinct from the regimented single-point perspective that Canaletto, for one, relied upon. The manipulation of space is possible through the use not only of color, which creates space for Hockney, but also of colored lights. Over the years Hockney has experimented with more and more complicated colored lighting systems. By the multiplicity of palette and instantaneity of response, visual space, which the audience perceives as physical space, can be shaped and reshaped by color, much like Jacobs discussed theoretically 60 years ago (M. Jacobs, 1924). Entire sections of a scene can be metamorphosed or made to vanish altogether. The best way to reveal Hockney's thoughts on color, light, and form is to let the conversation speak for itself.

REC: You've taken some joking for your "light box," which is actually a scale model of the Metropolitan Opera stage, complete with a colored lighting control system. You actually alter your design sketches while viewing them in the light box. Can you explain its importance?

DH: Not many people use color—real color—in the theater. If you're going to use color then you have to have colored lights, otherwise you'll never know what color to paint. You have to test it. I had that box made in London when we were doing the Ravel because of what happened when we were doing [*Satie's*] *Parade*.

When I finished the drops for *Parade* last year, John Dexter said "That's nice, we'll just put white lights on them." I said "No. You put red and blue lights on them because that's what will make it magic. That's what will make it sing." It took them some time to realize that I was right. In London, five months before we staged it, I lit it crudely, and then slowly we devised that machine so that I could time the color changes to fit the musical changes.

REC: Do you always work with the lights on your sketches?

DH: Constantly. I keep fiddling. Looking, listening, and playing with the lights and it simply takes you a long time because you keep hearing more and more in the music.

REC: During the matching task we did yesterday, you said that the "correct" color stood out when the music was played. How so?

DH: There's a shimmer so that one of the colors stands out at the moment that the music is on. When the sound is coming, there's an extra vibrancy to the color.

REC: A eureka feeling?

DH: Yes, an intuition that says "This is it!"

REC: Is this something that happens or are you deciding this?

DH: Well, it only happens when you look at this chart [*the Munsell color chips*]. It would be somewhat easier if these colors were bigger. If each color chip were a few inches big there would be a lot more of it and you could feel it more. It's a special characteristic of color, that the more you see it the more there is.

REC: You're the only one I've ever heard say that.

DH: I think it's common knowledge. To make blue bluer you simply add more space to it.

REC: This chip is red to me whether it's this big or this big. Its physical size doesn't change the color of it.

DH: If you make it bigger you make it redder. I know there's more of it, but it makes it *seem* redder. Light and dark is a factor, too. If it's bigger, then you know it's not dark. It becomes something else. Look at this color, which is much darker in tone than this one here. But if it was bigger, it wouldn't be dark because there would be more of it and it expands it a bit and it's not the same thing.

REC: So color can be used to control the sense of space?

DH: Blue has this quality to being spatial, which other colors do not. The more of it there is, the more you feel of it. I did the same thing with light and dark in *Oedipus Rex*.

At the end of the opera, Hockney projects gold light out onto the proscenium and the front of the house to incorporate the audience into the opera. Hockney's hand outlines a cross in the air as he speaks.

DH: The music is like this—horizontal and vertical, very geometric. I projected the gold onto the side of the proscenium to give it incredible weight and to make it big. Boom, boom. The first quality of *Rossignol* that caught my ear was of transparency. I listened first. I don't look at the score because I can't read music. When I first heard it it doesn't occur to you that it's Chinese. What one hears is a transparency. It's about transparent things, night, moonlight, water.

REC: Your set for *Rossignol* is also all blue, it's monochromatic.

DH: But there are a lot of different blues in it. It's not just all one blue.

[This infinite variety of a single color, the exactness of shade, is a typical synesthetic comment. The viewer does not notice the myriad nuances and merely perceives the design as blue.]

REC: How does the blueness fit in with the finished work of art?

DH: It's the blueness and this sense of transparency that's in the music that made me think of the very refined beautiful china of the 17th century. Not the overdone 19th century stuff with dragons, but much simpler, purer versions. I went to the Victoria and Albert Museum in London and in just two cases of pottery I took about 150 photographs and that's where the trees, mountains and people come from in the set. Since the three Stravinsky operas are all in some way ritualistic, each piece is united by a circle motif. John Dexter wanted a disc on the floor but I wanted a transparent blue circle. So I made it a blue china plate.

REC: What about revisions? How much of the color and shape comes to you from just hearing the music and how much do you bring to it by "intellectualizing" or intentionally revising?

DH: It's like the shimmer with the color chips. I know visually when the color or the lines fit the music. We made about 10 palace drops for *Rossignol* and I thought "It doesn't fit the music." The lines weren't right. Each time you listen, though, you hear more and more in the music. It's very complex. In the end, it looks like Chinese Cubism to me, but it fits the music. It looks three dimensional, too, because I've painted it on black velvet. But actually it's completely flat. Black has an enormous space to it. Once you grasp the illusion of three dimensions, you don't scrutinize it.

We went through 27 versions of *The Rite of Spring* sets before they fit the music too. Most of the problem there, however, was getting the color right.

REC: You say that you actually paint while the music is playing.

DH: It's very hard to describe because it's ineffable. With Ravel's tree music, for example, I remember drawing the lines of the tree to the music because it had a weight. You know how a tree has a volume and a weight. I drew it during the music.

For *Rossignol* and the others it was the same. When I'm working on it I will play the music constantly. Normally when I work I do not work to music. I don't like it as background because you find you either listen or you don't. It could be trashy music—a little ballet or something, *Swan Lake*—where you wouldn't be too distracted. But I couldn't possibly work and listen to a Beethoven quartet. I couldn't, because I would lose the lines of what I was drawing at the moment.

REC: Do you think it's hopeless for you to give an example of hearing something and then saying "This is what I've drawn to that specifically"?

DH: The problem is, the first thing I draw would not be quite right. Although lot of times they are. I put this down to the fact that music reveals a bit more to you when you hear it over and over. There's simply more there than you've thought at first.

See, you're asking me to describe verbally feelings, which in art you sometimes don't have to bother. You feel it. Verbalizing them is often impossible and unnecessary, of course. I'm not sure I would have thought about this at all except for the fact that you're going to do this in the theater. You begin to think in ways you wouldn't quite always think about the music. Maybe a musician would always think this way, but I wouldn't.

REC: Does the actual performance, the singing and musicians, influence the way your set looks to you?

DH: Yes, it works both ways. One has to be flexible, too, although I'm quite insistent on some points, particularly the color. There are many things to consider. You work with a director, and people have to move in your sets. John Dexter [*the director*] tends to make diagrams, that's his style. I said "Ok, but I'll make pictures of them since I like pictoral stuff." Then you're told that the chorus has to be there in the middle—36 of them—or they have to be in from the beginning. Well, that's ruined my picture, I think. Then I think, well there's no need to if you stick them in the middle right from the start, then you'll forget about them. They'll disappear. Then the musical people tell you there must be something behind the people otherwise you won't hear the sound, and you know if it doesn't sound right, it's going to look hideous. And so there's no point arguing. It's very complicated.

REC: Let's go back to your comment about Cubism. That Cubism is more real than reality and not just an intellectual idea.

DH: One-point perspective, like any photograph, is a view of the world from one exact point. It's a Renaissance machine, a little hole that you look through—an unnatural way to look at things. We really don't do that at all. You suddenly see that when you being to look at things—this table, for instance. Sometimes you see surfaces, the grain of the wood, the shine of your tape recorder, the blackness, it gets closer to the way you actually see things. It's a jumble all at first.

When you draw, you tend to look at relationships—and this is what's so difficult about drawing. You have to isolate a bit. A line of the table there, but while you're doing that that's all you're looking at and you didn't get the shape of everything else that's in the peripheral vision. So what you finish up with in the end is not quite real. You sight in bits that weld into one, but the Cubist way is to look one place but you might be painting what something in the peripheral visual field looks like.

I've just begun to try to examine this. When you look, what is it you really see? If you draw quickly it forces you to look. I have many methods of drawing, it's fascinating. I might be doing an academic drawing of a head. Well the moment you look into the eyes, the rest of the face goes away. Whereas when you draw quickly, you tend to be looking at the whole thing all the time. Of course it's harder to draw quickly. It's also harder to draw loosely, which is why people who can't draw very well draw very tight, always. If you draw slowly, all the time it's analysis. Whereas when you're drawing quickly, you're not really responding in an analytic way. You're not quite sure what it is you're doing. Your hand and mind are responding to whatever. . . . It's hard to say. Usually when you draw quickly a lot is hit and miss.

Line drawing is the hardest. I have to concentrate, it's the most tense work. A few lines have to represent weight, texture, flesh, many things, usually without chiaroscura. It's quite tense, I love the exercise. You never discover how to do it. Every drawing is just as hard. When you're doing line drawing you're not consciously thinking how to do it, you're thinking "What is it," trying to find out what's there—there's so much there— you're trying to throw away an awful lot. All drawing is throwing away, isn't it? You're always drawing much less than what is there. It's hard to find essences. Good drawing is knowing what to throw away.

I opened this chapter talking about the Pythagoreans, and will come full circle and mention Hockney's interest in geometry and fractals. Mathematics and science seem to have inspired him into the realm of mysticism, and Hockney's developing interest over the past few years is a preoccupation with creating new types of visual space in his photographic collages (Hockney, 1984). His art has shifted from painting to large ''Cubist''-style pictures made from collages of smaller snapshots. At the same time, Hockney talks about fractals, the geometric theory in which physical objects, like mountains or clouds, are conceived to be made of infinitely smaller and smaller identical shapes—like looking down a hall of mirrors. ''With the fractals, you look in, and in, and in and it always goes on being a fractal. The edges of things become blurred and that seems a good thing. Getting rid of borders seems a good thing. It's a way toward a greater awareness of unity'' (*New York Times,* September 13, 1986).

For Hockney not only does color have space, but sound does as well. Even one's own hearing gives a sense of personal space, and perhaps his gradual loss of hearing in recent years has triggered his preoccupation with creating new types of visual space in his photographic collages. ''It seems a natural thing to happen. You know, at the end of his life, Goya was deaf. In his last pictures all those screaming people were silent to him. But you seem to think the paintings are about noise, in a way.''

Hockney's current project at the time of this writing is *Tristan und Isolde* in Los Angeles (1987). He has in mind an entirely new blending of color and light, constructed scenery as opposed to painted flats and flexible space. He sees the depiction of space as far more than a technical device. ''I think that the way we depict space has a great deal to do with how we behave in it. When people go on about 'exploring outer space' I tell them that we're in outer space already if we know what to do with it. What I want to do is chop up space, and in *Tristan* we're going to do it'' (*New York Times,* December 6, 1987).

Hockney distrusted photography's claims of greater reality and authenticity. He believes photographs are extremely untrue. It is not just that lines bend in ways that they never do when one looks at the world. Rather, one's eye does not ever see that much in one glance. Photography's panorama is not true to life.

Thinking intensely about looking forced me to think more carefully about Cubism, because looking—perception—was the great theme of Cubism. I always love that phrase of Constable's where he says "I never saw an ugly thing," and doing these collages I think I have a better understanding of what he means: It's the very process of looking at something that makes it beautiful.

One can draw with a camera, however, and this is what Hockney does in using small single-point perspective photographs to create a larger image with multiple focal points.

Ordinary photography is obsessed with subject matter, whereas his photo collages are about the way things catch one's eye. Ordinary photographs present a world from which details can be elicited. Hockney suggests that this is the opposite of how we actually see the world. The general perspective is built up from hundreds of microperspectives. Vision is a continuous accumulation of details perceived across time and synthesized into a larger, continuously metamorphosing whole.

Hockney's photocollages explore the creation of deep space out of bits of pictures containing shallow space. A Mohave desert landscape, for example, telescopes 900 yards of road, cactuses, litter, and street signs into an image that seems everywhere in focus in front of the viewer. "In that picture, there was only one photograph that actually depicts space. Every other picture was made by the camera being close to the surface and almost parallel to it. And yet it looks like a landscape full of space. There's something happening that's a bit weird."

The treatment of space in Hockney's photo collages is reminiscent of the treatment of space in paintings by Piero della Francesca, one of Hockney's favorites (see Figure 8.6). "Everything we look at is in focus as we look at it. Now, the actual size of the zone the eye can hold in focus at any given moment is relatively small in relation to the wider visual field, but the eye is always moving through that field and the focal point of view, though moving, is always clear." The Renaissance artists went to great lengths to record each "object" at its moment of clearest focus. Every object on the canvas, whether near or far, can bear the weight of focused attention, but like the real world and precisely unlike the world as portrayed in conventional photography. Speaking of Piero della Francesca, Hockney says, "I've always loved the depiction of space in early Renaissance pictures, it's so clear. The definition of a bad picture for me is it's wooly. Those paintings aren't ever, no matter what's portrayed. If it's a mist, it's a clear mist and not a wooly mist. There has to be this clarity, which is the clarity of the artist who did it, the clarity of his vision, his sense of being" (Hockney, 1984).

Contemporary physics and mathematics texts by such scientists as David Bohm, Heinz Pagels, and Benoit Mandelbrot provide Hockney with metaphors that he has explored in artistic terms. The idea of fractals, according to which each discrete part of a whole is itself a whole universe of form, has its parallel in Hockney's photographic collages. Hockney hopes that this and similar work will unfold even wider human insights than those that are purely visual.

A lot of the early modern artists believed that art could change the world. A lot of artists today don't believe that. Well, I do. The revolution has been diluted to being just about art, instead of being about everything. And that trivializes art, in a way. It is beauty that will save us, it is.

The urge to depict and the longing to see depictions is very strong and deep within us. It's a 5,000 year old longing—we see it all the way back to the cave paintings—this need to render the real world. Art is about correspondences—making connections with the world and with each other.

Hockney's synesthesia helps to make this connection. The refinement of Hockney's synesthesia by his intellect and artistry has led him to see and develop these connections. This is the contribution of synesthesia to artistic perception and sensibility. The various spiritual movements that served as a background in the emergence of abstract art have in common the conviction that reality, whether one thinks of the cosmos, humanity, or both, is beyond the world as we directly experience it. All artworks, in general, transcend their sources. We are more than what we have read or what we have seen, and artists in particular strive for visions that transcend what we ordinarily know.

9
What Is Real?

In this chapter I look into the relationships among synesthesia, hallucinations, illusions, and imagery, and suggest that there is a spectrum of conditions that may share or display a common cognitive structure. I also examine the question of whether synesthesia is "real," and in doing so am forced to consider the larger issue of what is real.

The question of what is real also raises other *what* questions, such as "What is red?" or, even more difficult, "What is color?" As Sir Karl Popper points out (Popper, 1975; Popper & Eccles, 1977), "what is" questions "are never very fruitful, although they have been much discussed by philosophers. They are connected with the idea of *essences*." "What is" questions are liable to degenerate into a discussion of definitions or concepts. There are different difficulties in asking *where* questions. Where, for example, does vision occur? In the retina, the geniculate, the pulvinar, the striate cortex, or some higher construct, perhaps a place called mind? One recalls the anecdote of Hans Lucas Teuber who, rolling his eyes upward, said he had no objection to discussing higher functions as long as by the term "higher" one did not mean extracranial. These *what* and *where* questions are ones that are not easily answered by any kind of model. Popper's suggestion is to discuss not verbal issues (that is, definitions), but real issues.

To the extent that one believes that all psychological phenomena have physiological correlates, he could hope to discover those physical properties by increasing sophistication of examination. An example of this is blindsight, the ability to perceive and discriminate visual information in a field that is blind in conventional terms. The notion that monkeys without striate cortex could only respond to luminous flux and not the pattern of its distribution, a "fact" first demonstrated by Klüver (1942a), has given way with more finely dissected analysis so that we now know that animals (and humans) without striate cortex do in fact have discriminative visual capacity and, further, that it is mediated by brainstem pathways. In this analysis and resolution of these nongeniculate visual pathways, many new questions will certainly arise.

Positivists and rationalists may skip this chapter. One can throw up his hands and claim that the subjectivity of experiential phenomena is "unscientific," but ignoring it is worse than jumping in and finding at least some theoretical structure for the subjectivity. Once this is done observation is tidier and "objective" measurements more meaningful. The array of objective physiological changes that accompany perception include galvanic skin resistance; pupillary change; variation in temperature, pulse, and respiration; and electromyographic activity (body tonus). The bulk of these, one readily sees, are efferent manifestations of the autonomic nervous system. Changes in EEG, rCBF, and positron emission tomography (PET) are further objective measurements. We have already seen in Chapter 4 that objective changes occur during synesthesia in MW.

One must acknowledge, however, that there are no such things as sensory data. Although the term "sense datum" suggests immediacy, perception is the outcome of a most elaborate interaction between a stimulus and the apparatus of the brain. A visual experience is hardly a perfect replica of the retinal image: immense series of interactions begin in the retina and continue through stages of the cortex, building in complexity such that the hypercomplex cells of the inferotemporal lobe—feature detection neurons—respond *only* to certain geometric shapes, line orientations, or other *highly specific* attributes of a stimulus. However, even this does not reach consciousness as far as we understand the visual process.

The majority of knowledge does not reach consciousness (Kihlstrom, 1987; Rizzo & Hurtig, 1987). The neuron is a storyteller that accentuates some features, completely ignores others, and is our fragile link to the physical world.

We begin by looking at two illusions so common that only painters can avoid taking them for granted. We next examine the retinex theory of color vision, which shows that the *identical* flux of radiant energy reaching the eye can be perceived as *different* colors. A review of phantom vision and blindsight shows that the perception of vision does not require striate cortex or even photoreceptors, and that the system can "go on its own." Vision can be perceived by input from other systems, most likely proprioception. A review of the Gestalt school of von Hornbostel and Boernstein is followed by a discussion of microgenetics, a grand theory that has not had much experimental testing but that draws widely from other areas and is able to unite much of this material. As the gestaltists might say, being and perceiving are most closely related to vision because vision combines the perception of elementary bright-dark qualities with the faculty of high spatial *gestalten* in one process (Boernstein, 1967). Finally, there is a gesture to those who live in so concrete a world that they are unable to even conceive or imagine what synesthesia must be like. This incapacity of imagination is likened to alexithymia, a constriction or absence of emotion ("no words for feelings").

What the various overlaps show is that the function of seeing is not limited to the visual system. Astute humanists have commented on this, an excellent example being Aldous Huxley's *The Art of Seeing* (1942), a book that describes Huxley's blindness following punctate keratitis at age 16. This is an interesting analysis of developing an awareness for the ancillary nonoptic aspects of vision, particularly Huxley's chapters on "The Mental Side of Seeing," "Memory and Imagination," and "The Variability of Bodily and Mental Functioning." He appropriately chastised ophthalmologists who gave him spectacles and wrote him off as permanently blind. The book is a telling illustration of how dogma squelches the very creativity that is often the basis of much scientific discovery.

Colored Illusions: Color Constancy and Colored Shadows

An examination of illusions reveals that color is not perceived just by sensing the light from individual surfaces in a scene. It is a common belief that color is directly determined by a physical cause, the spectrum of the light that falls on the retina. The mistaken belief is that the eye, like a color television camera, senses the redness, greenness, and blueness at every point by measuring how much energy there is of the long wavelengths, medium wavelengths, and short wavelengths, respectively. Laboratory demonstrations wherein the observer sees one color when in fact he "ought" to see another are usually taken as proof that the eye does not work as well as it should based on the construction of its photoreceptors. For example, the retinex theory discussed below shows how the flux of radiant energy reaching the eye with identical triplets of short, medium, and long wavelengths can be perceived as two entirely different colors.

The correct explanation for color illusions, therefore, is that conventional theories are wrong if they are so easily and consistently violated. The color of objects does *not* depend on the spectral color of light reflected from them. Once it is seen that color can be dissociated from the visual means by which we see an object and determine it shape, we can then see how color can be separate in synesthesia and be attached to other objects with which it is not normally associated. Color can be independent of object recognition.

COLOR CONSTANCY

When asked if synesthesia is "real," I usually respond by asking what the questioner means by "real." Deep philosophical discussion is aborted by explaining the most common illusion of all, that of the constant color of objects in daylight. This helps put the notion of "reality" into its proper perspective. Reality is relative. The constant appearance of objects under widely varying conditions of illumination, intensity, and wavelength distribution is a well-known psychophysical issue, has an abundant literature, and is a central theme in an understanding of how we see (Hunt, 1967; Katz, 1935; von Helmholtz, 1866/1967).

Daylight is not fixed. It changes in brightness from dawn to its apex at high noon, when the sun is directly overhead, to dusk. The full moon (0.3 lux) is 3×10^{-6} as bright as the midday sun, yet the nervous system can adjust its sensitivity so that we can see effectively in either condition. We can, in fact, detect the flash of a single photon (Abell, 1969). Daylight also varies considerably in its spectrum, a feature few people seem to notice. The peak in the spectrum of diffuse daylight shifts 200 nanometers depending on the angular distance of the sun from the horizon (0°) and the zenith (90°) (Figure 9.1) (Henderson, 1977; Judd, MacAdam, & Wyszecki, 1964).

The morning light is reddish, the afternoon sun distinctly yellow-orange. The indirect northern light favored by artists peaks in the blue part of the spectrum. In the woods at springtime, when there is new leafy growth, the light is bright yellow-green; later in the summer when the leaves darken the light shifts to the green part of the spectrum; in a coniferous glen it appears more blue. Added to these fundamental changes in intensity and spectral shifts are the sun, the sky, moisture, and particulate matter, all sources that make defining daylight a problem. At any one point it is a mixture. Light is scattered, refracted, and reflected. In spite of this dynamic quality of daylight, a piece of paper will always look white, an apple, red, and a banana, yellow. This is called color constancy.

As I mentioned, artists seem to be the only people who note this daily dynamic. Artists know that color constancy is an illusion—the public does not. Claude Monet was heavily involved in the Impressionist movement, which was scientifically interested in how light is refracted and reflected, and impinges on the eye. One of his exercises was to paint the Cathedral at Notre Dame at different hours of the day to show how the color of the facade and entire ambience changed. Even today, many people respond as Monet's public did: thinking that he was depicting his emotional response to the cathedral at each time of day, and not understanding that he was simply trying to paint it the way it looked. This blindness to color change is not a recent phenomenon that accompanied the advent of electric light. Color theory is hardly discussed in formal art training any more; color constancy is rarely discussed in current texts on vision and even then only in passing instead of appropriately identifying it as a fundamental issue of color perception. Brou, Sciascia, Linden, and Letvin (1986) suggested a reason why we tend to dismiss the phenomenon. Living most of our modern life under artificial illumination,

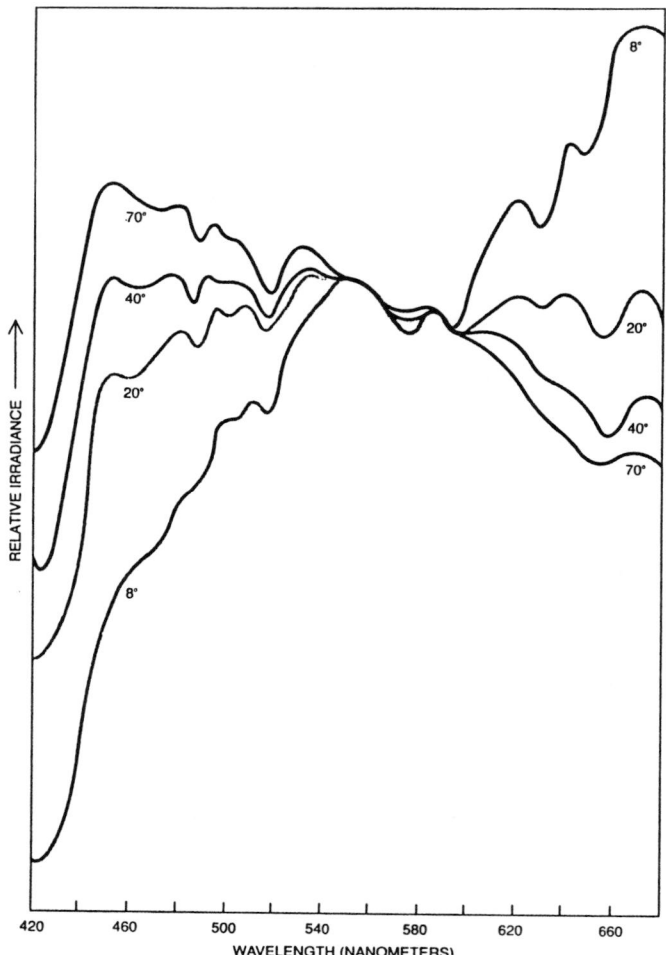

FIGURE 9.1. Daylight from sunrise to sunset varies considerably in both brightness and spectrum. Consequently, objects viewed at midday reflect more blue light than when seen in the evening, when they should appear redder. The four curves chart the spectrum at four times of day, when the sun is at various angular distances between the horizon (0°) and the zenith (90°). The 8° curve was measured half an hour before sunset: its peak at 660 nanometers is deep in the red part of the spectrum. Hours earlier, when the sun is high in the sky at 70°, the light's peak is some 200 nanometers shorter, well into the blue part of the spectrum. Although the colors of illuminated objects vary throughout the day, most people perceive them as the same at all times. From *Daylight and its spectrum* by S.T. Henderson, 1977, New York: John Wiley & Sons.

we have become inured to the experience that faces and cosmetics, for example, change color between incandescent and fluorescent lighting. Investigators of a century ago knew that color constancy poses a serious problem for efforts to understand perception. The constancy is so reliable that one routinely compares by memory the face color and lip color of someone who now stands under one form of daylight with the colors seen an hour ago, a day ago, a week ago, and under another form of daylight, and thus detects changes due to blushing or paling or signifying disease such as jaundice (which turns the skin yellow) or anoxia (which turns it blue). Such changes are much smaller than the possible changes in daylight color. It is as if, in the words of the 19th century physiologist Hermann von Helmholtz, we "discount the illuminant" when we perceive color.

We of course cannot discount the illuminant since we cannot tell what light illuminates a surface. The eye receives only that light reflected from the surface. Moreover, there is no such thing as a "sense datum." We are not aware of the processes occurring in the retina, only of the consequences of many processes applied to the flux of energy that reaches the retina. This is one reason why the analogy of the eye as a color television camera is poor. Once we have a different understanding of the psychophysical basis of color perception we can appreciate how the perception of color can be detached from object shape and exist independently or, as we might say in synesthesia, incongruously with other objects.

Consider the problem of visually distinguishing objects in one's environment. Imagine yourself in a natural setting such as the woods or a rock-strewn canyon. The objects in the environment are randomly distributed and reflect light according to their material composition and irregularities of their surfaces (texture). The task for detection is to distinguish one boundary from another. One region in the image is bounded by more than two, often many, regions and it would be helpful for the change in light across one boundary to predict some property across other boundary segments. *This is the problem of perceiving shape and form.*[1]

Color vision operates under dynamically changing daylight, varied reflectances, and a diversity of boundary arrangements. Color vision helps tell surfaces apart by supporting many more distinctions than monochromatic vision could. Yet variable distinctions are a meaningless signal equivalent to noise. Fidelity and uniqueness increase through color constancy. If boundary detection changed simply because there were a change in the illumination, we would be less able to distinguish objects.

Our ability to distinguish shape would also be impaired. There is a

---

[1]Form and shape are often incorrectly used interchangeably, especially by nonartists (e.g., Klüver's "form constants," when shape is really implied). Where possible I use form only to refer to the configuration of parts or abstractly as one of the elements of the plastic arts. Form includes shape.

strong link between color and shape perception, as is easily apparent by viewing monochromatic paintings or those executed with restricted palettes. An alternate demonstration is to examine the separation prints of the four-color printing process.

There are many means to print color: Ben Day, flat-zinc plates, lithography, offset, photogravure, woodcut, linoleum cut, mezzotint, aquatint, and colored etching. These are all variations on a theme. To print a color photograph, the original artwork is separated into four different plates. The color separations are known as halftone plates. The plates are reproduced from negatives made from the original artwork by using colored filters in front of the camera lens. A plate is sensitized so that only the complementary color is photographed; colors the same hue as the filter will not register on the plate. The filters are violet, green, and red. The inks used to print are cyan, magenta, and yellow. A fourth plate, called a key plate, is printed in black using a yellow-yellow-green filter.

An examination of the progressive proofs for such a printing process (that is, a picture printed in one ink from the plate taken through its complementary color filter) shows remarkable loss of detail, shape, contrast, edge, texture, and depth. It is not enough to imagine this; one must look at such photographs. It is then apparent how greatly color determines space. Color and shape perception are inextricably linked, and this process occurs not isolated in the eye but in the brain.

Since we are discussing illusions, it is interesting to note in passing that if care is taken in the color filters (violet not blue-violet, green instead of yellow-green, and red instead of scarlet) and the complimentary inks (yellow, crimson, and blue) then shadows and black can be produced much better than they can using the fourth black plate. The reproduction is also much truer to the original than in the four-color process. This "best way" is not done commercially because of expense. Nearly the same results can be obtained by a two-color printing method that uses true complementary colors: orange with blue-violet, red and blue, scarlet and blue-green, crimson and green, purple and yellow-green, and yellow and violet. The results with two such "bizarre" colors actually have a broader spectrum of color and better definition than printing in one color with black. These examples (from M. Jacobs, 1924) might be referred to as color illusions in which printers are able to reproduce a broad range of colors with a limited palette. The same result was produced photographically by Edwin Land, founder of the Polaroid Corporation. He could produce nearly the full range of colors present in the original scene by superimposing two black-and-white transparencies, one projected through a red filter and the other projected without a filter (white light) (Land, 1959).

Reflectance is a quality both intrinsic to a surface and independent of the variables that cause the dynamic changes in daylight. Reflectance is the ability of a surface to reflect light of each given wavelength. It is the ratio of light incident on a surface to the light that the surface reflects. Unfortunately, the eye receives only the latter, and, if one adheres to the old school dogma that the color of a surface depends on the light from that surface alone, then reflectance is useless in determining color. Comparisons of *adjacent* surfaces will be independent of the incident light if the surfaces are under the same illumination. This comparison is equivalent to the comparison to the reflectances, which are individually unknowable. Computer color displays have been devised by Brou et al. (1986) to illustrate this.

What the illustrations of color constancy show is this: surrounded by boundaries that are chromatically ordered, identical colors will appear different. Exchanging one of the boundaries for a small area that has marked spectral dissimilarity will induce the perception of color constancy.

COLORED SHADOWS

The phenomenon of colored shadows may be considered the opposite of color constancy. Shadows are not colorless. All shadows of any object will be a different color than the illuminated side, a color toward the complimentary color of the lighted side. For example, if an object is illuminated from one side by a colored light and from the opposite side by a white light, the shadow cast by the object blocking the colored beam will not be colorless, even though it contains only white light. The shadow, in fact, has a color that is complimentary to the colored light. The effect is striking.

If one photographed this experiment using colored lights from different parts of the spectrum and then compared the photographs, the shadows would appear quite different. However, by masking the shadows' surround (which is of colored light), one is surprised to see that the shadows are identical. This indicates that boundary and color perception are intimately related and suggests that if one were to perceive the phenomenon of a boundary, then he might experience color, such as often happens in synesthesia (recall Figure 4.3).

In both color constancy and colored shadows, the color attributed to a light is different from what it "really is." It is different from what the physical properties of the light lead one to expect and to predict. In color constancy, different spectral distributions (different physical stimuli) have the same color. In colored shadows, identical spectral distributions have different colors. To rephrase this, the same stimulus looks different (colored shadows) or different stimuli look the same (color constancy).

One could sit on his patio and talk about the lawn furniture. "Yes, I can see that the dawn's early light is rosy and that it's quite different from the golden glow of tea time, but my chaise longue is still yellow. It doesn't change with the color of the daylight because its yellowness is a physical property of the petrochemicals from which it's made. You can change the light all you want, even put a floodlight on it at night, and it won't change the fact that *I know in my mind that it's yellow*. It is a real, solid, physical object and real objects don't change.'' This insistence, in which the mind stubbornly refuses to acknowledge what the senses inform it, is a living example of color constancy illusion and shows how firmly ingrained it is.

Even if lit with colored floodlights for a party, many guests would insist that the chaise was "really yellow," and that any apparent change in color was "just an illusion," just as Monet's audience thought his paintings of the Cathedral of Notre Dame were an exercise of emotional expression and certainly could not reflect reality. Everybody knows that the stones of the cathedral, being "real objects," cannot change their color. It is not easy to understand that the color is in our brain and mind and not an intransmutable property of the bricks and mortar.

These examples show that daily experience is a fluid challenge of color constancy and colored shadows, illusions that are so firmly ingrained that many people fail to accept their illusory quality even when confronted with the facts. Only the artist seems undisturbed at the endless variation of color and at taking the physical world at its face value. Paradoxically, it is the artist who views the world as it "really is."

We have seen that colors are determined by boundaries. This is where a change in chroma is perceived. Since the 19th century we know that if the eye is immobilized so that the image does not move on the retina, then the subject is unable to see within about 2 seconds, the maximum time for retinal adaptation. A fundamental principle of neurophysiology is that neurons signal change and not a steady state. Normally the eyes are in constant movement (occular jitter) and the photoreceptors can thus constantly experience boundary changes. In mammalian vision, the retinal cones are very early elements in a series of neural apparatus that builds in complexity. Although much evidence indicates that detection of boundaries and vertices begins in the retina, one cannot argue that color is determined there as well. Exploration of the retinex theory and achromatopsia shows that color and shape are dissociable and subserved by different neural mechanisms.

Retinex Theory of Color Vision

There are always those who do not believe their senses but feel better about the "objective reality" of scientific measurement. For those more comfortable with the proof afforded by instrumentation, the numerical values of the retinex experiments should be more disturbing than were the visual examples of color constancy.

There is more to color constancy than meets the eye. Spectrophotometers cannot categorize color; only brains can do that. When viewing experiments that illustrate the principles of color constancy and colored shadows, one is tempted to ask, "What color is it really?" as if the eye were being fooled. The eye in fact is not being fooled but is functioning, as Land puts it, "exactly as it must with involuntary reliability to see constant colors in a world illuminated by shifting and unpredictable fluxes of radiant energy."

Because we all agree about the colors of objects, even down to the ability to match Munsell color chips that differ minutely in color, we assume that there is a stable *physical property* in a one-to-one correspondence that accounts for the color. This is not the case. It then seems a mystery how we can precisely agree on the colors we see when there is no obvious physical quantity at a point that enables us to specify the color of an object. Simple experiments make it abundantly clear that *the stimulus for the color of a point in an area is not the radiation from that point.* The psychophysical basis for the stimulus as a basis of a color lies elsewhere. Once this is understood, the detachment of color (or shape, or in fact any other derivative of a sense) in synesthesia will not seem so bizarre. An understanding of lightness, derived from the retinex theory, will bridge to a discussion of the gestalt psychologists.

History of the Study of Color

Newton (1730) stated that "every body reflects the rays of its own color more copiously than the rest, and from their excess and predominance in the reflected light has its color." Thomas Young (1802) suggested that there were three kinds of receptors with three different spectral sensitivities and that they worked together at a point. His idea was that the response of three detectors at a point determines color at that point. His first idea was correct, but the second is not. There are three kinds of receptors (P.K. Brown & Wald, 1963; W.B. Marks, Dobelle, & Mac-Nichol, 1964) but the receptors do not act together at a point, as is shown below.

James Clerk Maxwell (1855) and Hermann von Helmholtz (1866/1967) helped establish Young's ideas as a basis for color vision, and both held firmly to the idea that three energies at a point determine the color at that point. von Helmholtz noted that we saw the correct colors of objects in spite of variable illumination, but explained this anomaly in psychological terms, saying that "we are accustomed and trained to form a judgment of the colors" by "subtracting the illuminating color from colored surfaces."

The beauty of the physical world is fully matched by the beauty of the technical mechanisms that subserve vision and its derivative aspects. Land's experiments in color vision (1959) and the retinex theory of color vision (Land, 1977) are incontrovertible proof that the perception of color is not a property of what we call "the color" of light.

Newton separated sunlight into the spectrum with a prism in 1660. He even reversed this process and gathered the colored beams together with a second prism to reconstruct white light. This does not mean that color perception is a property of the spectrum of light.

One of Newton's experiments was to recombine only parts of the spectrum using a slit to cut off all but selected bands. When two such separate bands were mixed on a screen the color that appeared was one in between the bands of the spectrum he was mixing. In 1959, Land recreated this classic experiment. When slits were placed just inside the ends of the yellow bands of the spectrum, the yellowish beams combined on the screen to produce, in agreement with Newton, yellow light.

Land then modified this by placing black and white photographic transparencies of a scene of various colored objects in front of the slits. There was, of course, no color in the transparencies. There were only lighter and darker areas formed by black silver grains on transparent celluloid. The two transparencies, however, were not identical. Some objects in the scene were represented by areas that are lighter or darker in the first transparency than in the second, because one of the black and white transparencies was taken through a red filter and the second through a green filter. All that the transparency could do is pass more or less of the light falling on its different regions.

When the yellow beams passed through these transparencies and fell on the screen, the result was not yellow, as in Newton's experiment. The original colored scene was reproduced with a full array of colors, including black and white! This very simple experiment forces the astonishing conclusion that the rays themselves do not make the colors. At most, they can only bear information that *the nervous system uses to perceive as colors* of the various objects in the image. We can see that Aristotle was wrong about color being an absolute sense "peculiar to vision." We can see that color is more like an Aristotelian common sense and can exist independent of vision, as it does in synesthesia.

Land found that neither a colorless nor a colored image was determined by the flux of radiant energy reaching the eye. The ability of the eye to discover lightness values independent of flux is convincingly demonstrated when only a single photoreceptor system—the colorless rods—are operating. Whereas the initial signal in the electroretinogram is proportional to the light flux absorbed by the visual pigment, the final comprehensive response of the visual system is "lightness," which shows little or no relation to the light flux absorbed by the visual pigment.

Since the processing of flux to generate lightness could occur in the retina, the cortex, or partially in both, Land coined the term "retinex," a combination of retina and cortex to describe the ensemble of biological mechanisms that converts flux into a pattern of lightness. The term "lightness," which Land uses to mean sensation produced by a biological system, is a term that we will come back to in a discussion of Gestalt psychology and the modal and amodal attributes.

The three retinal-cortical systems each form a separate image of the world. The images are not mixed but are compared. Each system must discover independently, in spite of the variation and unknowability of the illumination, the reflectances for the band of wavelengths to which that system responds. "A retinex employs as much of the structure and function of the retina and cortex as is necessary for producing an image in terms of a correlate of reflectance for a band of wavelengths, an image as nearly independent of flux as is biologically possible" (Land, 1977).

RESEARCH ON LIGHTNESS

It is worth going into Land's work in some detail. We have already looked at the common but erroneous belief that the colors of the spectrum discovered by Newton are the colors of the world around us. By examining color constancy and colored shadows we have seen that everything in the world around us is unevenly illuminated. If the photoreceptors of the retina and other parts of the visual system behaved like spectrophotometers (as intensity meters with peaks in three different parts of the spectrum) the color of objects would change dramatically from one part of the field to another and also as the illumination changed. The fact that colors remain constant indicates that color cannot be perceived if the photoreceptors operated this way. The redness so evident in daylight film that is exposed in tungsten light never bothers us when we step indoors to a tungsten-lit room. Our nervous system does not perceive the extra red because it does not depend on the flux of radiant energy reaching it.

Land discovered the constancy of lightness values by first examining images completely devoid of color. The rod cells respond to light 10^3 times weaker than that required for cone response and can respond in isolation when one wears neutral-density goggles that reduce the incident light by 3×10^4 (Hecht & Hsia, 1945). After a half-hour dark adaptation, a colorless world emerges with an effective illumination of 1/1,500th foot-candles. Objects exhibit a range of lightness from white to black and maintain this lightness without significant change as they are moved about into regions of higher or lower flux. In fact the illumination can be easily altered to yield more flux from a region that continues to look very dark than from a region that looks light, whether viewing real objects or a montage of light and dark papers. In such a collage of various lightnesses (whether colored, black, white, or gray papers) the lightness of any element is not appreciably modified by relocating it to a new surround. Thus, the rod system is unable to produce a colored image, but does give one in terms of *lightness*.

McCann and Benton (1969) performed an experiment using two narrow-wave bands at 550 and 656 nanometers with levels adjusted so that only the rods and one of the cones (long wave) received enough light

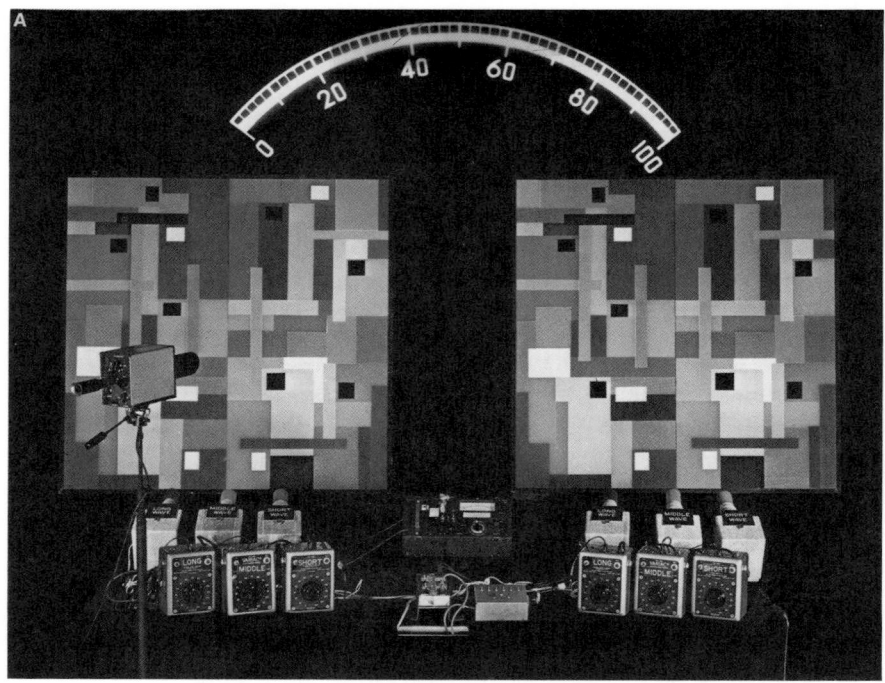

FIGURE 9.2. (A) Equipment setup for Land's "color Mondrian" experiment. The experiment employs two identical sheets of colored paper mounted on boards four and a half feet square. The colored papers have a matte finish to minimize specular reflection. Each "Mondrian" is illuminated with its own set of projector illuminators equipped with band-pass filters and independent brightness controls so that the long-wave ("red"), middle-wave ("green") and short-wave ("blue") illumination can be mixed in any desired ratio. A telescopic photometer can be pointed at any area to measure the flux, one wave band at a time, coming to the eye from that area. The photometer reading is projected onto the scale above the two displays. In a typical experiment the illuminators can be adjusted so that the white area in the Mondrian at the left and the green area (or some other area) in the Mondrian at the right are both sending the same triplet of radiant energies to the eye. The actual radiant-energy fluxes cannot be re-created here in this black and white reproduction. Under actual viewing conditions the white area continues to look white and the green area continues to look green, even though the eye is receiving the same flux triplet from both areas. From "The retinex theory of color vision" by E.H. Land, 1977. *Scientific American, 237*, p. 111. Copyright 1977 by E.H. Land. Reprinted by permission.

to function. The result was similar to the multicolored images produced by Land's duplex red-and-white system. McCann and Benton's experiment showed that lightness information collected at two wavebands by separate receptor systems is not averaged point by point or area by area

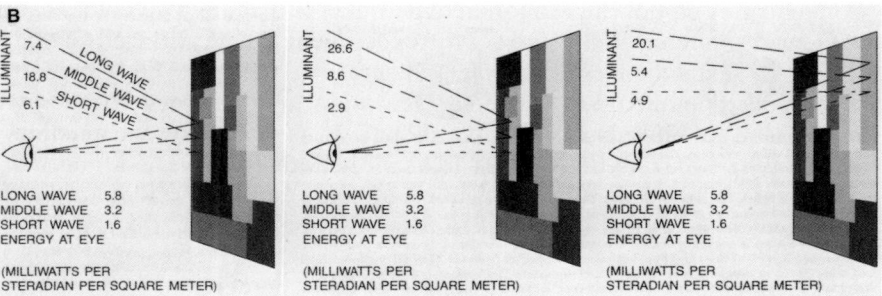

FIGURE 9.2. (B) Physics of Land's "color Mondrian" experiment. Identical energy fluxes at the eye provide different color sensations in the Mondrian experiments. In this example, with the illuminants from the long-wave, middle-wave and short-wave illuminators adjusted as indicated, an area that looks red continues to look red (*left*), an area that looks blue continues to look blue (*middle*) and an area that looks green continues to look green (*right*), even though all three are sending to the eye the same triplet of long-, middle- and short-wave energies. The same triplet can be made to come from any other area: if the area is white, it remains white; if the area is gray, it remains gray; if it is yellow, it remains yellow; and so on. From "The retinex theory of color vision" by E.H. Land, 1977, *Scientific American, 237,* p. 122. Copyright © 1977 by Scientific American, Inc. All rights reserved.

but is kept distinct and compared. Neither system alone (the rod or the long-wave cones) can produce colors. The appearance of a variety of colors (mainly reds, browns, yellows, blue-greens, grays, and blacks) suggests a process operating somewhere in the visual pathway that compares the lightness of separate images provided by the two retinex systems. When three independent images constituting the lightnesses of the short-, middle-, and long-wave sets of receptors are compared region by region, the full spectrum of color emerges. The reason, according to Land, that the color at any point in an image is essentially independent of the three fluxes on three wave bands is that color depends only on the lightness of each wave band, and lightness is independent of flux. The three lightnesses of an area determined by the three retinex systems is all that is necessary to characterize the color of any object in the field of view. For each and every trio of lightnesses there is a specific and unique color (some of which are not found in nature).

That this is so is shown by Land's "color Mondrian" experiments. This experiment uses two boards 4.5 feet square identically covered with about 100 pieces of paper of various colors and sizes. These Mondrians, named after the Dutch painter Piet Mondrian, to whose art the collage resembles, are arranged so that any piece of paper is surrounded by five or six papers of different color. (See Figure 9.2 for further details of the setup and measurement of the triplet of energy fluxes reaching the eye.)

The major point of the Mondrian experiment is that any two colors can be viewed simultaneously, and yet the experiment can be arranged so that each color sends the identical triplet of energies to the eye. The Mondrian experiment demonstrates that color sensation is not related to energy (reflectance × illumination) even though it is the only information reaching the eye from the various areas of the Mondrians. The Mondrian experiment is an in-depth investigation of color constancy. Radiant flux that reaches the eye is irrelevant to the sensation of color. Instead, it is the quality of lightness, which is perceived differently at each of three wavelengths, that is the ultimate source of color perception. It therefore makes no sense to speak of "color" reaching the eye.

THE RETINEX THEORY

Is there a physical correlate to the lightnesses of objects on three separate wavebands? The Mondrian experiment shows that each retinex system forms a separate lightness image of the world. The images are not mixed but compared, and the comparison of lightness at each area gives rise to the range of sensations we know as color. The physiological embodiment of Land's mathematical explanation could take various forms.

Imagine two light detectors positioned to measure the luminance at two different places on a sheet of white paper lighted strongly from one side. Since the illumination is not uniform, the luminances of the two detectors will be different. As the detectors move toward each other the luminances become equal and their ratio approaches 1. Now imagine any other hue next to the white. As the two detectors bridge the boundary between the two areas that differ abruptly in reflectance, the ratio of the outputs of the two detectors approaches the ratio of the two reflectances. This single process of taking the ratio beween two adjacent points both detects an edge and eliminates the effect of nonuniform illumination. (See Figure 4.3 regarding edge detection.)

The entire visual field can be processed as ratios of luminance at closely adjacent points, generating dimensionless numbers that are independent of the illumination. A computer program that does just this and computes lightness to detect edges was successfully constructed by Land (McCann, Land, & Tatnall, 1970). The location of the biological counterpart is unknown but calls for an arithmetic that covers the entire visual field, does not depend on eye movement, and can be seen in pulses of light less than 0.1 second.

If one looks at actual retinex records, there are large differences in lightness for most of the objects in the short-wave photograph and the photograph representing either of the other two systems. Yet, as Land pointed out, it is the comparatively small differences between the long-wave and middle-wave lightnesses that are responsible for experiencing vivid reds and greens.

This responsiveness to small differences in lightness also can explain the colors seen in highly unnatural situations: a spotlight in a void and Newton's spectrum produced by a prism. The perceived lightness changes little with enormous changes in flux. Of interest is what color the light is in a surrounding area devoid of light. A narrow band of 600 nanometers will produce a light reddish-orange, a color not ordinarily perceived.

The strikingly anomalous display of the spectrum is explained by the retinex theory as a series of three laterally displaced continuous gradients that share properties of both spots and areas. It is possible to predict the colors of the spectrum from these properties, whereas the color Mondrian experiments so simply demonstrate that it is not possible to assign a specific spectral composition to the radiance from a colored area in everyday life.

Objection could be raised that there is considerable psychophysical evidence for independent processing as well as an individual photoreceptor's restricted wavelengths (spectra). In the goldfish, horizontal cells are depolarized by long-wavelength light and hyperpolarized by middle-wavelength light (MacNichol, MacPherson, & Svaetichin, 1958; Svaetichin, 1956). Monkey lateral geniculate cells have receptive field center responses to one spectral region with antagonistic surround responses to another spectral region. Color opponent cells are also found in the ganglion and lateral geniculate cells (DeValois, 1965; DeValois & Pease, 1971; Wiesel & Hubel, 1966). In the ganglion cells of goldfish and the cortical cells of primates, one finds complex double-opponent cells having both red–on center and red–off surround combined with green–off center and green–on surround (Daw, 1968, 1972).

Such results may suggest opponent processing analogous to transmission of color television signals. A television camera uses three vidicon tubes, each responsive to one spectral region, and the intensity of light at each point of an image is determined separately for each waveband. A color television receiver has three electron guns for each of the three color-emitting phosphors. However, the signals that are transmitted from the TV station to the individual receivers are not three independent signals, but signals that are coded by a system similar to the opponent processing suggested by Hering (1964). Although the analogy is useful in illustrating how opponent processing can transmit signals over distances, it is poor in that television detects, transmits, and reproduces an equivalent set of radiances on the face of a cathode ray tube. A color television does not produce color sensations. One needs a visual system to do that. The signal transmitted to the cortex correlates with the reflectance of objects, not the radiance absorbed by the photopigments.

The retinex theory suggests that part of the reflectance calculation takes place in the retina and part in the cortex. The neurophysiological data suggest that there are intermediate levels in ganglion, geniculate, and cortical cells. At this intermediate level, which is also the level of neural processing at which synesthesia seems to occur, there is the opportunity for components of the processing to dissociate and for derivative aspects of perception to exist on their own. Whatever the actual properties of the physiological structures and their interactions, the color system as a whole works as a reflectance detecting device, as Land and colleagues demonstrated.

Land's experiments spanned 25 years and culminated in the three independent retinex systems and the Mondrian demonstration. The retinex theory states that color is determined by comparing the biological property of lightness. The three sets of ratios of integrals at edges and the product of these integrals within a set are the physical determinant between the visual system and areas in the physical world.

In relation to synesthesia, we see that the separate retinex systems usually work cohesively or congruently. Might it be possible that, in synesthesia, there is a spatial or temporal dissociation of one of the systems, giving rise to the perception of color where we do not normally expect it to occur? The analogy is with the desynchronization explanation for *déja vu*: a temporal desynchronization of the limbic component of a perception leads us to believe we have already experienced it.

Phantom Vision and Blindsight

Patients who are blind following cortical surgery or anterior lesions such as enucleation can perform a number of visual tasks in their "blind" visual field. When asked what they see they report "nothing," or "I was just guessing." Many parts of the brain are working in this example, although some system that generates reflective awareness seems to be removed. When a blind patient sees something and yet says he cannot see, this suggests two levels of seeing: one that consists of instrumental behavioral responses to optical information and other that refers to subjective awareness. The subjective awareness that can be mediated through nonoptic systems and still produce sensations that we regard as restricted to the visual mode is the subject of our interest.

PHANTOM VISION

David Cogan of the National Institutes of Health has collected a number of patients who have what he calls phantom vision. This is the perception of visual phenomena such as brightness, lights, and shape. These phenomena are seen mainly after enucleation or injuries that sever the optic nerves. He has a few examples in patients with cortical defects. Cogan has not published the material but has a collection of videotapes.

The cases cited here were presented to the Neurology Department of Washington Hospital Center on September 11, 1986.

Cogan notes that these patients do not readily volunteer this information and are ashamed of it because they know it is "not real."

Patient CH: Geometric Photisms with Cyclic Lightness

A few weeks after enucleation CH saw stars peripherally at 30° to 40°. He also noted a cycle of lightness and darkness, a variation in the sense of brightness that he perceived. This was not related to the diurnal photoperiod. The perception of stars was intensified by caffeine or increased mental activity (the patient was a stockbroker and continued to work).

Patient ER: Geometric Figures, Externally Projected

ER, a 50-year-old woman, had her left eye enucleated because of a melanoma. She saw geometric figures externally in front of her face and insisted that it was the "left eye" that saw them. This is contrary to conventional experience. One cannot tell which eye is seeing an object unless one covers each eye alternately to see that in fact only one eye is seeing the object (when, for example, one's nose gets in the way). ER insisted that the left eye caused the disturbance.

The geometric shapes were close to the face. She also complained of seeing "garbage," an assortment of blobs, spirals, and parallel lines that were grayish or metallic and seen in front of her face.

Her explanation is that "the brain is deprived and it's supplying its own stimulation. This is involuntary. The brain is doing it."

Patient JS: Synthesis of an Image

JS is a 20-year-old military recruit with severing of both optic nerves. He has no light perception, but closing the eyes dims the sense of brightness he perceives. Open areas, which he defines as "if there's not a solid object there," are described as a brightness.

He sees "objects" only where there is actually an object present, such as the sink when he shaves, the bed if he bumps into it, or parts of his own body. He palpates his legs when he says that he is able at times to see the outline of his legs. He is able to see his hand when he holds it up in front of his own face, but not Dr. Cogan's hand when Dr. Cogan holds it in front of the patient.

There is a conviction in his synthesis of an image. Cogan's interpretation is that he relies on other sensory input, perhaps proprioception, when he has a visual experience. This is particularly suggested in the patient seeing his own hand when he holds it in front of him, or seeing parts of his own body.

Patient CG: Image Analysis

This physicist is articulate and insightful. He has written about his phantom visions (Gillmor, 1980, 1981, 1982). He is able to see centrally things that are very much like Klüver's form constants. Sedatives and ethanol have no effect on his visions.

BLINDSIGHT

It is not difficult to find cases of residual vision in a field defect, but the blindsight monograph by Weiskrantz (1986) is chosen both because it is representative and because it may serve as a useful summary of previous cases for the interested reader.

An old presumption in studying vision was that we would uncover hierarchical layers of visual capacity; a further assumption is that all these layers resided in the striate cortex. Over half of all inputs into the brain are from visual fibers, making it theoretically plausible that other cognitive structures may be perceived as vision or in terms of vision. Much work with primates shows that visual discrimination can occur when the striate cortex is removed. This is not quite so surprising now because of our knowledge of extrastriate pathways (see Figure 9.3).

Klüver's work (1942a), initially indicating that monkeys lacked discrimination, was proven false by subsequent analysis. Monkeys lacking striate cortex can indeed detect stimuli of brief duration, can locate them in space, and can detect fine spatial separation between lines in a grating. Klüver did not originally publish the histology of his lesions. Later reconstruction of these brains by the Pasiks (cited in Weiskrantz, 1986, p. 9) showed the importance of the temporal lobes because Klüver's monkeys had temporal cortex anterior to the striate involved as part of their lesions. This would indicate the importance of temporal structures in the spatial qualities of vision, a quality that has been shown to be dissociable and of relevance to synesthesia.

Other cases show loss of specific attributes or classes of attributes of vision, such as achromatopsia with preserved form and the agnosias, which are analyzed below in the section on microgenetics. The well-known Riddoch phenomenon (Riddoch, 1917) is the inability to perceive stationary objects with preserved capacity to discriminate moving ones. I assume the anatomy of the extrageniculate pathways are well known to the reader and need not be reviewed here.

Reading Weiskrantz's detailed descriptions, it is evident how easily nonvisual perceptions are experienced during visual testing, particularly *movement and aspects of shape*. Weiskrantz found a double dissociation between the ability to detect a stimulus and to discriminate shape (that is, in that part of the field where the subject could not detect a stimulus, he

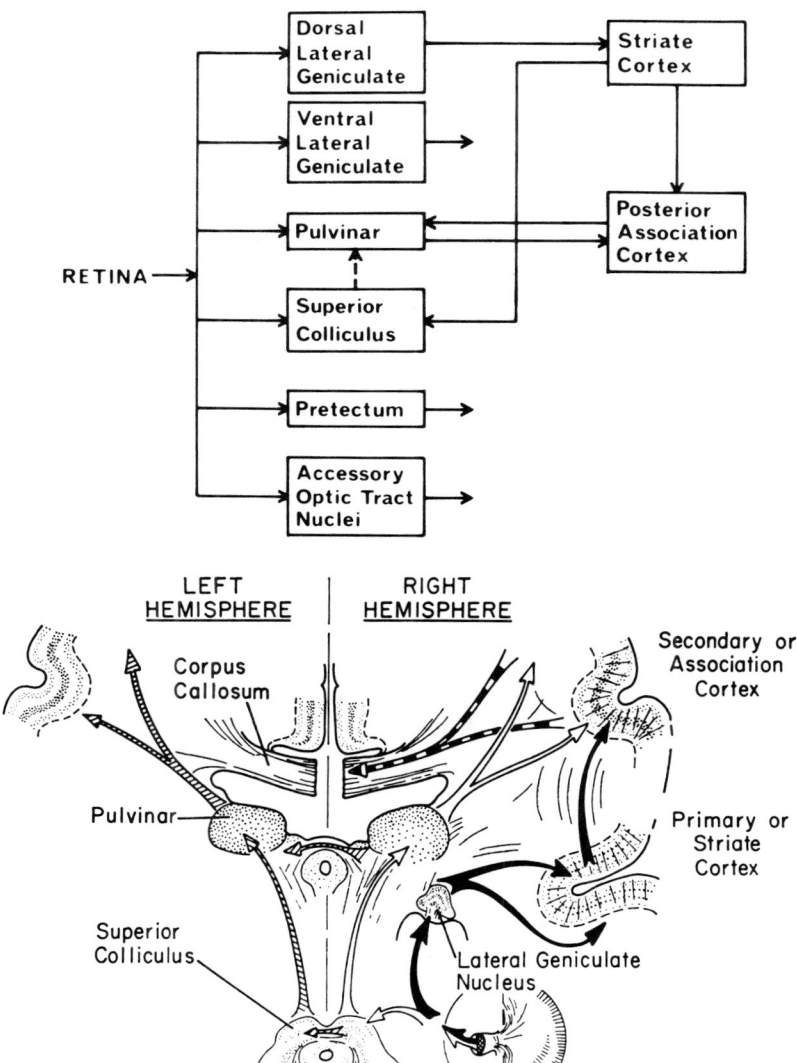

FIGURE 9.3. *Top:* Outputs from the primate retina. From *Blindsight. A case study and implications* (p. 5) by L. Weiskrantz, 1986, Oxford: Oxford University Press. Copyright 1986 by Oxford University Press. Reprinted by permission. *Bottom:* Subcortical visual pathways (*white arrows*) let objects in the far left visual field of the right eye be projected to visual cortices of both hemispheres in split brain patients via pulvinar and colliculus. From *The self and its brain* (p. 322) by K.R. Popper and J.C. Eccles, 1977. London: Springer-Verlag. Copyright 1977 by Springer-Verlag. Reprinted by permission.

nonetheless could discriminate shape well, and vice versa). In trying to discriminate movement thresholds, the experience was not veridical.

DB spoke of perceiving *complex patterns of radiating lines and grids, of shimmers and waves*. He has variously formed verbal descriptions: "a quick movement," "a sharp movement," or a "corner-shaped wave." These are the kinds of movements that may be perceived by synesthetes when they describe movement, lines, shapes, and things approaching and receding. Like patients with synesthesia, peduncular hallucinations, and phantom vision, DB also detected movement projected in front of him. He made such comments as:

. . . they all appeared to stand out in front of the screen. I felt I could push them back. . . . There was a definite movement. Something seemed to pop out a couple of inches. . . . I felt as if something was coming up to me. But I didn't *see* anything.

Among his residual capacities, DB's orientation was best preserved. As in synesthesia the *where* of a perception is separate from the *what*. And in both, the percept is believed to be external to the self, out in the real world.

Six patients with hemidecortication as a "treatment" for infantile seizures or hemiplegia (Perrenin, 1978; Perrenin & Jeannerod, 1978) had all of the neocortex and hippocampus and part or all of the caudate nucleus removed. Three cases had histological confirmation of ablated calcarine cortex. In a forced-choice response (guess where the target had appeared) there was a significant ability for subjects to localize targets by pointing in the blind fields. Subjects did better with moving targets than with stationary ones. Two subjects could also discriminate patterns better than chance.

The question of conscious awareness of vision naturally arises in blindsight, and I think is best expressed in comments on fatigability. Psychophysical testing is tedious for both subject and examiner. DB was attentive and conscientious with testing of the intact field and manifested typical fatigue. He commented on his lack of fatigue when the blind field was being tested: "But I'm not *doing* anything in my blind field—I am just guessing." Compare this to a typical comment of synesthetes that "it just happens. I don't do anything to cause it."

Multiple parallel routes are a feature of many sensory systems and may have a bearing on synesthesia. Other interesting observations that fall under the rubric of subception can only be mentioned here. Marcel (1983a, 1983b) noted that the adjustments made by the hands when blindsighted patients reached for an object were appropriate to the object. They were also able to tell which of a group of words was semantically related to a word flashed into the blind visual field. Palliard, Michael, and Stelmach (1983) showed tactile dissociation in a patient with a parietal anesthesia who nonetheless could localize deep touch and the direction of graphesthesia on her arm. Travel and Damasio (1985) demonstrated electrodermal response in prosopagnosic patients when shown familiar faces that they could not recognize.

Concerning the neural level at which blindsight and similar phenomena of subception might operate, there is, in general, a reasonable correspondence between properties of nonstriate visual systems and the residual vision seen in patients with field defects due to striate lesions. Dissociation between performance and awareness (knowledge) occurs in many areas of perception, and various functions can be dissociated. Midbrain pathways are only one of many candidates and are of particular interest because of peduncular hallucinations (discussed below). There is a relationship between collicular single unit activity and saccadic eye movements in localization (Pöppel, Held, & Frost, 1973). There is also a topological map of the visual field in the superior colliculus that could allow for spatial localization.

Optic Imagery and the Gestaltists

Walter Boernstein was a student of von Hornbostel and also knew well the work of Jaensch. I will relate his views of that school of psychology and in particular the work on imagery (Boernstein, 1967, 1970). We will also examine the nonvisual, amodal qualities of lightness and darkness.

Boernstein was very interested in the relationship between perceiving and thinking and approached it from three biological aspects: psychology, comparative physiology, and phylogenetics. The synthesis of phylogenetics with human psychology is a postulate going back some 100 years to Wilhelm Wundt. There are three main thrusts to Boernstein's analysis.

The first is that neither perceiving nor thinking is an isolated activity; each is correlated with other organismic functions. Boernstein criticized long-held notions that each faculty is homogeneous, that what was found to be characteristic of one sense would be valid for all senses, or that vision could correctly serve as the paradigm for all senses (see comments in Chapter 1).

Second, Boernstein believed that perceiving and thinking are arranged hierarchically, and extend from archaic, *purely somatic* processes that are inaccessible to consciousness to the highest differentiated mental functions. He believed that the transition from low to high processes could be demonstrated within the single individual and also in the course of evolution.

Finally, the hierarchical order could be traced in phylogenesis by encephalization (in the "psychologization of functions") and by a close fusion of primitive functions with highly differentiated ones. The fusion of high with low functions is more realized with vision than any other human sense, and an example of a persistent primitive mechanism is the responsiveness of all living organisms to bright and dark stimuli. Erich von Hornbostel (1931) showed that nonvisual sensory stimuli were also perceived as "light" or "dark." In light of what has been discussed with color constancy and the retinex theory—the role of the biologic quality of *lightness* in the perception of color and shape—the psychophysical perception of lightness and darkness in other modalities is of particular interest. In his unsuccessful efforts to explain synesthesia as just an amplification of language-based cross-modal associations, L.E. Marks (1974) did demonstrate a regular mapping of auditory to visual brightness in nonsynesthetes.

Much of von Hornbostel's theory rests on his deductions rather than on experimental material. von Hornbostel's theory is that each percept is characterized by two categories of sensory qualities: its specific quality and its nonspecific one. The specific one varies according to its modality (color in vision, taste in gustation, pitch in hearing) and other "amodal" qualities such as brightness, darkness, and roughness. Note the similarity to Aristotle's common senses.

The concept of von Hornbostel's amodal sensory qualities, that is, the theory that brightness-darkness is a basic sensory function, was not well received by contemporaries, who either misinterpreted it as dealing with analogies, symbols, or "mere" associations, or else simply ignored it. It achieved some recognition later when the specific and nonspecific afferents of the mammalian brain were discovered.

What von Hornbostel did was show that percepts of all modalities are characterized by nonspecific amodal qualities of bright and dark. The bright stimuli of nonoptic modalities influence the faculty of seeing in the same direction as physical light, whereas dark nonoptic stimuli influence it in the same direction as physical darkness. This is brought about by the action of the amodal nonoptic modalities on body tonus.

Boernstein emphasized the role of *structure* (shape, configuration of parts) in perceiving and thinking. Perceiving high *gestalten* is not a pure sensory function but requires integration of body tonus. His term was "specific sensoritonic sense synergies" underlying perceptual processes. In later years Heinz Werner and Jean Piaget applied the term sensu-tonus to all sensory systems. Although the optic system is most highly correlated with body tonus and therefore the highest "spatial sense," the other senses, such as olfaction, taste, and temperature discrimination, do have a spatial dynamic structure with little contour. Boernstein termed this "prespatial."

It is the high spatial structure that vision carries that makes it capable of "syn-opsis," the perceiving "at one glance" a dynamic structure both in exteroception and in imagery. This spatial sense, in all sensory modes, permits one to perceive transposable "invariants," which is a precondition for perception and discursive thinking. This arrangement, proposed by Boernstein and his predecessors, also allows for a dissociation of the elements, particularly the spatial component. One can suppose that the quality of lightness can also be dissociated.

Boernstein proposed synergistic sensorimotor synergies in perceptual processes together with von Hornbostel's theory of bright-dark perception as a common amodal quality of all senses in man, and probably lower animals, and showed the correlation between sensory and allied motor functions as a basis for the ability of the organism not only to perceive bright and dark sensory stimuli but also to experience accompanying emotions. Substantial support for the theory came from his experiments on induced optic imagery, that is, the additive effects of nonoptic processes on visual perception (Boernstein, 1939).

More specifically, Boernstein dealt with physiological mechanisms underlying the psychophysical perception of bright and dark qualities. He showed that gestalt concepts such as "stability," "constancy," "figure-ground organization," and "spatial perception," once held to be requisites of perception, were in fact not necessary: perception could still occur without any one of those gestalt properties. Boernstein was probably right in suggesting that the only way to understand the basic facts of perception in man was by tracing them back to their development during phylogenesis and to replace the popular "sense psychology with sense biology."

Boernstein cited, for example, his own evidence that the cortical taste area in man was in the parietal operculum. This ran counter to the dominant view that taste would involve rhinencephalic structures that are in the anatomical neighborhood of olfaction. Together with J.F. Fulton, Boernstein showed gustatory impairment only after removal of *both* sensory and motor cortical face areas. This supported his theory of a sensorimotor synergy. He further proposed that the cortical taste area in man would be in the neighborhood of the area subserving the related motor functions—all lingual, masticatory motor, and sensory cortices as opposed to the rhinencephalic structures.

How might this analysis address movement in synesthesia? The movement of simple photisms would not be so difficult, but what about the tactile senses approaching and receding in MW, the movement of geometric shapes and oscilloscope lines in the various patients with colored hearing, and the relative movement of spatial maps and forms in those subjects with number forms? The gestaltists trace the phyletic evolution of thinking from intended movements. "What originally in fish is a combination of reflexes ('taxis') becomes an intended movement in the course of phylogenesis; and, finally, in primates, including man, an internalized movement; i.e., a movement is first anticipated, and then carried out" (Boernstein, 1970).

The internalization of a spatial problem can be called either visual imagery or deliberating the solution. Anticipating the solution "in imagined space" before acting is the beginning of thinking.

The principle of specific sensoritonic sense synergies states that the sensory component of each sensory system is correlated with a tonic component on the same level of differentiation and, through it, with the body tonus as a whole. The sensory correlation is particularly developed in the optic system, and one may influence the other. The amodal nonoptic stimuli that increase body tonus can induce optic imagery and vice versa. Spatial orientation, based on the spatial senses and the body tonus ("mortorium"), is the root from which thinking evolves. Finally, Boernstein distinguished somatopsychological types that manifest themselves in different degrees of thinking (empirical versus rational) as well as in the degree of integration of perceiving, feeling, and thinking.

There is a stage of experiencing the external environment at which "perceiving" and "feeling" are not yet distinguishable. Color (translucent), appearance (soft), affect tone (lovely, friendly) are but different aspects of the same global psychophysiological state in individuals of this type—individuals who are well integrated according to Jaensch (Boernstein 1967, p. 165).

Boernstein cited Jaensch's (1931) personality types—the integrated (i.e., those who have optic imaginative thinking (*anschaulishes denken*)) and the disintegrated—suggesting that there are in fact personalities that are prone to imagery and those who are not, just as there are those prone to synesthesia and those who are not. The disintegrated person does not integrate seeing and thinking, whereas in the integrated personality visual perception, visual imagery, and visual imagination, based on "optic motor dynamism," constitute a dynamically integrated unit (*anschauliches denken*).

Regarding synesthesia, this may shed some light on a possible continuum between synesthetes, who perceive additional and changing qualities of a stimulus that the majority of people do not, versus those who "think visually" but do not have projected percepts nor other defining criteria of synesthesia. These two groups stand out from a third nonvisual group who find the entire topic incredulous. The analogy is with alexithymia, patients who have an emotional constriction (literally "no words for feelings") (Cytowic, 1985; Lesser, 1985).

Is There a Continuum with Imagery?

Are synesthesia, number forms, and the outcome of electrical stimulation of the brain a perception, a memory, or an image? Undoubtedly there are features of each, and a firm answer may not be possible. The reason I ask this is that number forms, which are possessed by some synesthetes or can exist by themselves, are often *not* projected externally (see Table 7.1). The memory maps of MLP (Chapter 7) demonstrate this. What is clear, however, is that these number forms and spatial organizations are extremely helpful to these patients in memory retrieval. What is missing is the affective component.

Induced Optic Images

Light and dark optic images can be elicited by bright and dark nonoptic stimuli. Sounds, tastes, scents, and touches can be induced in dark-adapted subjects (Boernstein, 1967). The induced optic images run the gamut from phosphenes to well-structured dream images that have a temporal sequence.

In discussions of imagery, the question of the relationship of images to perceiving and thinking is usually the center of interest. Many philosophers suggest that images in the strictest sense are products of language, a self-intentioned phantasm. The confusion characteristic of the literature on intrinsic optic imagery is reviewed by Holt (1964). There is a paucity of phenomenonological and taxonomic studies.

People will "see things" distinct from pure imagery during dark adaptation (Boernstein, 1967, p. 166 ff). Boernstein's experiments illustrate that subjects react quite differently to the same process of dark adaptation with regard to the frequency, vividness, and elaboration of the visual images. In some, an external nonvisual stimulus, such as the slamming of a door, will cause a momentary increase in brightness; others will have spontaneous images before complete dark adaptation is reached.

Boernstein could induce visual imagery with inhalation of "dark" and "bright" odorants. Of interest with regard to synesthesia, subjects saw discrete, generic patterns, except for a few "highly integrated subjects," whose images were more interpretive and metaphoric. That is, the intrinsic images of integrated subjects would have perceptual aspects. The approximately 30% negative results of Boernstein and von Hornbostel's experiments may have to do with Jaensch's personality types toward visualization.

Under appropriate conditions, stimulus agents inadequate for seeing are adequate stimuli for visual imagery, precisely because they do not enter the brain through retinocortical pathways.

The relationship among seeing, feeling, and thinking is well expressed in Indo-European languages, where the root *"vid"* gives rise to eidetic and vision (both meanings), as well as idea, idol, ideation, and so forth.

Electrical Stimulation of the Brain

What is elicited in electrical stimulation of the brain (ESB) is more than a memory. Penfield showed that there is the full-fledged participation of all the somatic and emotional feelings in their normal temporal sequence. Yet the patient does not forget that he is simultaneously on an operating table in Montreal. After ablation of the temporal cortex that was stimulated to produce the memory, it is clear that the memory is not lost by physical removal of the tissue. That is, the same memory (minus the emotional component that accompanied the electrical stimulation) is available to the patient postoperatively. However, the ancillary emotional and somatic sensations, the vividness of it all, is missing compared to the same memory that was evoked by application of the stimulating electrode.

Finally, there can sometimes be an affective state associated with imagery. Imagery, in distinction from ESB and synesthesia, is voluntary rather than elicited, and it is never projected externally. Memories either can serve to facilitate imagery or can become part of the conscious imagery itself (i.e., be incorporated).

One could speculate whether these three issues containing elements of perception, memory, and imagery share a common brain mechanism. However, one does not really need a unitary hypothesis for these conditions. Just as disparate genotypes can give identical phenotypes, what we are always looking at is the end product of one of these three psychophysical states. Similarly, many begged the question in the split brain experiments, asking "what side" or "what part" was contributing to behavior X, when obviously all mental events require bihemispheric participation despite the fact of "localization"—which really means maximal contribution of a focal brain mechanism. An obvious example is that the left angular gyrus is known to be necessary for arithmetical manipulation, yet one cannot argue that while calculating the rest of the brain is doing "nothing." To do so would be an extreme reductionism. Contribution to varying degrees of different kinds of brain mechanisms may be responsible for these three behavioral states. The "phenotypic" manifestation may then depend on how much of each of these is operating.

SUMMARY

We discussed Boernstein's theory of specific sensorimotor sense synergies in perceptual processes, and their growth from von Hornbostel's theory of light and dark perception as being common to all senses in man, and probably animals; we then set this as a background for the correlation between sensory and motor functions in perceiving light and dark qualities of nonoptic stimuli together with emotions, and how this can be expressed in optic imagery. The induction of optic images by nonoptic stimuli and the experience of other senses induced by changes in body tonus and lightness perception are compatible with the facts of synesthetic perception, particularly in perceiving many of the sensations as outside of the body. Finally, Boernstein traced the phyletic structure of perception in an effort to replace "sense psychology with sense biology." He criticized standard gestalt concepts of perception as unnecessary.

Microgenetics

The theory of microgenetics is rooted in the analysis of aphasic errors but is coherent across modalities. Rather than argue that language is the basis for synesthesia, we can examine the other side of the coin and see how a *failure of language* could be responsible for the synesthete misspeaking something seen as something heard. Related to this is an investigation of perceptual errors that we call agnosia. Synesthesia is neither an aphasia nor an agnosia in the conventional sense, since the object is not substituted or replaced; rather, the synesthetic object is seen *in addition* to the stimulus.

Another important feature is the left hemispheric residence of synesthesia and the multiple evidence for defects in language and language-related skills such as acalculia, finger gnosis, and right-left orientation. The kind of error made is fundamental to the dynamic microgenesis theory, which can explain dynamic errors in a way that the Wernicke model cannot. One cannot map a dynamic psychology onto a rigid anatomy. In synesthesia one has a stimulus-dependent change in focal cerebral metabolism—a metabolic lesion, if you will.[2]

As seen from the foregoing chapters, the parallel synesthetic sensation is not a fully developed object. It is generic and never elaborated. It never assumes a pictorial or dream-like quality, although it may possess movement and in this sense have a temporal sequence as dreams do. The synesthetic percept is more like a *moment* of an incomplete object rather than the unfolding of a dream-like story with subject-object relations. Syensthesia has both color and form, which can be dissociated from one another—just as form and meaning can be dissociated in visual agnosia, and form and color can be dissociated in achromatopsia.

Finally, we will develop further in this chapter the issue of illusions, which were introduced in Chapter 4, as one of the phenomena that are similar to synesthesia. Microgenetic theory is quite revealing in its analysis of hallucinations and visual illusions. This is particularly so in that microgenesis holds that objects unfold out of limbic structures and memory toward their analysis in the external world, where they become externalized. The temporal-limbic structures serve as the fundamental layers of processing in microgenesis.

It is possible in this theory to see how during this unfolding from the limbic level, which communicates with all sensory modalities, a de-

---

[2]Task-dependent elements in determining the size of metabolic lesions are known, for example, in PET scanning. For example, in linguistic versus tambour processing the PET lesion is larger than the computed tomography lesion and the "reality" and detection of lesions can be task dependent (Jason Brown, MD, personal communication).

veloping object that is externalizing in the real world could carry with it an attenuated object or feature of that object, such as shape or color, that we then call synesthesia.

SOME DEFINITIONS USED IN MICROGENETICS

Phylogenesis and Ontogenesis

In ontogeny, one sees development of the brain as a whole. Everything is developing. In the cognition of the child or the developing organism, one grasps cognition or behavior as an ontogenetic whole, expressing development of all systems as whole. When one looks at pathology in the adult, however, he is looking at a slice of processing sequence in a cognitive structure.

The triune brain concept of Paul MacLean should help us think about vertical organization of brain function: a vertical, evolutionary, hierarchical point of view. These different levels of brain organization are not superimposed like a stack of coins, but are internested and emerge stereodynamically over the entire neuraxis, being laid in parallel all the way down. MacLean derived many of his ideas from Paul Yakovlev.

Symptom

In a microgenetic model a symptom is a normal but preliminary behavior. It is a piece of the subsurface of the structural behavior that is prematurely displayed. Assume a patient calls a table a chair. In the microgeny of word finding there is a zeroing in on the kind of word to a point where "table" and "chair" have a covalence and either one could come out. Then finally the word "table" pops out. If "chair" comes out by error, it is really normal in that stage of the unfolding of the word.

Hallucination

Hallucinations are attenuated or truncated object perceptions. They reveal a normal stage that is embedded in a final object, a stage that is given up in the final object.

Awareness

Another issue involves awareness of both our actions and perceptions and questions such as, "What is volition?" Questions such as this are not easily answered by anyone with any model. The issue of being an agent of an action goes back to the Wilhelm Wundt–William James debate and is possibly related to the recurrent collaterals that Teuber wrote about; an in-depth discussion of this would take us beyond the point, but it should be noted that intactness of the perceptual system may allow one to be aware that one's actions are erroneous, such as occurs in patients with frontal confabulation.

I will not say much about the microgenetic view of the frontal aphasias since they relate more to action than to perception, but I do want to point out the mentation of frontal cofabulation. Some patients are aware that they confabulate. Frontal patients can have an awareness of their errors yet somehow be unable to correct them. This is another example of the dissociation between knowledge and action. Patients with frontal lesions can verbalize the correct performance but cannot in fact perform correctly on, for example, the Wisconsin Card Sorting Test. Defects in awareness tend to be seen in patients with posterior lesions, suggesting a more frontal location for synesthesia, since synesthetes are aware of both worlds.

The illusive nature of awareness is beautifully shown in Kornhüber's work of the readiness potential (*bereitschaftspotential*; see Figure 9.4) (Kornhüber, 1974; Kornhüber & Deecke, 1965). For those not familiar with this work, the subject is instructed to move a finger when he feels like it. Negative slow potentials, predominantly frontal, build up bilaterally and then zero in on the supplementary motor area, then the motor area contralateral to the finger movement. This readiness potential occurs 800 milliseconds before the finger movement, far in excess of the time required for an action potential to traverse the known polysynaptic circuitry. In other words, the readiness potential far antedates the decision of the subject to make a movement. *We are deceived that we are a free agent in deciding to make a movement.* The decision is an interpretation we give to a behavior that has been initiated someplace else by another part of ourselves. The logical extreme of this interpretation is that nothing is real. Kornhüber's work has been extended by Libet (1985; Libet, Alberts, Wright, & Feinstein, 1967; Libet, Gleason, Wright, & Pearl, 1983).

There is a configurational quality of brain states mediating behavior. Just as gravity describes the relationship between masses, so too "mind," "consciousness," and similar terms refer to relationships between the organism and its environment. This view suggests that we cannot discover mind either by digging into the brain, as the neuropsychologists hope, or by searching the environment, as the behaviorists do. Eccles (1970) is separate in seeing mind and consciousness as everywhere, a suprastructure surrounding us. Pribram suggested that sensory input addressed networks, and patterns within the network constituted features. No one knew, however, what constituted those patterns. Eccles (1970) proposed an answer: since many synapses fire simultaneously one could consider them as a wavefront. This idea is disturbing to neurophysiologists, who are used to recording from one neuron at a time, as Eccles started out doing. Pribram had a holographic theory of memory as well as

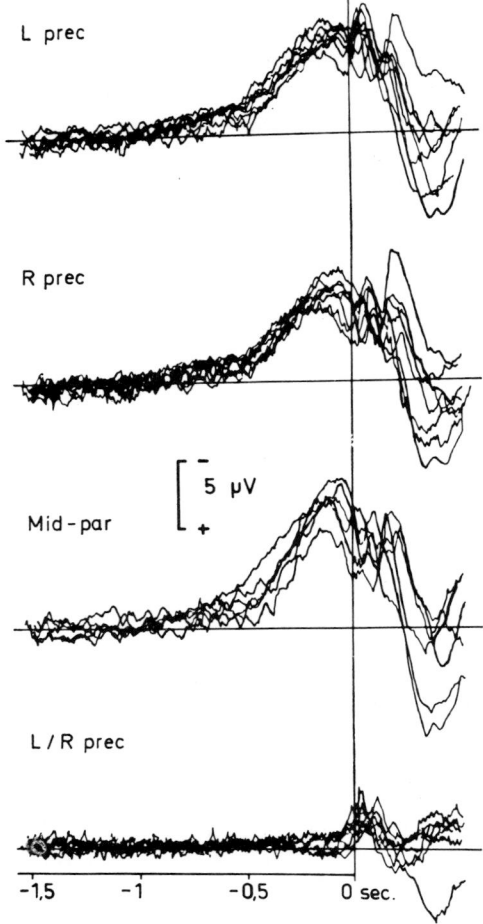

FIGURE 9.4. Readiness potentials from various cortical regions in response to voluntary finger movements. Time zero is onset of finger movement. Graphs represent averages of 250 responses. From *The self and its brain* (p. 284) by K.R. Popper and J.C. Eccles, 1977. London: Springer-Verlag. Copyright 1977 by Springer-Verlag. Reprinted by permission.

mind that said that mind was not located in a place. The brain produces images that are outside of itself; the reference was to a hologram that produces images that we can perceive as being three-dimensional and outside of the film and laser beam that produce it. Like a rock in a stream that slows down the flow, a lesion in a configurational scheme causes a slowing down at a point in cognitive processing. Eccles argued that cognition is mediated by wavefronts.

OBJECT PERCEPTION

The egocentric unfolding of primitive archaic space into a perception of an external object as represented by migrogenetic theory fits nicely with the perception of objects externally in synesthesia.

Microgenetics relates the qualitative errors in fluent aphasia to visual object perception. In the evocation of a word, a perceptual representation of the word "chair" goes through a series of levels in the mental representation of a word, from limbic to parietal to Wernicke's area toward auditory cortex. In this sequence, it goes from experiential or affective relations to categorical relations toward a phonological representation. There is an analogous situation in visual object perception and hallucination. In the perception of an object, there is the emergence of an object from a system of limbic structures where objects are selected out of experientially, symbolically, and affectively related objects toward a final stage of feature analysis.

This is different from the conventional direction of visual perception. Normally, afferents come into visual cortex and relay to inferotemporal cortex for matching to memory images or to parietal lobe for updating with the environment. That is, there are successive levels of shape construction. Conventionally, we think that an object is constructed and then matched to memory. The reverse is true in microgenesis. The object unfolds out of memory toward its analysis in the external world. It unfolds from within the observer, within the subject, from a primitive archaic space through a dream-like system of experiential, symbolic stages toward a representation as a holistic object and object relations in a three-dimensional Euclidean space. It unfolds out of a volumetric or egocentric space within the body, a space of hallucination, out toward the space of the external world, and finally detaches as an independent object "out there" in the world around us.

This is a different epistemological stand about the nature of the world that we see: The world around us is like a concentric layer of space representation. It is an image, but just an image in a different space, a space "out there" that we see as public shared space. An image is an object in private space. The argument of microgenetics is that objects unfold through stages of image formation and finally exteriorize as objects. To put it differently, a real object in the real world around us is an image that has undergone further processing. A real object is an image that is exteriorized, whereas an image is an object that is attenuated in its development.

A perception consists of a series of levels of space representation leading from a two-dimensional space map within the body organized around the brainstem-tectal system.

Thirty percent of the optic nerve fibers go to the brainstem and certainly not all of them subserve pupillary response. An autonomous two-dimensional spatial map builds up in the brainstem, passes to the limbic system (to egocentric, volumetric, dream-like space), to the parietal system (to a three-dimensional Euclidean object space, a space that is still part of the body), and finally to a stage of feature analysis and selective focal attention—those features of an object that are independent, detached, and have lives of their own. There is sensory input at each of these levels. There is a heavy brainstem input to modulate this early stage; there are limbic collaterals of the optic radiations; there is a heavy parietal input through the pulvinar; and, of course, there is input from the main geniculostriate system.

HALLUCINATIONS

The argument in microgenetics is that object representation is an enclosed, autonomous system of cognitive representation and that objects are not built up from sensations, not constructed from "sense data," but rather sensation constrains this process to model the object out there. There is input at successive levels and successive levels of constraint on an autonomously developing object representation. If one eliminates some of these sensory levels the system goes on its own and one has a hallucination. A common experience would be hallucinating one's name called or the telephone ringing while surrounded by the white noise in the shower.

A hallucination is an object development that is not constrained to model an object out there in the real world that we think exists beyond our perceptions. This is the microgenetic orientation. This model supposes that objects and images share the same mechanisms and that they are part of the same process.

This has been the recent thrust of cognitive science in its study of imagery, but it is an old story in neuropsychology. For example, recall Klüver's eidetic images (Chapter 4). He noted pupillary constriction during visualization of a bright eidetic image and dilatation with dark eidetic images. There are other examples of the relationship between hallucination and object perception in the older literature.

For example, organic hallucinations tend to invade a defective visual field. In the older literature, when the fashion was to look at the evolution of a hemianopia, visual hallucinations occurred early in the development of the field defect and later in its recovery (Seguin, 1886). In patients with scotoma, the hallucination affects the scotomatous part of the field (release hallucinations). This is true not only in vision but also in audition. Morel (1936) showed that schizophrenic patients had "scotoma"—gaps where they could not hear—in their audiograms during auditory hallucinations.

One might intuit that a patient cannot attend to a hallucination and a perception at the same time—but in fact one *can* perceive and attend simultaneously. Patients can have a visual perception and a hallucination side by side. They can see both. It is not a problem of attending to both. The important fact is that in vision one cannot hallucinate and perceive in the same space, in the same locus, at the same time.

Hallucinations replace the object. The hallucination replaces that part of the visual field where it occurs. It is not superimposed on the perception, but replaces it, and it does so because it is a preliminary object. Even hallucinations that seem real to the perceiver are not really object-like in their sense of realness. Hallucinations are fluid and dynamic, like synesthesia. Colors melt off object boundaries and the space of a hallucination is a tangible, almost viscous, space, not the empty space of object perceptions. In both hallucination and synesthesia, space itself is an object.

There is a continuum between the object and the space around it so that objects seem to be in a fluid medium. (That fluid medium is the space around the object.) In his demonstration of an achromatopic field, Damasio illustrated a spatial "gap" between the hemiachromatopic field and the normal field. The space of patients having visual hallucinations is lacking in depth, a foreshortened attenuated space. The whole point is that even in those hallucinations that seem real, hallucinatory space is a primitive archaic space that replaces the perception in that part of the field where it occurs. This is so because, as microgenetic theory argues, the hallucination is a preliminary object. One cannot have an object and a hallucination in the same place at the same time because the hallucination is part of the structure of the object.

There is very little evidence for this kind of thinking, but one example is a well-known PET scan from UCLA that shows right posterior hypometabolism in a patient with left-sided seizures and hallucinations in the left field. During a seizure there is hypermetabolism in the previously hypometabolic area, correlating with the hallucination, suggesting that the hallucination and the perception are bound up in the same part of the brain—they use the same neural real estate.

Visual Images

There is a hierarchy in image formation leading from a stage of brainstem-organized dreamless sleep through a stage of dreaming with increasing resolution and clarity to a memory image. This then becomes a quite clear image, not just an image in the mind's eye, like a memory image, but a picturable image, an eidetic image. It is almost, but not quite, like an object. Then come afterimages (see Figure 9.5).

This is a normal hierarchy of imagery. We know that there are transitions (see Chapter 3) between these states, for example, waking up from a dream and having a memory image of the dream. Old studies of eideticism show relationships between eidetic images and memory im-

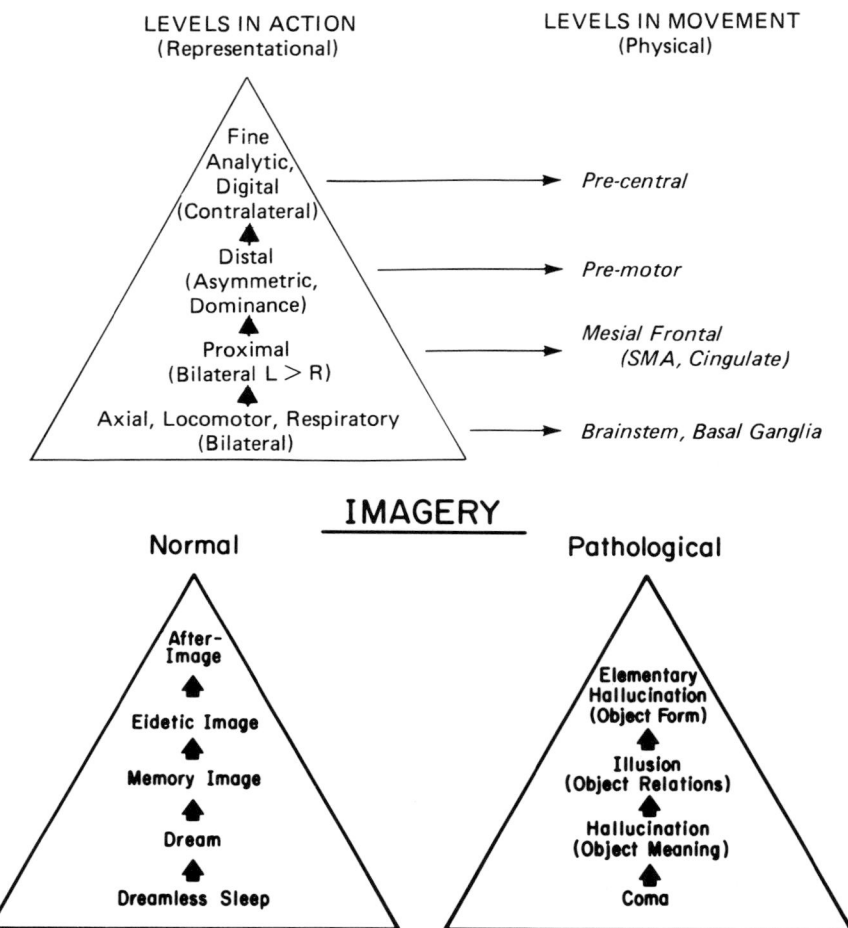

LEVELS IN ACTION
(Representational)

LEVELS IN MOVEMENT
(Physical)

Fine
Analytic,
Digital
(Contralateral)   ⟶   *Pre-central*

Distal
(Asymmetric,
Dominance)   ⟶   *Pre-motor*

Proximal
(Bilateral L > R)   ⟶   *Mesial Frontal
(SMA, Cingulate)*

Axial, Locomotor, Respiratory
(Bilateral)   ⟶   *Brainstem, Basal Ganglia*

IMAGERY

Normal

After-
Image

Eidetic Image

Memory Image

Dream

Dreamless Sleep

Pathological

Elementary
Hallucination
(Object Form)

Illusion
(Object Relations)

Hallucination
(Object Meaning)

Coma

FIGURE 9.5. Microgenetic hierarchy of action and imagery. Each level has an anatomical correlate. See text for further description. (Courtesy of Jason Brown, MD)

ages. Over time eidetic images begin to fade and become more like memory images.

The argument is that levels of imagery are constrained by perceptual sensory input at successive levels so that the image substrate eventually models the object. These images form like the substance of an object perception if under the control of sensation. With suspension of sensory input, one has successive levels of image formation (see Figure 9.5) and their pathological correlates would be coma from dreamless sleep; dream-like hallucination (where object meaning, experience, and symbolic relationships are important) for temporal lobe lesions; parietal lesions giving disruptions within an image causing illusory phenomena (distortions of shape and size of objects "out there"); and finally occipital elementary hallucinations and photisms that are similar to afterimages.

Neural Levels of Visual Images

Brainstem

Normally, one thinks that the upper brainstem mediates dreamless sleep. Lesions give either akinetic mutism or coma. However, there are disorders of object perception here that are characterized by ballistic misreaching, neglect in the immediate limb space, and peduncular hallucinations.

Supranuclear palsy (Steele-Richardson-Olchewsky syndrome) involves the upper brainstem, basal ganglia, and cerebellum, but spares the cortex. Patients have a dementia with axial rigidity and severe spatial difficulties. They have ballistic misreaching and primitive space perception. Peduncular hallucinations involve lesions of the peduncles at the level of the colliculi and red nucleus. These can be full field and polysensory and tend to be crepuscular (i.e., occurring at twilight when there is reduction of visual input). Patients tend to be amused by the visions, but eventually develop a hallucinatory psychosis and are unable to tell if they are awake or dreaming. Images are close to the subject, as in synesthesia, and categorical, not having a strong historical or developmental dream-like quality (Albessar, 1934; DeMorsier, 1938; Geller & Bellur, 1987; J. L'hermitte, 1922; Schilder, 1953).

Temporal Lobe

The kinds of experiences one sees in synesthesia are most consistent with the kinds of hallucinations and illusory phenomena that one sees in the more temporal kinds of lesions. In the temporal lobe there are a group of agnosias and a group of hallucinations that have common features (see Figure 9.5).

Agnosia for Faces, Objects, and Routes. Bilateral lesions of the mesial temporal lobes give an object agnosia and problems of face recognition and route identification. Posterior temporal occipital lesions are required bilaterally to produce this. Damasio has recent CT evidence for this anatomic necessity.

The association between route finding and face recognition disorders is very strong, and both are similar in a way to object recognition problems. If one shows such an agnostic a glass, he or she might call it a plate. The problem is with the semantic category of the object and is not a naming problem. Patients grasp the class of the object but not the object concept itself. There is a similar defect in face agnosia and route recognition problems. Patients with this type of agnosia (and who have normal form perception) have difficulty in selecting an instance from a class of overlearned objects. They may have trouble telling their car from other cars in the parking lot. There are stories of farmers not being able to distinguish their cows, and World War II pilots who can verbalize structural characteristics of various aircraft but cannot identify their photographs or silhouettes. This is good evidence that there is not a module in the brain for face recognition but that the defect is similar to what one sees for object and route recognition problems.

These kinds of errors are similar to those one sees in monkeys with bilateral temporal lobe lesions who have problems with visual recognition that are not due to memory or perceptual discrimination problems but, as Teuber argued long ago, are due to difficulty in selecting an object out of an array of other objects related to it. Their problem is analyzing an object out of a group of similar objects. *The generic qualities take over.*

In synesthesia, we have a stimulus causing a regression to earlier, more generic, features of perception, features that belong to another mode. One can see this as an arrested unfolding at the generic level.

Hallucinations and Experiential Responses During Electrical Stimulation of the Temporal Lobe. For information on these hallucinations, refer to the discussion in Chapter 4.

Organic Hallucinations. Organic hallucinations tend to be large and scenic, and progress moment to moment. They have a dream-like, historical quality. One tends not to see this kind of pictorial hallucination with brain tumors (at least not today with much earlier diagnosis; in the past, physicians would follow growth of the lesion by evolution of symptoms), where more banal visual phenomena are seen. However, the temporal lobe lesion patient who hallucinates will tend to have a more dream-like hallucination.

Summary. We can now ask what is the relationship among a hallucination, a dream, and an agnosia for objects or faces as described above?

In a dream one actually sees the object that is misidentified or perceived in a dream; but in agnosia we do not suppose that a subject who calls a glass a plate actually sees a plate. We suppose that he actually sees the glass but, in his mind, he believes it to be a plate. The displaced image survives in the agnosia as the symptom of the agnosia. The semantic error (in the agnosia) is the symptom of that kind of agnosia where, in the hallucinating patient, cognition only reaches a certain point and does not unfold further. The endpoint of the whole series of percept formation actualizes as a kind of perception that we call a hallucination. Whereas the hallucinating patient actually sees the objects that he misconceives, the agnostic buries the hallucinatory symptom. Misrecognition is the price the agnostic pays to avoid having hallucinations. Agnosia and hallucination can be seen as two sides of the same coin.

Hallucinations in Parietal Lobe Syndromes

Most parietal syndromes involve manipulospatial defects because they involve interaction in the space of the limb perimeter. Drawing tasks, misreaching, neglect of body space—all are related to objects in the immediate surround.

The kinds of hallucinatory phenomena in parietal lesions also involve spatial distortions: things getting bigger or smaller; acceleration of time; inversion phenomena (people standing on their heads) (Klopp, 1951; Mouren & Tatossian, 1963; Pötzl, 1943; I. Steiner, Shanin, & Melamed, 1987); and micropsia and macropsia. All of these collectively are known as metamorphopsia. *These are illusory phenomenon,* not true hallucinations, because they involve objects that are really out there undergoing distortion. Microgenesis interprets this as a stage giving rise to dream-like images and the peculiar visual agnosias described above. The whole constellation in the microgeny of an object has come up one more level to resolution toward a spatial image. It is a spatial image out there in the world just immediately around the subject, not quite independent because of its relation to limb action. Synesthesia is like this in being close up in the subject's immediate personal space. One can have image phenomena, even spatial defects, that involve distortion of objects or deficits in interaction with the objects.

Palinopsia is also a parieto-occipital lobe syndrome. It is a visual perseveration (Critchley's term). In some sense it is related to abnormal eidetic imagery, and abnormal persistence of an object perception. One might think of its as a released eideticism.

Occipital Lobe

In occipital lobe lesions, one finds problems with the analysis, discrimination, and fine featural segmentation of an object. The selective attention to component features of the object yields *form-based deficits.* Scotomas, agnosias, alexias, color agnosia, face recognition, and route identification problems are all based on form discrimination, and not on object meaning.

There are, therefore, two kinds of face, route, and object agnosias: those based on form and those based on meaning. The older literature talks about apperceptive and associative agnosia; these really refer to agnosias based on object meaning (temporal lesions) and others based on object form (occipital and parietal lesions). These different kinds of agnosia refer to a different level in the object.

Thus we see that there are a series of levels leading from dream to memory images to eideticism to afterimages, with a pathological correlate at each of these levels, leading from a limbic to a parietal to an occipital stage. The evolution of the brain leads in this direction, not the other way around. The sequence of defects in visual imagery and visual perception correspond to the mode of the posterior aphasias. There are deep-level problems of language perception related to experiential and word meaning effects; surface-level problems involving categorical object relational effects; and, finally, phonological defects linked to more recent levels of evolution. To perceive a word phonologically is similar to analyzing an object into its features, because one has an abstract lexical representation that comes in and up and has to be segmented.[3]

So microgenesis suggests that a lot of these syndromes can be understood as *moments* in the process of object formation, the process of lexical realization linked to levels in the evolution of the brain. It is a theory that tries to be coherent across different cognitive domains.

The model of action is the same as that for the anterior aphasias; the model of the posterior aphasias is a model of visual perception. There is an inner bond between image problems and object defects. The relationship between imagery and object perception is complex. It is an attempt to explain the diversity of phenomena in terms of a unitary model in which diversity is captured through the concept of changes at successive levels rather than separate models or different local theories for every symptom that one sees. That, after all, is what an evolutionary theory does. When Darwin saw the diversity of the world he tried to develop some principle that would explain diversity. Microgenesis is an evolutionary-based model.

J.W. Brown (1977, 1982, 1983) defined microgenesis theory as a theory that tries to explain diversity but maintain consistency across different modes of perception. Microgenesis accounts for diversity in a unitary unfolding process through unfolding over levels and disruption at successive levels as it distributes itself over different sensory modalities or into action. All of the symptoms one sees are clinically explicable in terms of moments in normal processing within each of these different components of the unitary process.

MICROGENETIC EXPLANATION OF DIFFERENT TYPES OF SYNESTHESIA

The microgenetic notion of regression or the arrested unfolding at the generic level can be used to explain MW's geometric taste, the audiomotor synesthesia of Devereaux (1966) in which there are axial and ballistic movements in response to nonsense verbal stimuli, and the many patients with colored hearing in which shape is represented in the parallel sensation. However, what about more restricted forms such as colored letters and numbers that may or may not be projected? There are really two questions here: the first is about projection, while the second asks

---

[3]Peter MacNeilage has written persuasively about the process of a lexical representation being a kind of spatial image, with slots for the phonemes, where one has to insert the phonemes into the right slot in that spatial image. It is similar to what is involved in the analysis of an object gestalt into its featural elements.

how one reconciles the notion that isolated colored letters or numbers represent an attenuation at the generic level.

The first question has already been answered in previous chapters. There are instances of synesthesia in which the parallel sense is clearly projected onto the external world and replaces the object in the field that it occupies. In other cases, the patient is not certain "where it is" that he perceives the synesthetic sense. The analogy is with the spectrum of illusions and hallucinations, which also occur at various levels—such as the dream-like states, memory images, eidetic images, and afterimages, visual distortions (metamorphopsia), and peduncular hallucinations that are seen with disturbances at various levels in the limbic, temporal, parietal, and occipital lobes as well as at the brainstem level. The kinds of analysis that one performs in microgenesis are consistent with the degree to which the synesthetic sense is externalized, or "projected" as we used the terminology earlier.

The second question is answered by again noting that there is a spectrum of synesthetic performance that ranges from a vivid polysensory *Gewebe* (web) to highly restricted forms. The instance of colored letters or colored numbers (which are really the same thing, a lexical representation) has to do with the levels of lexical and phonemic representation of digits and letters. When synesthetes hear letters and numbers they say that they visualize them. Certainly when they are reading they have the shape there in front of them on the page; when they hear or spell they image it. Then there is the case of EW, for whom the sound determines the color of the letter. In EW's case it is the phonemic and not the lexical quality that has a color attached to it. This suggests that morphic, lexical, phonemic, and chromic attributes are all derivative elements of a deeper or larger cognitive structure.

In the case of colored letters, the morphology is that which belongs to the lexical representation of the letter, a morphic structure that is more developed as an external object rather than having a more generic shape that then arises because it is attenuated from an earlier or deeper level.

In considering the dissociation between form-based and meaning-based errors that microgeny explores, one sees that the form-based defects occur with structures in the occipital lobe, whereas the temporal-limbic area shows errors in object meaning. This is consistent with the proposal that synesthesia involves temporal limbic operation in that one has preservation of the form without any meaning in synesthesia. The semantic vacuity is such an obvious feature of synesthesia. What survives is the *form*.

SUMMARY

What microgenesis lends to support synesthesia is its explanation of object formation and hallucination. In microgenesis, object formation is an autonomous process arising from limbic and brainstem levels, constrained by sensory input operating at higher levels of isomodal and heteromodal cortex. We are in agreement that the cortex is not primarily involved with object formation or object perception. Support comes from classic experiments involving removal of some or all of the neocortex in monkeys. Although logic says that one has profoundly altered the nervous system by removing the neocortex, the animals behave quite normally and it is difficult to tell grossly that one has done anything to them. The cortex, therefore, seems to provide a finer grain of discrimination, such as feature analysis, and its operation is not required in the level of perception necessary for everyday survival. Detailed and sophisticated analysis will, of course, show that deficits do exist.

It also seems to me that there is an analogy between the kinds of errors made in aphasia, particularly frontal aphasics who have awareness of their errors, and the form constants and kinds of generic perceptions one finds in synesthesia. Synesthetes too have awareness of their "errors," if one will allow that the symptom of synesthesia is like any other symptom: it is part of a normal behavior that is prematurely displayed. Just as frontal patients who can verbalize the correct performance on the Wisconsin Card Sorting Test yet are unable in fact to perform correctly, so too are synesthetes aware that the parallel sense that they perceive is a hallucination but are simultaneously convinced by what they see. As in the dissociation between knowledge and performance in the frontal lobe patients, there is a dissociation between knowledge and perception in synesthesia.

In this regard, synesthesia fits in nicely with the question of what is a symptom as answered by the microgenetic model. In this theory, a symptom is a normal but preliminary behavior, a piece of the substructure of an action, or a perception that is prematurely displayed. Just as in the microgeny of word finding there is a point at which "table" and "chair" have a covalence, and either one could come out in a task of naming a four-legged piece of furniture, so too in the normal unfolding of object perception the generic form may be inadequately constrained such that it carries additional information that detaches into reality and becomes externalized as a perception in another mode, hence synesthesia.

In microgenesis there is a unity across modalities. It is quite useful as a theory in explaining the various combinations of synesthesia. However, the same kinds of relationships that underlie visual synesthesia can apply to synesthesia in other senses.

10
Conclusions

We do not have the final word on synesthesia yet. I have provided much material for cogitation and future work by interested students who may be fortunate enough to meet a 5-point synesthete. I have some suggestions for future work and how that might be best carried out.

But first let us look at what we have accomplished. Foremost is a clear definition of synesthesia for the first time in 200 years. The importance of this cannot be underestimated. Most of the messiness in trying to get a grip on synesthesia over the years has stemmed precisely from the lack of well-articulated inclusion criteria. The change in conceptualization of cognitive theory has contributed much less to this confusion. This intellectual sloppiness persists even today, as I pointed out in the work of Raeder and Marks (p. 184). If we expect to make further headway in this phenomenon, then we are going to have to insist on comparing apples to apples.

Hand in hand with a strong definition we also have a categorization of types of synesthesia, and it is equally as important to distinguish these types because of their different etiologies. Moreover, each etiology sheds a different light on the underlying brain mechanism of synesthesia. The most important type is idiopathic synesthesia, the involuntary stimulus-induced union of the senses, which is present in childhood and persists for a lifetime. The remaining types are simple synesthesia (which does not necessarily require a deafferented sensory field), epileptic synesthesia, and induced synesthesia (both electrically induced and drug induced).

I do not foresee significant changes in nosology. The stories of true synesthetes are too similar to predict this should occur. It will be important that the psychophysical testing is replicated and for this it is necessary that the testing and future technological probes be done on subjects whose synesthesia is projected. A further requirement is that an appropriate stimulus is used that is repeatable and does not fatigue. Although there is no evidence that any of the current cases of idiopathic synesthesia are due to a seizure, the hypothesis should be cleanly refuted. We have such a refutation in subject MW, whose EEG, which included nasopharyngeal and T1–T2 temporal electrodes, was normal. Refuting the hypothesis in more subjects would be welcome.

The many people who wrote to me about their desire to write laser music computer programs and the like will now understand fully why I am unable to oblige their request for help. A secret formula simply does not exist. However, this brings me to my final point. It is my sincere hope that 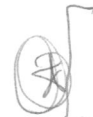 scientists and artists will stop seeing themselves as separate persons. If there is a symbol in synesthesia it is one of integration, not just of how we sense the world around us but of who we are. It is an appreciation for the many facets that make up both the person and the life as they grow through this physical world. We would all benefit, I think, from unlearning the restrictions that have been taught to us, the shoulds and oughts, what is permissible and what is not, what is proper for a scientist and what is the realm of the artist.

We are laden with values. Neither art nor the artist is mysterious and inaccessable. Mary Hambidge [1975] often said, "the way is beauty." It is a fine mantra. Both science and art examine parts of the physical universe, and in relating the part to the whole seek to find meaning. So they are both analytical in the Cartesian sense, but they are also both a song and a dance.

It is certain that the New Age will appropriate synesthesia, and I do not have strong misgivings. I would point out that the New Age is not a product of the 1980s. This type of thinking has been going on for over 70 years. It goes back to Ernest Holmes' Church of Religious Science and Mary Baker Eddy's Christian Science, which gave form to the idea of a holistic existence. It is what prompted Mary Hambidge to create her Center for Creative Arts and Sciences in 1934. It is what has prompted a study of subjectivity in science, of value that is hidden in theory, and of mathematical relationships in art. It is also the kind of thinking that leads me to see that "my soul is full of stars, my heart of colored music."

Appendix
Index of Specific Synesthetes' Perceptions

References

Abell, G. (1969). *Exploration of the universe* (2nd ed., chap. 2). New York: Holt Reinhart.

Adey, W.R. (1977). The sensorium and the modulation of cerebral states: Tonic environmental influences on limbic and related systems. *Annals of the New York Academy of Sciences, 290*, 396–420.

Adler, N. (1972). *The underground stream. New lifestyles and the antinomian personality*. New York: Harper & Row.

Alajouanine, Th. (1948). Aphasia and artistic realization. *Brain, 74*, 229–241.

Albessar, R. (1934). *L'Hallucinose pédonculaire*. Paris: Doin et Cie.

Altura, B.T., & Altura, B.M. (1981). Phencyclidine, lysergic acid diethylamide, and mescaline; cerebral artery spasms and hallucinogenic activity. *Science, 212*, 1051–1052.

Amoore, J.E. (1977). Specific anosmia and the concept of primary odors. *Chemical Senses and Flavor, 2*, 267–281.

Anderson, J. (1886). On sensory epilepsy: A case of basal cerebral tumor, affecting the left temporosphenoidal lobe, and giving rise to a paroxysmal taste-sensation and dreamy state. *Brain, 9*, 385–395.

Arden, G.B., & Soderberg, U. (1959). The relationship of lateral geniculate activity to the electrocorticogram in the presence or absence of the optic tract input. *Experientia, 15*, 163–164.

Argelander, A. (1927). *Das Farbenhören und der synästhetische Faktor der Wahrnehmung*. Jena (Germany): Fischer.

Arnheim, R. (1986). The artistry of psychotics. *American Scientist, 74*, 48–54.

Assai, G., Eisert, H.G., & Hecaen, H. (1969). Analyse des resultats du Farnsworth D15 chez 155 malades atteints de lesions hemispheriques droites ou gauches. *Acta Neurologica et Psychiatrica Belgica, 69*, 705–717.

Atweh, S.F., Banna, N.R., Jabbur, S.J., & Tómey, G.F. (1974). Polysensory interactions in the cuneate nucleus. *Journal of Physiology, 238*, 343–355.

Bachman, D.M. (1984). Formed visual hallucinations after metrizamide myelography. *American Journal of Ophthalmology, 97*, 78–81.

Bader, A., & Navratil, L. (1976). *Zwischem Wahn und Wirklichkeit: Kunst, Psychose, Kreativität*. Lucerne: Bucher.

Bagshaw, M.H., & Pribram, K.H. (1953). Cortical organization in gustation (*Macaca mulatta*). *Journal of Neurophysiology, 16*, 499–508.

Bailey, P., & Bonin, G. (1951). *The isocortex of man*. Urbana, IL: NP

Baizer, J.S., Robinson, D.L., & Dow, B.M. (1977). Visual responses of area 18 neurons in awake, behaving monkey. *Journal of Neurophysiology, 40,* 1024–1037.

Bear, D.M. (1983). Hemispheric specialization and the neurology of emotion. *Archives of Neurology, 40,* 195–202.

Bear, D.M., & Fedio, P. (1977). Quantitative analysis of interictal behavior in temporal lobe epilepsy. *Archives of Neurology, 34,* 454–467.

Beatty, W.W., & Tröster, A.I. (1987). Gender differences in geographical knowledge. In *Sex roles.* NP

Bencze, K.S., Troupin, A., & Prockop, L.D. (1988). Reflex absence epilepsy. *Epilepsia, 29,* 48–51.

Bender, M.B. (1945). Polyopia and monocular diplopia of cerebral origin. *Archives of Neurology and Psychiatry, 54,* 323–338.

Bender, M.B., Feldman, M., & Sobin, A.J. (1968). Palinopsia. *Brain, 91,* 321–338.

Bente, D., Itil, T., & Schmid, E.E. (1957). EEG studies concerning the action of LSD-25. *Electroencephalography and Clinical Neurophysiology, 9,* 359.

Berrios, G.E., & Brook, P. (1982). The Charles Bonnett syndrome and the problem of visual perceptual disorders in the elderly. *Age and Aging, 11,* 17.

Bexton, W.M., Heron, W., & Scott, T.H. (1954). Effects of decreased variations in the sensory environment. *Canadian Journal of Psychology, 8,* 70–76.

Bishop, M.P., Elder, S.T., & Heath, R.G. (1963). Intracranial self-stimulation in man. *Science, 140,* 394–396.

Bleuler, E., & Lehmann, K. (1881). *Zwangsmassige Lichtempfindungen durch Schall und verwandte Erscheinungen.* Leipzig: Fues Verlag.

Boernstein, W.S. (1939). Uber die physiologischen Grundlagen des Wahrnehmens: Der Einfluss "heller" und "dunkler" Reize und den Melanophoren Zustand in Amphibien. *Archives Internationales de Pharmacodynamie et de Therapie, 61,* 387–414.

Boernstein, W.S. (1967). Optic perception and optic imageries in man: Their roots and relations studied from the viewpoint of biology. *International Journal of Neurology, 6*(2), 147–181.

Boernstein, W.S. (1970). Perceiving and thinking: Their interrelationship and organismic organization. *Annals of the New York Academy of Sciences, 169,* 673–682.

Bogen, J.E. (1969a). The other side of the brain I: Dysgraphia and dyscopia following cerebral commissurotomy. *Bulletin of the Los Angeles Neurological Society, 34*(2), 73–105.

Bogen, J.E. (1969b). The other side of the brain II: An appositional mind. *Bulletin of the Los Angeles Neurological Society, 34*(3), 135–162.

Bogen, J.E. (1969c). The other side of the brain III: The corpus callosum and creativity. *Bulletin of the Los Angeles Neurological Society, 34*(4), 191–220.

Boring, E.G. (1942). *Sensation and perception in the history of experimental psychology* (p. 27). New York: Appleton.

Bos, M.C. (1929). Über echte und unechte audition coloree. *Zeitschrift fur Psychologie, 3,* 321–401.

Bowers, H., & Bowers, J.E. (1961). *Arithmetical excursions.* New York: Dover.

Bowker, R.M., & Morrison, A.R. (1976). The startle reflex and PGO spikes. *Brain Research, 102,* 185–190.

Bridger, W.H. (1960). Signaling systems in the development of cognitive functions. In M. Brazier (Ed.), *The central nervous system and behavior* (pp. 425–461). New York: Josiah Macy Jr. Foundation.

Brindley, C.S., & Lewin, W.S. (1968). The sensations produced by electrical stimulation of the visual cortex. *Journal of Physiology, 196,* 479–493.

Broca, P. (1878). Anatomie comparée des circonvolutions cerebrales. Le grand lobe limbique et la scissure limbique dans la série des mammifères. *Revue d'Anthropologie, 1,* 385–432.

Brodal, A. (1969). *Neurological anatomy in relation to clinical medicine.* London: Oxford University Press.

Brou, P., Sciascia, T.R., Linden, L., & Letvin, J. (1986). The colors of things. *Scientific American, 255*(3), 84–91.

Brown, J.W. (1977). *Mind, brain and consciousness.* New York: Academic Press.

Brown, J.W. (1982). Hierarchy and evolution in neurolinguistics. In M. Arbib, D. Caplan, & J. Marshall (Eds.), *Biology of mental processes.* New York: Academic Press.

Brown, J.W. (1983). The microstructure of perception: Physiology and patterns of breakdown. *Cognition and Brain Theory, 6,* 145–184.

Brown, J.W. (in press). The nature of voluntary action. *Brain and Cognition.*

Brown, P.K., & Wald, G. (1963). Visual pigments in human and monkey retinas. *Nature, 37*–43.

Brust, J.C.M., & Behrens, M.M. (1977). "Release hallucinations" as the major symptom of posterior cerebral artery occlusion, a report of two cases. *Annals of Neurology, 2,* 432–436.

Buser, P., & Imbert, M. (1961). Sensory projections to the motor cortex in cats: A microelectrode study. In W.A. Rosenblith (Ed.), *Sensory communication* (pp. 607–626). New York: John Wiley & Sons.

Byrne, R.W. (1982). Geographical knowledge and orientation. In A.W. Ellis (Ed.), *Normality and pathology in cognitive functions* (pp. 239–264). New York: Academic Press.

Calkins, M.W. (1893). A statistical study of pseudo-chromasthesia and of mental forms. *American Journal of Psychology, 5,* 439–464.

Calkins, M.W. (1895). Synesthesia. *American Journal of Psychology, 7,* 90–107.

Cascino, G.D., & Adams, R.D. (1986). Brainstem auditory hallucinosis. *Neurology, 36,* 1042–1047.

Caskey, L.D. (1924). *The geometry of Greek vases.* Boston: NP

Castel, L-B. (1725). Clavecin par les yeux, avec l'art de peindre les sons, & toutes sortes de pieces de musique. *Mercure de France, 1725,* 2552–2577.

Castel, L-B. (1735). Nouvelles experiences d'optique & d'acoustique. *Mémoires pour l'Historie des Sciences et des Beaux Arts, 1735,* 1444–1482, 1619–1666, 1807–1839, 2018–2053, 2335–2372, 2642–2768.

Charcot, J-M. (1987). *Charcot the clinician: the Tuesday lessons* (C.G. Goetz, trans.). New York: Raven Press.

Cocteau, J., Schmidt, G., Steck, H., & Bader, A. (1961). *Insania Pingens.* Basel: CIBA.

Cogan, D.G. (1973). Visual hallucinations as release phenomenon. *Albrech von Graefes Archiv fur Klinische und Experimentelle Ophthalmologie, 188,* 139–150.

Cohen, M.J., Landgren, S., Strom, L., & Zotterman, Y. (1957). Cortical reception of touch and taste in the cat. *Acta Physiologica Scandinavica Supplement, 135,* 1–50.

Cohen, S. (1970). Seeing with all three eyes. In S. Cohen (Ed.), *The beyond within: The LSD story* (2nd ed., pp. 45–63). New York: Antheneum.

Coleman, W.S. (1894). Hallucinations in the sane associated with local organic disease of the sensory organs, etc. *British Medical Journal, 1,* 1015–1017.

Corales, R.L., Maull, K.I., & Becker, D.P. (1980). Phencyclidine abuse mimicking head injury. *Journal of the American Medical Association, 243,* 2322.

Critchley, M. (1977). Ecstatic and synaesthetic experience during musical perception. In M. Critchley & R.A. Henson (Eds.), *Music and the brain: Studies in the neurology of music.* Springfield, IL: Charles C. Thomas.

Crowell, G.F., Stump, D.A., Biller, J., McHenry, L.C., Jr., & Toole, J.F. (1984). The transient global amnesia-migraine connection. *Annals of Neurology, 41,* 75–79.

Cunningham, T.J. (1972). Sprouting of the optic projections after cortical lesions. *Anatomical Record, 172,* 298.

Cushing, H. (1909). *Brain, 32,* 44.

Cytowic, R.E. (1975). Anton Chekhov: A physician-genius in spite of himself, Parts I–III. *North Carolina Medical Journal, 36,* 612–614, 679–681, 733–735.

Cytowic, R.E. (1976a). Anton Chekhov: A physician-genius in spite of himself, Part IV. *North Carolina Medical Journal 37,* 29–31.

Cytowic, R.E. (1976b). Aphasia in Maurice Ravel. *Bulletin of the Los Angeles Neurological Society, 41,* 109–114.

Cytowic, R.E. (1985). Alexithymia—or stupidity? (letter). *New England Journal of Medicine, 313,* 53.

Cytowic, R.E., & Stump, D.A. (1985). *Reduced cortical blood flow in geometrically-shaped taste synesthesia.* Paper presented at the meeting of the International Neuropsychological Society, February 6–9.

Cytowic, R.E., Stump, D.A., & Larned, D.C. (1987). Closed head trauma: Somatic, ophthalmic and cognitive impairments in nonhospitalized patients. In H.A. Whitaker (Ed.), *Neuropsychological studies of non-focal brain damage: Dementia and trauma.* New York: Springer-Verlag.

Cytowic, R.E., & Wood, F.B. (1982). Synesthesia I: A review of theories and their brain basis. *Brain and Cognition, 1,* 29.

Cytowic, R.E., & Wood, F.B. (1982). Synesthesia II: Psychophysical relationships in the synesthesia of geometrically shaped taste and colored hearing. *Brain and Cognition, 1.*

Dahl, H. (1965). Observations on a "natural experiment": Helen Keller. *Journal of the American Psychoanalytical Association, XIII*(3), 533–550.

Damasio, A.R. (1985). Disorders of complex visual processing: Agnosias, achromatopsia, Balint's syndrome, and related difficulties of orientation and construction. In M-M. Mesulam (Ed.), *Principles of behavioral neurology.* Philadelphia: F.A. Davis Co.

Damasio, A.R., Yamada, T., Damasio, H., Corbet, J., & McKee, J. (1980). Central achromatopsia: Behavioral, anatomic and physiologic aspects. *Neurology, 30,* 1064–1071.

D'Andrade, R., & Egan, M. (1974). The colors of emotion. *American Ethnologist, 1,* 49–63.

Darwin, E. (1790). *The botanic garden, Pt 2. The loves of the plants, with philosophical notes.* London: J. Johnson. [reprinted (1978) New York: Garland Publishers.]

Daw, N.W. (1968). Color-coded ganglion cells in goldfish retina: Extension of their receptive fields by means of new stimuli. *Journal of Physiology (London)*, *197*, 567–592.

Daw, N.W. (1972). Color-coded cells in goldfish, cat, and rhesus monkey. *Investigative Ophthalmology*, *11*, 411–417.

Dejerine, J. (1892). Contributions a l'etude anatomo-pathologique et clinique des differentes varietes de cecite verbale. *Memoires de la Societe Biologique, 4*, 61–90.

Delbrück, M. (1986). *An essay on evolutionary epistemology* (G.S. Stent et al., Eds.). Oxford: Blackwell Scientific Publications.

DeMorsier, G. (1938). Les hallucinations. *Revue Oto-neuro-ophthalmologique, 16*, 244–702.

Denereoz, A. (1931). *L'harmonie des nombres: Rhythmes humains, rhythmes cosmiques*. Laudanne: G. Vaney-Burnier.

De Renzi, E., & Faglioni, P. (1967). Impaired performances on color tasks in patients with hemispheric damage. *Cortex, 3*, 194–216.

Desimone, R., & Gross, C.G. (1979). Visual areas in the temporal cortex of the macaque. *Brain Research, 178*, 363–380.

DeValois, R.L. (1965). Behavioral and electrophysiological studies of primate vision. *Contributions to Sensory Physiology, 1*, 137–178.

DeValois, R.L., & Pease, P.L. (1971). Contours and contrast: Responses of monkey lateral geniculate nucleus cells to luminance and color figures. *Science, 171*, 694–696.

Devereaux, G. (1966). An unusual audio-motor synesthesia in an adolescent. *Psychiatric Quarterly, 40*(3), 459–471.

Diamond, I.T., & Neff, W.D. (1957). Ablation of temporal cortex and discrimination of auditory patterns. *Journal of Neurophysiology, 20*, 300–315.

Dobelle, W.H., & Mladejovsky, M.G. (1974). Phosphenes produced by electrical stimulation of human occipital cortex, and their application to the development of a prosthesis for the blind. *Journal of Physiology, 243*, 553–576.

Donath, H. (1922). Synesthesia. *Archiv für Psychiatrie und Neurologie, 29*, 112–119.

Douglas, R.J., & Marcellus, D. (1975). The ascent of man: Deductions based on a multivariate analysis of the brain. *Brain, Behavior and Evolution, 11*, 179–213.

Downey, J.E. (1911). A case of colored gustation. *American Journal of Psychology, 22*, 528–539.

Downey, J.E. (1912). Seeing sounds and hearing colors. *Independent, 78*, 315–318.

Dräger, U.C., & Hubel, D.H. (1975). Responses to visual stimulation and relationship between visual, auditory, and somatosensory inputs in mouse superior colliculus. *Journal of Neurophysiology, 38*, 690–713.

Dubner, R. (1967). Interaction of peripheral and central input in the main sensory trigeminal nucleus in the cat. *Experimental Neurology, 17*, 186–202.

Dudycha, G.J., & Dudycha, M.M. (1935). A case of synesthesia: Visual-pain and visual-audition. *Journal of Abnormal and Social Psychology, 30*, 57–69.

Dunn, D.W., Weisberg, L.A., & Nadell, J. (1983). Peduncular hallucinations caused by brainstem compression. *Neurology 33*, 1360–1361.

Duplessis, Y. (1975). *The paranormal perception of color* (P. Von Toal, transl.). New York: Parapsychology Foundation, Inc.

Eccles, J.C. (1970). *Facing reality: Philosophical adventures of a brain scientist.* New York: Springer-Verlag.

Echlin, F.A., & McDonald, J. (1954). The supersensitivity of chronically isolated and partially isolated cerebral cortex as a mechanism in focal cortical epilepsy. *Transactions of the American Neurological Association, 79,* 75–79.

Essman, W.B. (1977). Serotonin in learning and memory. In W.B. Essman (Ed.), *Serotonin in health and disease, Vol. 3, The central nervous system* (Chap. 3). New York: Spectrum.

Ettlinger, G., & Blakemore, D.B. (1969). Cross modal transfer set in the monkey. *Neuropsychologia, 7,* 41–47.

Evarts, E.V. (1957). A review of the neuro-physiological effects of lysergic acid diethyamide (LSD) and other psychomometic agents. *Annals of the New York Academy of Sciences, 66,* 479–495.

Fanchamps, A. (1978). Some compounds with hallucinogenic activity. In B. Berde & H.O. Schild (Eds.), *Handbuch der experimentallen Pharmakologie, Vol 49 (new series), Ergot alkaloids and related compounds* (Chap. 8). New York: Springer-Verlag.

Fessard, A. (1961). The role of neuronal networks in sensory communication within the brain. In W.A. Rosenblith (Ed.), *Sensory communication* (pp. 585–606). New York: John Wiley & Sons.

Fibiger, H.C., Lepaine, E.G., & Phillips, A.G. (1978). Disruption of memory produced by stimulation of the dorsal raphe nucleus: Mediation by serotonin. *Brain Research, 155,* 380–386.

Fincham, E.F. (1963). Monocular diplopia. *British Journal of Ophthalmology, 47,* 705–712.

Finkel, M. (1976). Experimentally induced psychosis in man. In H.A. Abramson (Ed.), *Neuropharmacology, transactions of the Second Conference of the Josiah Macy Foundation, May 25–27* (p. 235). New York: Macy Foundation.

Flechsig, P. (1901). *Lancet, 2,* 1027.

Flournoy, Th. (1893). *Des phenomenes de synopsie* (pp. 98 ff.). Paris: Alcon.

Forster, F.M. (1977). *Reflex epilepsy, behavioral therapy and conditional reflexes.* Springfield, IL: Charles C. Thomas.

Freedman, S.J., & Marks, P.A. (1965). Visual imagery produced by rhythmic photic stimulation: Personality correlates and phenomenology. *British Journal of Psychology, 56,* 95–112.

Fuller, J.L., & Thompson, W.R. (1960). Behavior genetics. Westport: Greenwood.

Furst, C.J., Fuld, K., & Pancoe, M. (1974). Recall accuracy of eidetikers. *Journal of Experimental Psychology, 102*(6), 1133–1135.

Galton, F. (1869). *Hereditary genius.* London: Macmillan.

Galton, F. (1907). *Inquiries into human faculty and its development.* London: J.M. Dent & Sons.

Gatter, K.C., Winfield, D.A., & Powell, T.P.S. (1980). An electron microscopic study of the types and population of neurons in the cortex of the motor and visual areas of the cat and rat. *Brain, 103*(2), 245–258.

Geller, T.J. & Bellur, S.N. (1987). Peduncular hallucinosis: Magnetic resonance imaging confirmation of mesencephalic infarction during life. *Annals of Neurology, 21,* 602–604.

Gengerelli, J.A. (1976). Eidetic imagery in two subjects after 46 years. *Journal of General Psychology, 95,* 219–225.

Geschwind, N. (1964). In C.J.J.M. Stuart (Ed.), *Monograph series on language and linguistics, No. 17* (p. 155). Washington, D.C.: Georgetown Unviersity.

Geschwind, N. (1965a). Disconnection syndromes in animals and man. *Brain, 88,* 237–294.

Geschwind, N. (1965b). Disconnection syndromes in animals and man, Part II. *Brain, 88,* 585–644.

Geschwind, N., & Galaburda, A.M. (1985a). Cerebral lateralization. Biological mechanisms, associations, and pathology: I. A hypothesis and a program for research. *Archives of Neurology, 42,* 428–459.

Geschwind, N., & Galaburda, A.M. (1985b). Cerebral lateralization. Biological mechanisms, associations, and pathology: II. A hypothesis and a program for research. *Archives of Neurology, 42,* 521–552.

Geschwind, N., & Galaburda, A.M. (1985c). Cerebral lateralization. Biological mechanisms, associations, and pathology: III. A hypothesis and a program for research. *Archives of Neurology, 42,* 634–654.

Geschwind, N., & Levitsky, W. (1968). Human brain: Left-right asymmetries in temporal speech region. *Science, 161,* 186–187.

Ghika, M.C. (1927). *Esthetique des proportions.* Paris.

Ghika, M.C. (1930). *Le nombre d'or.* Paris.

Gillmor, C.S. (1980). Visual images observed following an enucleation. *Perception, 9,* 493–502.

Gillmor, C.S. (1981). Visual images observed after enucleation. *Archives of Ophthalmology, 99,* 1468.

Gillmor, C.S. (1982). Further remarks concerning visual images observed following unilateral enucleation. *Perception, 11,* 47–51.

Ginsberg, M.D., Chang, J.Y., Kelly, R.E., et al. (1988). Increases in both cerebral glucose utilization and blood flow during execution of a somatosensory task. *Annals of Neurology 23,* 152–160.

Gloor, P., Olivier, A., Quesney, L.F., et al. (1982). The role of the limbic system in experiential phenomena of temporal lobe epilepsy. *Annals of Neurology, 12,* 129–144.

Goethe, J.W. von. (1810). *Zur Farbenlehre.* Tübigen: JG Gotta.

Gogan, P. (1970). The startle and orienting reactions in man: A study of their characteristics and habituation. *Brain Research, 18,* 117–135.

Golgi, C. (1883). Recherches sur l'histologie des centre nerveaus. *Archives of Italian Biology, 3,* 285–317.

Golgi, C. (1884). *Archives of Italian Biology, 4,* 92–123.

Goodman, D.G., & Horel, J.A. (1966). Sprouting of the optic tract projections in the brain stem of the rat. *Journal of Comparative Neurology, 127,* 71–83.

Goodman, L.S., & Gilman, A. (1975). *The pharmacological basis of therapeutics* (5th ed.). New York: Macmillan.

Gowers, W.R. (1901). *Epilepsy and other chronic convulsive diseases* (2nd ed.). London.

Gray, C.R., & Gummerman, C.R. (1975). The enigmatic eidetic image: A critical examination of methods, data and theories. *Psychological Bulletin, 82,* 383–407.

Greenwald, M.J., Greenwald, S.L., Arch, M., et al. (1983). Long-lasting visual after effect from viewing a computer video terminal display. *New England Journal of Medicine, 309,* 315.

Groves, P.M., Wilson, C.H., & Boyle, R.D. (1974). Brainstem pathways, cortical modulation, and habituation of the acoustic startle response. *Behavioral Biology, 10,* 391–418.

Haber, R.N. (1969). Eidetic images. *Scientific American, 220,* 36–44.

Haber, R.N. (1979). Twenty years of haunting eidetic imagery: Where's the ghost? *Behavioral and Brain Sciences, 2,* 583–629.

Haber, R.N. (1983). The impending demise of the icon: A critique of the concept of iconic storage in visual information processing. *Behavior and Brain Sciences, 6,* 1–54.

Haber, R.N., & Haber, R.B. (1964). Eidetic imagery. I: Frequency. *Perceptual and Motor Skills, 19,* 131–138.

Hachinski, V. (1987). The nature of migraine (editorial). *Archives of Neurology, 44,* 327.

Halgren, E., Walter, R.D., Cherlow, D.G., & Crandall, P.H. (1978). Mental phenomena evoked by electrical stimulation of the human hippocampal formation and amygdala. *Brain, 101,* 83–117.

Hambidge, J. (1920). *Dynamic symmetry.* New Haven, CT: Yale University Press.

Hambidge, J. (1924). *The Parthenon.* New Haven, CT: Yale University Press.

Hambidge, J. (1926). *The elements of dynamic symmetry.* New York: Brentano's.

Hambidge, M. (1975). In A. Voulis (Ed.), *Apprentice in creation.* Rabun Gap, GA: The Hambidge Center.

Hartman, A.M., & Hollister, L.E. (1963). Effect of mescaline, LSD and psilocybin on color perception. *Psychopharmacologia, 4,* 441–451.

Hausser-Hauw, C., & Bancaud, J. (1987). Gustatory hallucinations in epileptic seizures: Electrophysiological, clinical and anatomical correlates. *Brain, 110,* 339–359.

Hayek, E.A. (1952). *The sensory order* (pp. 19 ff.). London: Routledge & Kegan Paul.

Hecht, S., & Hsia, Y. (1945). Dark adaptation following light adaptation to red and white light. *Journal of the Optical Society of America, 35,* 261–267.

Henderson, S.T. (1977). *Daylight and its spectrum.* New York: John Wiley & Sons.

Hering, E. (1964). *Outlines of a theory of the light sense* (L.M. Hurvich & D. Jameson, trans.). Cambridge, MA: Harvard University Press.

Heron, W., Doaene, B.K., & Scott, T.H. (1956). Visual disturbances after prolonged perceptual isolation. *Canadian Journal of Psychology, 10,* 13–18.

Herskowitz, J., Rosman, N.P., & Geschwind, N. (1984). Seizures induced by singing and recitation. A unique form of reflex epilepsy in childhood. *Archives of Neurology, 41,* 1102–1103.

Hilbert, R. (1895). Zur Kenntnis der sogennanten Doppelempfindungen. *Archiv für Augenheilkunde, 31,* 44–48.

Hockney, D. (1984). *Cameraworks.* New York: Knopf.

Holden (1891). Color association with numerals. *Nature, 64,* 223.

Hollister, L.E. (1968). *Chemical psychoses, LSD and related drugs.* Springfield, IL: Charles C. Thomas.

Holmes, G. (1918). Disturbances of visual orientation. *British Journal of Ophthalmology, 2,* 449–486, 506–516.

Holmes, G. (1919). Disturbances of spatial orientation and visual attention with loss of stereoscopic vision. *Archives of Neurology and Psychiatry, 1,* 385.

Holt, R.R. (1964). Imagery: The return of the ostracized. *American Psychologist, 19*, 254–264.

Horn, G. (1965). The effect of somaesthetic and photic stimuli on the activity of units in the striate cortex of unanesthetized, unrestrained cats. *Journal of Physiology, 179*, 263–277.

Horowitz, M.J. (1964). The imagery of visual hallucinations. *Journal of Nervous and Mental Diseases, 138*, 513–523.

Horowitz, M.J. (1975). Hallucinations: An information processing approach. In R.K. Siegel & L.J. West (Eds.), *Hallucinations: Behavior, experience and theory*. New York: John Wiley & Sons.

Horrax, G. (1923). Visual hallucinations as a cerebral localizing phenomenon: With especial reference to their occurrance in the temporal lobes. *Archives of Neurology and Psychiatry, 10*, 532.

Hubel, D. (1982). Exploration of the primary visual cortex. *Nature, 299*, 515–524.

Hubel, D.H., & Wiesel, T.N. (1962). Receptive fields, binocular interaction and functional architecture in the cat's visual cortex. *Journal of Physiology, 160*, 106–154.

Hubel, D.H., & Wiesel, T.N. (1968). Receptive fields and functional architecture of monkey striate cortex. *Journal of Physiology, 195*, 215–243.

Hubel, D.H., & Wiesel, T.N. (1972). Laminar and columnar distribution of geniculo-cortical fibers in the Macaque monkey. *Journal of Comparative Neurology, 158*, 267–294.

Hume, P. (1979, December 23). Messiaen's grandest canyon suite. *Washington Post*.

Hunt, R.W.G. (1967). *The reproduction of color*. London: Wiley.

Huxley, A. (1942). *The art of seeing*. New York: Harper & Bros.

Ingvar, D.H., & Soderberg, U. (1956). Effect of LSD upon cerebral blood flow and EEG in cats. *Experientia, 12*, 427.

Ionasescu, V. (1960). Paroxysmal disorders of the body image in temporal lobe epilepsy. *Acta Psychiatrica Scandinavica, 35*, 171–181.

Isaacson, R.L. (1982). *The limbic system* (2nd ed.). New York: Plenum Press.

Itten, J. (1971a). *Kunst der Farbe: Subjektives Erleben und objektives Erkennen als Wege zur Kunst*. Ravensburg: O. Maier.

Itten, J. (1971b). *Johannes Itten*. Bern: Kunsthalle.

Itten, J. (1973). *Der Unterricht: Farben, Formen, textiles Gestalten*. Krefeld: Vereinigte Seidenwebereien AG.

Jackson, H. (1898). *Lancet, 1*, 79–87.

Jacobs, B.L. (1977). Dreams and hallucinations: A common neurochemical mechanism mediating their phenomenological similarities. *Neuroscience and Behavioral Reviews, 2*, 59–60.

Jacobs, B.L., & Trulson, M.E. (1979). Dreams, hallucinations and psychosis—the serotonin connection. *Trends in Neuroscience, 2*, 276–280.

Jacobs, L., Karpick, A., Bozian, D., et al. (1981). Auditory-visual synesthesia: Sound induced photisms. *Archives of Neurology, 38*, 211–216.

Jacobs, M. (1924). *The art of colour*. New York: Doubleday.

Jacome, D.E., & Gumnit, R.J. (1979). Audioalgesic and audiovisuoalgesic synesthesias: Epileptic manifestation. *Neurology, 29*, 1050–1053.

Jaensch, E.R. (1930). *Eidetic imagery and typological methods of investigation*. (2nd ed., O. Oeser, trans.). New York: Harcourt, Brace.

Jaensch, E.R. (1931). *Über die Grundlagen der Menschlichen Erkentniss.* Leipzig: J.A. Barth.

Jakobson, R. (1941). *Kindersprache, Aphasie und Allgemeine Lautgesetze.* Uppsala: Almquist & Wiksells Boktryckeri.

James, W. (1901). *The varieties of religious experience.* New York: Colliers.

Jasper, H. (1958). Reticular-cortical systems and theories of the integrative action of the brain. In: *Biological and biochemical bases of behavior* (pp. 37–61). Madison: University of Wisconsin Press.

Judd, D.B., MacAdam, D.L., & Wyszecki, G. (1964). Spectral distribution of typical daylight as a function of corrected color temperature. *Journal of the Optical Society of America, 54,* 1031–1040.

Julesz, B. (1964). Binocular depth perception without familiarity cues. *Science, 145,* 356–362.

Jung, R. (1964). Neurologische Grundlagen der optischen Wahrnehmung. *Zeitblatt fur die Gesamtes Neurologie und Psychiatrie, 180,* 209–210.

Kandel, E.R. (1979). Psychotherapy and the single synapse. The impact of psychiatric thought on neurobiologic research. *New England Journal of Medicine, 301,* 1028–1037.

Kandinsky, V. (1881). Zur Lehre von den Hallucinationen. *Arkiv für Psychiatrie und Nervenkrankheiten, 11,* 453–464.

Kandinsky, V. (1885). *Kritische und klinische Betrachtungen im Gebiere der Sinnestäuchungen* (p. 170). Berlin: Friedländer.

Kandinsky, V. (1910). *Über das geistige in der Kunst, inbesondere in der Malerei.* Munich: Piper & Co. (First complete English translation, 1946, *On the spiritual in art* (Baroness Rebay con Ehrenweisen, trans.). New York: Solomon R. Guggenheim Foundation, for the museum of nonobjective paintings.)

Karwoski, T.F., Gramlich, F.W., & Arnot, P. (1944). Psychological studies in semantics: I. Free association reactions to words, drawings, and objects. *Journal of Social Psychology, 20,* 233–247.

Karwoski, T.F., & Odbert, H.S. (1938). Color-music. *Psychological Monographs, 50,* No. 2 (whole No. 222).

Karwoski, T.F., Odbert, H.S., & Osgood, C.E. (1942). Studies in synesthetic thinking II: Role of form in visual responses to music. *Journal of General Psychology, 26,* 199–222.

Katz, D. (1935). *The world of color* (R.B. MacLeod & C.W. Fox, trans.). London: Kegan Paul, Trench, Trubner.

Kawamura, M., Hirayama, K., Shinohara, Y., et al. (1987). Alloaesthesia. *Brain, 10,* 225–236.

Keeler, M.H. (1970). Klüver's mechanisms of hallucinations as illustrated by the paintings of Max Ernst. In W. Keup (Ed.), *Origin and mechanisms of hallucinations.* New York: Plenum Press.

Kennedy, F. (1911). The sympatomology of temporo-sphenoidal tumors. *Archives of Internal Medicine, 8,* 317–350.

Kihlstrom, J.F. (1987). The cognitive unconscious. *Science, 237,* 1445–1452.

Kinsbourne, M., & Warrington, E.K. (1963). A study of visual perseveration. *Journal of Neurology, Neurosurgery, and Psychiatry, 26,* 468–475.

Klein, A.B. (1926). *Color music, the art of light.* London: Crosby, Lockwood & Son.

Kling, L.W., Clark, M.A., Compton, H.R., et al. (1987). The 1986 Lake Nyos gas disaster in Cameroon, West Africa. *Science, 236,* 169–175.

Kloos, G. (1931). Synäesthesien bei psychich Abnormen Auch. *Psychiatrie und Neurologie, 94,* 417–469.

Klopp, H. (1951). Über umgekehrt- und verkehrtsehen. *Deutsche Zeitschrift fur Nervenheilkunde, 165,* 230.

Klüver, H. (1928). Studies on the eidetic type and on eidetic imagery. *Psychological Bulletin, 25*(2), 69–104.

Klüver, H. (1931). The eidetic child. In C. Murchison (Ed.), *A handbook of child psychology* (pp. 643–668). Worcester, MA: Clark University Press.

Klüver, H. (1932). Eidetic phenomena. *Psychological Bulletin, 29,* 181–203.

Klüver, H. (1942a). Functional significance of the geniculo-striate system. *Biology Symposia, 7,* 253–299.

Klüver, H. (1942b). Mechanisms of hallucinations. In Q. McNemar & M.A. Merrill (Eds.), *Studies in personality.* New York: McGraw-Hill.

Klüver, H. (1965). In P.H. Hoch & J. Zubin (Eds.), *Psychopathology of perception.* New York: Grune & Stratton.

Klüver, H. (1966). *Mescal and mechanisms of hallucinations.* Chicago: University of Chicago Press.

Klüver, H., & Bucy, P.C. (1939). Preliminary analysis of functions of the temporal lobes in monkeys. *Archives of Neurology and Psychiatry, 42,* 979–1000.

Kornhüber, H.H. (1974). Cerebral cortex, cerebellum and basal ganglia: An introduction to their motor function. In F.O. Schmitt & F.G. Worden (Eds.), *The neurosciences third study program* (pp. 267–280). Cambridge, MA: MIT Press.

Kornhüber, H.H., & Deecke, L. (1965). Hirnpotentialänderungen bei Wilkürbewegungen und passiven Bewegungen des Menschen: Bereitschaftspotential und reafferente Potentiale. *Pflüger's Archiv fur die Gesamte Physiologie, 284,* 1–17.

Kubie, L.S. (1943). Use of induced hypnagogic reveries in recovery of repressed anmesia data. *Bulletin of the Menninger Clinic, 7,* 172–182.

Kubie, L.S. (1966). *Neurotische deformationen des Schopferischen prozisses.* Hamburg: Rorwhet.

Kubie, L.S., & Margolin, S. (1942). Physiological method for induction of states of partial sleep, and securing free association and early memories from such states. *American Neurological Association, 68,* 136–139.

LaBarre, W. (1975). Anthropological perspectives on hallucination and hallucinogens. In R.K. Siegel & L.J. West (Eds.), *Hallucinations: Behavior, experience and theory* (pp. 9–52). New York: John Wiley & Sons.

Laignel-Lavastine (1901). Audition calorée familiale. *Revue Neurologique, 9,* 1152–1162.

Lance, J.W. (1976). Simple formed hallucinations confined to the area of a specific visual field defect. *Brain, 99,* 719–734.

Lance, J.W., & McLeod, J.G. (1981). *A physiological approach to clinical neurology* (3rd ed., chap. 13). London: Butterworths.

Land, E.H. (1959). Experiments in color vision. *Scientific American, 200,* 84–89.

Land, E.H. (1977). The retinex theory of color vision. *Scientific American, 237*(6), 108–128.

Land, E.H., & McCann, J.J. (1971). Lightness and retinex theory. *Journal of the Optical Society of America, 61*(1), 1–11.

Landgren, S. (1957). Convergence of tactile, thermal, and gustatory impulses on single cortical cells. *Acta Physiologica Scandinavica, 40,* 210–221.

Langenbeck, K. (1913). *Zeitschrift für sinnesphysiologie, XLVII,* 162. Cited by Jakobson, 1941.

Langfeld, H.S. (1926). Synesthesia. *Psychological Bulletin, 23,* 599–602.

Lashley, K.S. (1949). Persistent problems in the evolution of mind. *Quarterly Review of Biology, 24,* 28–42.

Lauritzen, M., Balslev Jøgensen, M., et al. (1982). Persistent oligemia of rat cerebral cortex in the wake of spreading depression. *Annals of Neurology, 12,* 469–474.

Leao, A.P.P. (1944). Spreading depression of activity in cerebral cortex. *Journal of Neurophysiology, 7,* 359–390.

Lende, R.A. (1963). Cerebral cortex: Amalgam in the marsupial. *Science, 141,* 730–732.

Lessell, S. (1975). Higher disorders of visual function: Positive phenomenon. In J.S. Glaaser & J.L. Smith (Eds.), *Neuroophthalmology* (vol. 8, pp. 27–43). St. Louis: C.V. Mosby Co.

Lesser, I.M. (1985). Alexithymia. *New England Journal of Medicine, 312,* 690–692.

Levine, D.N., Warach, J., & Farah, M. (1985). Two visual systems in mental imagery: Dissociation of "what" and "where" in imagery due to bilateral posterior cerebral lesions. *Neurology, 35,* 1010–1018.

L'hermitte, J. (1922). Syndrome de la calotte du pédoncule cérébral. *Societie de Neurologie,* November 9.

L'hermitte, F., Chain, F., Aron, D., Leblanc, M., & Jouty, O. (1969). Les troubles de la vision des couleurs dans les lesions posterieures du cerveau. *Revue Neurologique, 121,* 5–29.

Libet, B. (1985). Unconscious cerebral initiative and the role of conscious will in voluntary action. *The Behavioral and Brain Sciences, 8,* 529–566.

Libet, B., Alberts, W.W., Wright, E.W., & Feinstein, B. (1967). Responses of human somatosensory cortex to stimuli below threshold for conscious sensation. *Science, 158,* 1597–1600.

Libet, B., Gleason, C.A., Wright, E.W., & Pearl, D.K. (1983). Time of conscious intention to act in relation to onset of cerebral activity (readiness-potential). The unconscious initiation of a freely voluntary act. *Brain, 106,* 623–642.

Livingstone, M. (1987). *Parallel processing of form, movement, color, and depth in humans and other primates: Anatomy, physiology, demonstrations, and illusions.* Paper presented at the 69th annual meeting of the Association for Research in Nervous and Mental Diseases Inc., "Vision and the brain: The organization of the central visual system," New York, December 4–5. (Abstracted in *Archives of Neurology, 44,* 1211.)

Livingstone, M.S. (1988). Art, illusion and the visual system. *Scientific American, 258,* 78–85.

Livingstone, M.S., & Hubel, D.H. (1984). Anatomy and physiology of a color system in the primate visual cortex. *Journal of Neuroscience, 4,* 309–356.

Lorente de No, R. (1943). Cerebral cortex: Architecture, intracortical connections, motor projections. In J.F. Fulton (Ed.), *Physiology of the nervous system* (2nd ed., pp. 274–301). Oxford, England: Oxford Unviersity Press.

Lorenz, K. (1965). *Über Tierisches und Menschliches Verhalten; aus dem Werdegang der Verhaltenslehre* (Bd I, II). Munich: Peiper.

Luria, A.R. (1968). *The mind of a mnemonist*. New York: Basic Books.

MacLaine, S. (1983). *Out on a limb*. New York: Bantam.

MacLean, P.D. (1949). Psychosomatic disease and the "visceral brain": Recent developments bearing on the Papez theory of emotion. *Psychosomatic Medicine, 11*, 338–353.

MacLean, P.D. (1970). The triune brain, emotion and scientific bias. In F.O. Schmitt (Ed.), *The neurosciences, second study program* (pp. 336–349). New York: Rockefeller University Press.

MacLean, P.D. (1972). Cerebral evolution and emotional processes. *Annals of the New York Academy of Sciences, 193*, 137–149.

MacLean, P.D. (1973). *A triune concept of the brain and behavior*. Toronto: University of Toronto Press.

MacLean, P.D. (1975). Sensory and perceptive factors in emotional functions of the triune brain. In L. Levi (Ed.), *Emotions—their parameters and measurements*. New York: Raven Press.

MacLean, P.D. (1977). An evolutionary approach to brain research on prosemantic (nonverbal) behavior. In J.R. Rosenblatt & B. Komisarus (Eds.), *Reproductive behavior and evolution* (pp. 137–164). New York: Plenum.

MacLean, P.D. (1978a). A mind of three minds: Educating the triune brain. In *Seventy-seventh Yearbook of the National Society for the Study of Education*. (pp. 308–342). Chicago: University of Chicago Press.

MacLean, P.D. (1978b). Why brain research on lizards? In N. Greenberg & P.D. MacLean (Eds.), *Behavior and neurology of lizards* (pp. 1–9). Bethesda: National Institute of Mental Health.

MacLean, P.D. (1978c). Challenges of the papez heritage. In K. Livinston & O. Hornkiewicz (Eds.), *Limbic mechanisms* (pp. 1–15). New York: Plenum.

MacLean, P.D. (1980). Role of transhypothalamic pathways in social communication. In P.J. Morgane & J. Panksepp (Eds.), *Handbook of the hypothalamus, Vol. 3, Part 3: Behavioral studies of the hypothalamus* (pp. 259–287). New York: Marcel Dekker.

MacLean, P.D. (1985). Brain evolution relating to family, play, and the separation call. *Archives of General Psychiatry, 42*, 405–417.

MacNichol, E.F., MacPherson, L., & Svaetichin, G. (1958). Studies on spectral response curves from the fish retina. In: *Symposium on visual problems of color* (Vol. 2, pp. 529–538). London: Her Majesty's Stationery Office.

Madachy, J.S. (1979). *Madachy's mathematical recreations*. New York: Dover.

Malkinson, T.J., Cooper, K.E., & Veale, W.L. (1985). Induced changes in intracranial pressure in the anesthetized rat and rabbit. *Brain Research Bulletin, 15*, 321–328.

Mandell, A.J. (1980). Toward a psychobiology of transcendence: God in the brain. In J.M. Davidson & R.J. Davidson (Eds.), *The psychobiology of consciousness*. New York: Plenum Press.

Marcel, A.J. (1983a). Conscious and unconscious perception: Experiments on visual masking and word recognition. *Cognitive Psychology, 15*, 197–237.

Marcel, A.J. (1983b). Conscious and unconscious perception: An approach to the relations between phenomenal experience and perceptual processes. *Cognitive Psychology, 15*, 238–300.

Marks, L.E. (1974). On associations of light and sound: The mediation of brightness, pitch and loudness. *American Journal of Psychology, 87*, 173–188.

Marks, L.E. (1975). On colored-hearing synesthesia: Cross-modal translations of sensory dimensions. *Psychological Bulletin, 82*(3), 303–331.

Marks, L.E. (1978). *The unity of the senses: Interrelations among the modalities.* New York: Academic Press.

Marks, W.B., Dobelle, W.H., & MacNichol, E.F. (1964). Visual pigments of single primate cones. *Science,* March 13, 1181–1182.

Marshack, A. (1975). Exploring the mind of ice age man. *National Geographic 147*(1), 62–89.

Maxwell, J.C. (1855). *Scientific Papers of James Clerk Maxwell* (W.D. Niven, Ed.). New York: Dover Publications.

McCann, J.J., & Benton, J.L. (1969). Interaction of the long-wave cones and the rods to produce color sensations. *Journal of the Optical Society of America, 59*(1), 103–107.

McCann, J.J., Land, E.H., & Tatnall, S.M. (1970). *American Journal of Optometry, 47,* 845.

McKellar, P. (1957). *Imagination and thinking.* New York: Basic Books.

Merril, E.G., & Wall, P.D. (1978). Plasticity of connection in the adult nervous system. In C.W. Cotman (Ed.), *Neuronal Plasticity* (pp. 97–111). New York: Raven Press.

Messiaen, O. (1956). *Technique de mon language musicale.* Paris: Alphonse Leduc.

Messiaen, O. (1977). *Des Canyons Aux Etoiles.* Liner notes, Erato STU70974/975 (recording). Paris: Alphonse Leduc.

Messing, R.B., Pettibone, D.J., Kaufman, N., et al. (1978). Behavioral effects of serotonin neurotoxins, an overview. *Annals of the New York Academy of Sciences, 305,* 480–496.

Mesulam, M-M. (Ed.). (1985). *Principles of behavioral neurology.* Philadelphia: F.A. Davis Co.

Micheloyannakis, J., & Ionnidou, A. (1986). Reflex epilepsy. *Journal of Child Neurology, 1,* 382–383.

Miller, S., & Peacock, R. (1982). Evidence for the uniqueness of eidetic imagery. *Perceptual and Motor Skills, 55,* 1219–1233.

Miller, T.C., & Crosby, T.W. (1979). Musical hallucinations in a deaf elderly patient. *Annals of Neurology, 5,* 301–302.

Miner, H. (1956). Body ritual among the Nacirema. *American Anthropologist, 58,* 503–507.

Molliver, M.E, Grazanna, R., Morrison, H., & Coyle, J.T. (1977). Immunohistological characterization of noradrenergic innervation in the rat neocortex: A regional and laminar analysis. *Neuroscience Abstracts.*

Monnier, M. (1959). Hallucinogenic, psychotonic and analeptic stimulants of the CNS. In: *XXI International Congress of Physiological Sciences. Symposia and Special Lectures* (p. 149). Buenos Aires, August, 1959.

Monnier, M. (1975). *Functions of the nervous system, Vol. 3, Sensory functions and perception.* Amsterdam: Elsevier.

Monroe, R.R., Heath, R.G., Mickle, X., et al. (1957). Correlation of rhinencephalic electrograms with behavior. *Electroencephalography and Clinical Neurophysiology, 9,* 623–642.

Moore, R.F. (1935). Subjective lightning streaks. *British Journal of Ophthalmology, 19,* 545–547.

Moore, R.Y., & Bloom, F.E. (1978). Central catecholamine neuron systems: Anatomy and physiology. *Annual Review of Neuroscience, 1*, 129–169.

Morel, F. (1936). Des bruits d'oreille, des bourdonnements, des hallucinations auditivs élémentaires, communes et verbales. *Encéphale, 31*, 81–95.

Mössel, E. (1927). *Die Proportionen in Antike un Mittelalter.* Munich: NP

Mountcastle, V.B. (1957). Modality and topographic properties of single neurones of cat's somatic sensory cortex. *Journal of Neurophysiology, 20*, 408–434.

Mountcastle, V.B. (Ed.). (1962). *Interhemispheric relations and cerebral dominance.* Baltimore: Johns Hopkins Press.

Mountcastle, V.B. (1979). An organizing principle for cerebral function: The unit module and the distributed system. In F.O. Schmitt & F.G. Worden (Eds.), *The neurosciences fourth study program* (pp. 21–42). Cambridge, MA: MIT Press.

Mountcastle, V.B., & Powell, T.P.S. (1959). Neural mechanisms subserving cutaneous sensibility, with special reference to the role of afferent inhibition in sensory perception and discrimination. *Bulletin of the Johns Hopkins Hospital, 105*, 201–232.

Mouren, P., & Tatossian, A. (1963). Les illusions visuospatiales. Etude clinique. *Encéphale, 5*, 438–480.

Mulder, D.W., & Daly, D. (1952). *Journal of the American Medical Association, 150*, 173–176.

Murata, K., Cramer, H., & Bach-y-Rita, P. (1965). Neuronal convergence of noxious, acoustic and visual stimuli in the visual cortex of the cat. *Journal of Neurophysiology, 28*, 1123–1239.

Myers, C.A. (1911). A case of synesthesia. *British Journal of Psychology, 4*, 228–238.

Myers, R.E. (1962). Commissural connections between occipital lobes of the monkey. *Journal of Comparative Neurology, 118*, 1–16.

Nabokov, V. (1949, April 9). Portrait of my mother. *New Yorker*, pp. 33–37.

Nabokov, V. (1966). *Speak, memory: An autobiography revisited.* New York: Dover. (First published in 1951 as *Conclusive evidence.*)

Nashold, B.S., Jr. (1970). Phosphenes resulting from stimulation of the midbrain in man. *Archives of Ophthalmology, 84*, 433–435.

Newton, I. (1730). *Optiks* (4th ed., 1952). New York: Dover Publications.

Noordhout, A.M., Timsit-Berthier, M., Timsit, A., et al. (1987). Effects of beta blockade on contingent negative variation in migraine. *Annals of Neurology, 21*(1), 111–112.

Odbert, H.S., Karwoski, T.F., & Eckerson, A.B. (1942). Studies in synesthetic thinking I: Musical and verbal associations of color and mood. *Journal of General Psychology, 26*, 153–173.

Ojemann, G.A., & Whitaker, H.A. (1978). Language localisation and variability. *Brain and Language, 6*, 239–260.

O'Keeffe, G. (1987). National Gallery of Art, Washington, DC, November 1–February 21.

Olds, J., & Milner, P. (1954). Positive reinforcement produced by electrical stimulation of septal area and other regions of rat brain. *Journal of Comparative and Physiological Psychology, 47*, 419–427.

Oleson, J. (1987). The ischemic hypothesis of migraine. *Archives of neurology, 44*, 321–322.

Ortmann, O. (1933). Theories of synesthesia in the light of a case of colored hearing. *Human Biology, 5,* 155–211.

Osgood, C.E. (1956). *Method and theory in experimental psychology.* New York: Oxford Unviersity Press.

Osgood, C.E. (1960). The cross-cultural generality of visual-verbal synesthetic tendencies. *Behavioral Science, 5,* 146–149.

Osgood, C.E., Suci, G.J., & Tannenbaum, P.H. (1957). *The measurement of meaning.* University of Illinois

Palliard, J., Michael, F., & Stelmach, G. (1983). Localization without content: A tactile analogue of 'blind sight.' *Archives of Neurology, 40,* 548–551.

Papez, J.W. (1937). A proposed mechanism of emotion. *Archives of Neurology and Psychiatry, 38,* 725–743.

Peiper, A. (1951). Instinkt und angeborene scheme beim saugling. *Zeitschrift fur Tierpsychologie, 8,* 449–456.

Penfield, W. (1958). The role of the temporal cortex in recall of past experience and interpretation of the present. In *Ciba Foundation Symposium, Neurological basis of behaviour* (pp. 149–174). London: Churchill.

Penfield, W., & Jasper, H. (1954). *Epilepsy and the functional anatomy of the human brain.* Boston: Little, Brown.

Penfield, W., & Perot, P. (1963). The brain's record of auditory and visual experience. *Brain, 86,* 595–696.

Penfield, W., & Roberts, L. (1959). *Speech and brain mechanisms.* Princeton: Princeton University Press.

Peroutka, S.J., Lebovitz, R.M., & Snyder, S.H. (1981). Two distinct central serotonin receptors with different physiological functions. *Science, 212,* 827–829.

Perrenin, M.T. (1978). Visual function within the hemianopic field following early cerebral hemidecortication in man. II: Pattern discrimination. *Neuropsychologia, 16,* 696–708.

Perrenin, M.T., & Jeannerod, M. (1978). Visual function within the hemianopic field following early cerebral hemidecortication in man. I: Spatial localization. *Neuropsychologia, 16,* 1–13.

Pierce, A.H. (1912). Synesthesia. *Psychological Bulletin, 9,* 179–181.

Plummer, H.C. (1915, April 10). Color music—a new art created with the aid of science. The color organ used in Scriabin's symphony "Prometheus." *Scientific American.*

Pollen, D.A., & Trachtenberg, M.C. (1972). Alpha rhythm and eye movements in eidetic imagery. *Nature, 237,* 109–112.

Pöppel, E., Held, R., & Frost, D. (1973). Residual visual function after brain wounds involving the central visual pathways in man. *Nature 243,* 295–296.

Popper, K.R. (1975). *Objective knowledge, an evolutional approach.* Oxford: Clarendon Press.

Popper, K.R., & Eccles, J.C. (1977). *The self and its brain.* London: Springer-Verlag.

Pötzl, O. (1943). Über Verkehrtsehen. *Zeitschrift für die Gesamte Neurologie und Psychiatrie, 176,* 780.

Prinzhorn, H. (1919). Das bildnerische Schaffen der Geisteskrankheiten. *Zeitschrift für die Gesamte Neurologie und Psychiatrie, 52,* 307–326.

Prinzhorn, H. (1922). Gibt es schizophrene Gestaltungsmerkmale in der Bildnerei der Geisteskranken? *Zeitschrift für die Gesamte Neurologie und Psychiatrie, 78,* 512–531.

Prinzhorn, H. (1972). *Artistry of the mentally ill* (E. von Brockdorff, transl.). New York: Springer-Verlag.

Profita, J., & Bidder, H. (1988). Perfect pitch. *Journal of Medical Genetics, 29*(4), 763–771.

Purpura, D.P. (1956a). Electrophysiological analysis of psychotogenic drug action. I: Effect of lysergic acid diethylamide (LSD) on specific afferent systems in the cat. *Archives of Neurology and Psychiatry, 75,* 122–131.

Purpura, D.P. (1956b). Electrophysiological analysis of psychotogenic drug action. II: General nature of lysergic acid diethylamide (LSD) action on central synapses. *Archives of Neurology and Psychiatry, 75,* 132–143.

Purpura, D.P. (1957). Experimental analysis of the inhibitory action of LSD on cortical dendritic activity. *Annals of the New York Academy of Sciences, 66,* 515–536.

Purpura, D.P., Pool, J.L., Ranshoff, J., et al. (1957). Observations on evoked dendritic potentials of human cortex. *Electroencephalography and Clinical Neurophysiology, 9,* 453–459.

Quincke, X. (1890). *Synesthesia.* Zeitschrift für Klinische medizin, XVII.

Rader, C.M., & Tellegen, A. (1987). An investigation of synesthesia. *Journal of Personality and Social Psychology, 52,* 981–987.

Rakic, P. (1971). Guidance of neurons migrating to the fetal monkey cortex. *Brain Research, 33,* 471–476.

Rakic, P. (1972). Mode of cell migration to the superficial layers of fetal monkey neocortex. *Journal of Comparative Neurology, 145,* 61–84.

Rakic, P. (1974). Neurons in rhesus monkey visual cortex: Systematic relation between time of origin and eventual disposition. *Science, 183,* 425–427.

Rakic, P. (1975). Timing of major ontogenetic events in the visual cortex of the rhesus monkey. In J. Buchwald & M. Brazier (Eds.), *Brain mechanisms in mental retardation.* New York: Academic Press.

Ramón y Cajal, S. (1911). *Histologie du systeme nerveux de l'homme et des vertebres* (Vol. II, p. 993). Paris: Maloine.

Reder, A.T., & Wright, F.S. (1982). Epilepsy evoked by eating: The role of peripheral input. *Neurology, 32,* 1065–1069.

Reichard, G., Jakobson, R., & Werth, E. (1949). Language and synesthesia. *Word, 5,* 224–233.

Reznikoff, G.A., Manaker, S., Rhodes, C.H., et al. (1986). Localization and quantification of beta adrenergic receptors in human brain. *Neurology, 36,* 1067–1073.

Richter, I. (1932). *Rhythmic form and art: Investigation of the principles of composition in the works of the great masters.* London: John Lane The Bodley Head Limited.

Riddoch, G. (1917). Dissociation of visual perception due to occipital injuries, with especial reference to appreciation of movement. *Brain, 40,* 15–57.

Ries, H.A. (1969). The elicitation of mediators and colors as a function of stimulus tone frequency. *Dissertation Abstracts International, 30*(6A), 2395.

Riggs, L.A., & Karwoski, T. (1934). Synesthesia. *British Journal of Psychology, 25,* 29–41.

Rizzo, M.R. (1988). *Seeing contour and color. Proceedings of the third international symposium of the Northern Eye Institute.* London: Pergamon Press.

Rizzo, M.R., & Esslinger, P.J. (1988). *Colored hearing synesthesia: Investigation of neural factors in a single subject.* Unpublished manuscript.

Rizzo, M.R., & Hurtig, R. (1987). Looking but not seing: Attention, perception and eye movements in simultanagnosia. *Neurology, 37,* 1642–1648.

Rizzo, M.R., Kritchevsky, M., & Damasio, A. (1986). The role of luminance, saturation, and hue in achromatopsia (abstract). *Proceedings of the Annual Meeting of the American Neurological Asociation,* p. 68.

Rockel, A.J., Hiorns, R.W., & Powell, T.P.S. (1974). Numbers of neurons through full depth of neocortex. *Proceedings of the Anatomic Society of Great Britain and Ireland, 118,* 371.

Rolak, L.A., & Baram, T.Z. (1987). Charles Bonnet syndrome (letter). *Journal of the American Medical Association, 257,* 2036.

Rosenbaum, F., Harati, Y., Rolak, L., et al. (in press). Visual hallucinations in sane people: Charles Bonnet syndrome. *Journal of the American Geriatric Society.*

Ross, E.D., Jossman, P.B., Bell, B., et al. (1975). Musical hallucinations in deafness. *Journal of the American Medical Association, 231,* 620–622.

Rubin, M.L. (1974). The woman who saw too much. *Surgical Ophthalmology, 16,* 382–383.

Samuel, C. (1976). *Conversations with Olivier Messiaen* (F. Aphrahamian, transl.). London: Steiner and Bell.

Sarnat, H.B., & Netsky, M.G. (1981). *Evolution of the nervous system.* New York: Oxford University Press.

Schatzman, M. (1981, January). Ghosts in the machine. *Psychology Today,* p. 99 (citing Shatzman, M. *The story of Ruth.* New York: Putnam's.).

Scheerer, R. (1924). Die entoptische Sichtbarkeit der Blutbewegung im Auge und ihre klinische Bedeutung. *Klinische Monatsblatter fur Augenheilkunde, 73,* 67–107.

Scheibel, M., Scheibel, A., Mollica, A., & Moruzzi, G. (1955). Convergence and interaction of afferent impulses of single units of reticular formation. *Journal of Neurophysiology, 18,* 309–331.

Schilder, P. (1953). *Medical psychology.* New York: International University Press.

Schultze, X. (1912). Krankhafter Wandertrieb, räumlich beschrankte Taubheit für bestimmte Töne und "tertiare" Empfindungen bei einem Psychopathen. *Zeitschrift für die Gesamte Neurologie Psychiatrie, 10,* 399.

Scotti, G., & Spinnler, H. (1970). Colour imperception in unilateral hemisphere-damaged patients. *Journal of Neurology, Neurosurgery and Psychiatry, 33,* 22–28.

Seguin, L.E. (1886). A clinical study of lateral hemianopsia. *Journal of Nervous and Mental Diseases, 13,* 445–454.

Sharpless, S.K. (1969). Isolated and deafferented neurons: Disuse supersensitivity. In H.H. Jasper, A.A. Ward, & A. Pope (Eds.), *Basic mechanisms of the epilepsies* (pp. 329–348). Boston: Little, Brown.

Sherrington, C.S., & Grünbaum, A.S. (1902). *British Medical Journal 2,* 784.

Shirahashi, K. (1960). Electroencephalographic study of mental disturbances experimentally induced by LSD-25. *Folia Psychiatrica et Neurologica (Japan) 14,* 140.

Siegel, R.K. (1977). Hallucinations. *Scientific American, 237*(4), 132–140.

Siegel, R.K., & West, L.J. (1975). *Hallucinations: Behavior, experience and theory.* New York: John Wiley & Sons.

Silverstein, A.B., & Klee, G.D. (1957). Effects of lysergic acid diethylamide on intellectual function. *Archives of Neurology and Psychiatry, 80,* 477–480.

Singer, W. (1977). Control of thalamic transmission by corticofugal and ascending reticular pathways in the visual system. *Physiological Reviews, 57,* 386–420.

Skyhøj-Olsen, T., Friberg, L., & Lassen, N.A. (1987). Ischemia may be the primary cause of the neurologic deficits in classic migraine. *Archives of Neurology, 44,* 156–161.

Sloper, J.J. (1973). An electron microscope study of the termination of afferent connections to the primate motor cortex. *Journal of Neurocytology, 2,* 361–368.

Smith, G.E. (1907). A new topographical survey of the human cerebral cortex, being an account of the distribution of the anatomically and physiologically distinct cortical areas and their relationship to the cerebral sulci. *Journal of Anatomy (London) 41,* 237–254.

Smith, H.L. (1905). Synesthesia. *Bulletin of the Johns Hopkins Hospital, 16,* 258–263.

Smythies, J.R. (1960). The stroboscopic patterns. III. Further experiments and discussion. *Journal of Psychology, 51,* 247–255.

Snow, C.P. (1959). *The two cultures and the scientific revolution.* New York: Pantheon.

Sokoloff, L. (1981). Review: Localization of functional activity in the central nervous system by measurement of glucose utilization with radioactive deoxyglucose. *Journal of Cerebral Blood Flow and Metabolism, 1,* 7–36.

Spiers, M.A., Schomer, D.L., Blume, H.W., & Mesulam, M-M. (1985). Temporolimbic epilepsy and behavior. In Mesulam, M-M. (Ed.), *Principles of behavioral neurology.* (pp. 289–326). Philadelphia: F.A. Davis Co.

Stein, B.C., & Arigbede, M.O. (1972). Unimodal and multimodal response properties of neurons in the cat's superior colliculus. *Neurology 36,* 179–196.

Steiner, I., Shanin, R., & Melamed, E. (1987). Acute "upside down" reversal of vision in transient vertebrobasilar ischemia. *Neurology, 37,* 1685–1686.

Steiner, J.E. (1973). The gustofacial response: Observation on normal and anencephalic newborn infants. In *Symposium on oral sensation and perception* (pp. 254–278). Bethesda, MD: National Institutes of Health.

Stimmel, B. (1979). *Cardiovascular effects of mood altering drugs.* New York: Raven Press.

Stromeyer, C.F., & Psotka, J. (1970). The detailed texture of eidetic images. *Nature, 225,* 346–349.

Stump, D.A., & Williams, R. (1980). The noninvasive measurement of regional cerebral circulation. *Brain and Language, 9,* 35–46.

Suarez de Mendoza, F. (1890). *L'audition colorée.* Paris: Octave Donin.

Sullivan, J.W.N. (1914, February 21). An organ on which color compositions are played. The new art of color music and its mechanism. *Scientific American.*

Svaetichin, G. (1956). Spectral response curves of single cones. *Acta Physiologica Scandinavica Supplement, 134,* 18–46.

Szentagothai, J. (1969). Architecture of the cerebral cortex. In H.H. Jasper, A.A. Ward, & A. Pope (Eds.), *Brain mechanisms of the epilepsies* (pp. 13–28). Boston: Little, Brown.

Szentagothai, J. (1972). The basic neuronal circuit of the neocortex. In H. Petsche & M.A.B. Brazier (Eds.), *Synchronization of EEG activity in epilepsies* (Symposium of the Austrian Academy of Sciences, Vienna, Austria, Sept 12–13, 1971) (pp. 9–24). New York: Springer-Verlag.

Szentagothai, J. (1974). A structural overview. In J. Szentagothai & M.A. Arbib (Eds.), *Conceptual Models of Neural Organization* (Neurosciences Research Program Bulletin, 12) (pp 354–410).

Szentagothai, J., & Arbib, M.A. (1975). The "module-concept" in cerebral cortex architecture. *Brain Research, 95,* 475–496.

Teuber, H-L. (1961). Sensory deprivation, sensory suppression and agnosia: Notes for neurologic theory. *Journal of Nervous and Mental Diseases, 132,* 32–40.

Tömböl, T. (1974). An electron microscope study of the neurons of the visual cortex. *Journal of Neurocytology, 3,* 525–531.

Towe, A.L. (1973). Somatosensory cortex: Descending influences on ascending systems. In A. Iggo (Ed.), *Handbook of sensory physiology, Vol 2, Somatosensory system* (pp. 701–718). Berlin: Springer-Verlag.

Travel, D., & Damasio, A.R. (1985). Knowledge without awareness: An autonomic index of facial recognition by prosopagnosics. *Science, 220,* 1453–1455.

Trevarthen, C.B., & Sperry, R.W. (1973). Perceptual unity of the ambient visual field in human commissurotomy patients. *Brain, 96,* 547–570.

Valens, E.G. (1964). *The number of things: Pythagorus, geometry, and human strivings.* New York: E.P. Dutton.

Van Essen, D.C., Maunsell, J.H.R., & Bixby, J.L. (1981). The middle temporal area in the macaque: Myeloarchitecture, connections, functional properties and topographic organization. *Journal of Comparative Neurology, 199,* 293–326.

Vernon, P.E. (1930). Synesthesia in music. *Psyche, 10,* 22–40.

Verrey, D. (1888). Hemiachromatopsie droite absolute. *Archives d'Ophthalmologie (Paris) 8,* 289–300.

Vike, J., Jabbari, B., & Maitland, C.G. (1984). Auditory-visual synesthesia. Report of a case with intact visual pathways. *Archives of Neurology, 41,* 680–681.

Vogt, M., Gunn, C.G., & Sawyer, C.H. (1957). EEG effects of intraventricular 5-HT and LSD in the cat. *Neurology, 7,* 559.

von Helmholtz, H. (1866/1967). Physiological optics (J.P.C. Southall, trans.). New York: Dover.

Von Hornbostel, E.M. (1926). Unity of the senses. *Psyche, 7,* 83–89.

Von Hornbostel, E.M. (1931). Über Geruchshelligkeit. *Pfluger's Archiv fur die Gesamten Physiologie, 227,* 517–538.

Voss, W. (1930). Das Farbhören bei Erblindeten. (Cited by Critchley, M. (1977). Ecstatic and synaesthetic experience during musical perception. In M. Critchley & R.A. Henson (Eds.), *Music and the brain: Studies in the neurology of music* (p. 226). Springfield, IL: Charles C. Thomas.)

Walraven, J. (1985). Prolonged complimentary chromatopsia in users of video display terminals. *American Journal of Ophthalmology 100,* 350–352.

Weil-Malherbe, H. (1977). Serotonin and schizophrenia. In W.B. Essman (Ed.), *Serotonin in health and disease, Vol 3, The central nervous system* (chpt 69). New York: Spectrum.

Weinstein, E.A., Cole, M., & Mitchel, M.S. (1963). *Transactions of the American Neurological Association, 88,* 172.

Weinstein, E.A., Kahn, R.L., & Slote, W.H. (1955). Withdrawal, inattention and pain asymbolia. *Archives of Neurology and Psychiatry, 74,* 235–248.

Weiser, H.G. (1983). Depth recorded limbic seizures and psychopathology. *Neuroscience and Biobehavioral Reviews, 7,* 427.

Weiskrantz, L. (1980). Varieties of residual experience. *Quarterly Journal of Experimental Psychology, 32,* 365–386.

Weiskrantz, L. (1986). *Blindsight. A case study and implications.* Oxford: Oxford University Press.

Welch, K.M.A. (1987). Migraine. A biobehavioral disorder. *Archives of Neurology, 44,* 323–327.

Weller, A. (1931). Zur Geschichte und Kritik der Synästhesia—Forschung. *Archiv für dei Gesamten Psychologie, 79,* 325–384.

Werner, H. (1948). *Comparative psychology of mental development.* Chicago: Follet.

West, L.J. (1962). A general theory of hallucinations and dreams. In L.J. West (Ed.), *Hallucinations.* New York: Grune & Strantton.

West, L.J. (1975). A clinical and theoretical overview of hallucinatory phenomena. In R.K. Siegel & L.J. West (Eds.), *Hallucinations: Behavior, experience and theory* (pp. 287–311). New York: John Wiley & Sons.

Wheeler, R.H. (1920). *The synesthesia of a blind subject.* University of Oregon publications No. 5.

Wheeler, R.H., & Cutsforth, T.D. (1922). Synesthesia, a form of perception. *Psychology Review, 29,* 212–220.

Whitaker, H.A. (1979). Electrical stimulation mapping of language cortex. In O. Creutzfeld, H. Scheich, & C. Schreiner (Eds.), *Experimental brain research supplementum II: Hearing mechanisms and speech.* Berlin: Springer-Verlag.

Whitaker, H.A., & Ojemann, G.A. (1977). Graded localization of naming from electrical stimulation mapping of left cerebral cortex. *Nature, 270,* 50–51.

White, C.S., Humm, J.H., Armstrong, E.D., et al. (1952). Human tolerance to exposure to carbon dioxide; 6% carbon dioxide in air and oxygen. *Aviation Medicine, 1,* 439–455.

Wiesel, T.N., & Hubel, D.H. (1966). Spatial and chromatic interaction in the lateral geniculate body of the rhesus monkey. *Journal of Neurophysiology, 29,* 1115–1156.

Wiesendanger, M. (1969). The pyramidal tract. Recent investigations on its morphology and function. *Ergebnisse der Physiologie, 61,* 1122–1124.

Williams, J.E., & Jackson, W.F. (1968). Connotative meanings of color hues. *Perceptual and Motor Skills, 26,* 499–502.

Wishaw, I.Q. (1987). Hippocampal, granule cell and CA304 lesions impair formation of a place learning-set in the rat and induce reflex epilepsy. *Behavioral Brain Research, 24,* 59–72.

Wood, T. (1936). *True Thomas.* London: Cape.

Woolsey, C.N. (1952). *Biology of mental health and disease* (p. 52). New York: Hoeber.

Yakovlev, P.I. (1948). Motility, behavior and the brain. Stereodynamic organization and neural co-ordinates of behavior. *Journal of Nervous and Mental Diseases, 107*(4), 313–335.

Yakovlev, P.I. (1962). Morphological criteria of growth and maturation of the nervous system in man. *Research Publications of the Association for Nervous and Mental Disorders, 39,* 3–46.

Yakovlev, P.I. (1970). The structural and functional "trinity" of the body, brain and behavior. In H.T. Wycis (Ed.), *Current research in neurosciences, topical problems in psychiatry and neurology* (Vol. 10, pp. 197–208). New York: Karger.

Yakovlev, P.I., & Lecours, A-R. (1967). The myelogenetic cycles of regional maturation of the brain. In A. Minkowski (Ed.), *Regional development of the brain in early life* (pp. 3–70). Oxford: Blackwell Scientific.

Yamamoto, T. (1984). Taste responses of cortical neurons. *Progress in Neurobiology, 23,* 273–315.

Young, T. (1802). *Philosophical Transactions, 92,* 12–48.

Zeising, A. (1854). *Die neue Lehre von den Proportionen des menschlichem Körpers.*

Zeki, S.M. (1973). Colour coding in rhesus monkey prestriate cortex. *Brain Research, 53,* 422–427.

Zeki, S.M. (1977). Colour coding in the superior temporal sulcus of rhesus monkey visual cortex. *Proceedings of the Royal Society of London (Biology) 197,* 195–223.

Zialko, H.U. (1959). Psychotropic drugs and initial psychic state (neurosis). In P.B. Bradley, P. Denikev, & C. Radvoco-Thomas (Eds.), *Neuropsychopharmacology* (p. 711). Amsterdam: Elsevier.

Zigler, M.J. (1930). Tone shapes: A novel type of synesthesia. *Journal of General Psychology, 3,* 277–287.

Index